Anticoagulants, Antiplatelets, and Thrombolytics

METHODS IN MOLECULAR MEDICINE™

John M. Walker, SERIES EDITOR

Anticoagulants, Antiplatelets, and Thrombolytics

Edited by

Shaker A. Mousa

Albany College of Pharmacy, Albany, NY

HUMANA PRESS ✳ TOTOWA, NEW JERSEY

This publication is printed on acid-free paper. ∞
ANSI Z39.48-1984 (American Standards Institute) Permanence of Paper for Printed Library Materials.

Production Editor: Mark J. Breaugh.

Cover design by Patricia F. Cleary.

Cover illustration: Potent inhibition of FGF2-induced angiogenesis by r-TFPI in the chick chorioallantoic membrane (CAM) model. See Fig. 4 on page 146.

Printed in the United States of America. 10 9 8 7 6 5 4 3 2 1

E-ISBN: 1-59259-658-4

Library of Congress Cataloging in Publication Data

Anticoagulants, antiplatelets, and thrombolytics / edited by Shaker A. Mousa.
      p. ; cm. -- (Methods in molecular medicine ; 93)
Includes bibliographical references and index.
  ISBN 1-58829-083-2 (alk. paper)
  1. Anticoagulants (Medicine) 2. Blood platelets. 3. Thrombolytic therapy. 4. Fibrinolytic agents.
  [DNLM: 1. Anticoagulants--therapeutic use. 2. Thrombolytic Therapy--methods. 3. Fibrinolytic Agents--therapeutic use. 4. Heparin--therapeutic use. 5. Platelet Aggregation Inhibitors--therapeutic use. 6. Thrombocytopenia--drug therapy. QZ 170 A629 2003] I. Mousa, Shaker A. II. Series.
  RM340.A566 2003
  615'.718--dc22
                                    2003017231

Preface

During the past decade, remarkable progress has been made in the development of newer drugs to treat thrombotic and cardiovascular diseases. Over this last 10 years, concentrated efforts were made to discover new drugs and to develop novel uses for such traditional antithrombotic drugs as aspirin, heparin, and oral anticoagulants. Biotechnology, molecular biology, combinatorial approaches, isolation and characterization of natural products with antithrombotic activity, and a reassessment of traditional drugs have been the key factors behind these developments.

Some 1 million Americans die of thrombotic and cardiovascular disorders every year. On a global level, the relative proportion of mortality is even higher. Thus, thrombosis and related disorders represent the number one cause of mortality. The understanding of the mechanisms behind the pathogenesis of venous thromboembolism, acute coronary syndromes, cerebral vascular ischemic and thrombotic events, and diseases associated with thrombotic disorders has provided additional insights toward the development of various therapeutic approaches to control these pathogenic events. The roles of plasmatic proteins, blood cells, vascular endothelium, and target organs in both thrombogenesis, such as antithrombin III, Tissue Factor Pathway Inhibitor (TFPI), protein C, prostacyclin, nitric oxide, and physiologic activators of fibrinolysis has led to the development of both direct and indirect modalities to treat thrombosis. On the other hand, the knowledge of the proteases involved in thrombogenesis, including tissue factors, coagulation factors, adhesion molecules, and fibrinolytic inhibitors have provided insights into the mechanisms by which thrombogenesis can be pharmacologically controlled.

The pharmaceutical industry has played a key role, not only in the development of new drugs, but also in providing sizable resources to academic institutions to foster the development and clinical validation of the uses of these drugs. Such drugs as low molecular weight heparins, antithrombin agents, the hirudins, such antiplatelet drugs as the GPIIb/IIa inhibitors, and the ADP receptor antagonists have emerged as improved therapeutic strategies over conventional drugs. The development of these drugs required a major undertaking by the pharmaceutical industry with allocation of sizable resources. Beside fiscal considerations, an objective assessment of the newer drugs at both the preclinical and clinical levels was mandatory for optimal applications.

Anticoagulants, Antiplatelets, and Thrombolytics provides a comprehensive update on many of the critical in vitro and in vivo models of thrombosis and hemostasis. Additionally, this book highlights the novel use of low molecular weight heparins, the newer applications of GPIIb/IIIa antagonists, aspirin, and clopidogrel, and the expanded usage of thrombolytics and polytherapeutic approaches. The recent approval of antiplatelet drugs for intermittent claudication, the aspirin–dipyridamol combination for ischemic stroke, and thrombolytic agents in cerebral ischemia represent some of the

v

concepts that will be highlighted. Similarly, aspirin combinations with oral anticoagulants and other drugs have been in discussion for improved management of arterial thrombosis.

The recognition of heparin-induced thrombocytopenia as a catastrophic complication of heparin therapy necessitated the development of such alternate anticoagulant drugs as the antithrombin agents. Today, hirudins can be used to achieve comparable anticoagulation in heparin-compromised patients. The variation in aspirin tolerance and increased susceptibility to gastric toxicity from this drug led to the development of such ADP receptor antagonists as ticlopidine and clopidogrel. The oral anticoagulant drugs, however, have remained the only orally bioavailable agents that can be used for an extended period of time despite their inherent limitations. These drugs remain unchallenged by low molecular weight heparins, antithrombin agents, and antifactor Xa drugs. Thus, the impact of new drug development on traditionally used drugs has added a fresh dimension. It is interesting to note that many of the polytherapeutic approaches now combine traditional drugs with newer drugs.

The novel developments in antithrombotic drugs include such monotherapeutic approaches as the antiproteases (factors IIa, Xa, and VIIa), tissue factor targeting, platelet receptor targeting, and antithrombin III modulation. Despite the clear mechanisms of action of some of these agents, the recognition of the modulatory effects of aspirin and heparin has led to the development of a multitarget approach. Interestingly, all of the traditional drugs, such as heparin, aspirin, and warfarin, are multitargeting drugs. The recognition that thrombotic disorders represent a syndrome rather than a disease is of crucial importance in the development of newer drugs. Either a polytherapeutic approach with drug combinations or a drug with multiple actions will likely be more appropriate for the management of thrombotic disorders.

Shaker A. Mousa

Contents

Contributors

HIKMAT ABDEL-RAZEQ • *King Fahd Armed Forces Hospital, Jeddah, Saudi Arabia*

JAMES P. ABULENCIA • *Department of Chemical and Biomolecular Engineering, Johns Hopkins University, Baltimore, MD*

OMAR AL-AMOUDI • *King Abdul-Aziz University Hospital, Jeddah, Saudi Arabia*

ABDEL-AZIZ AL-HUMIADI • *King Faisal Specialist Hospital and Research Center, Jeddah, Saudi Arabia*

HUSSEIN ALIZEIDAH • *Tawam Hospital, Al Ain, United Arab Emirates*

ABDULAZIZ ALZEER • *King Khalid University Hospital, Riyadh, Saudi Arabia*

FAISAL AL-SAYEGH • *Health Sciences Center, Kuwait University, Kuwait*

LARRY R. BUSH • *Sepracor Inc., Marlborough, MA*

LIGUO CHI • *Cardiovascular Pharmacology, Pfizer Global Research and Development, Ann Arbor Laboratories, Ann Arbor, MI*

JAWED FAREED • *Department of Pathology, Loyola University Medical Center, Maywood, IL*

ALISON GAGNON • *Incyte Genomics, Beverly, MA*

DEBRA HOPPENSTEADT • *Department of Pathology, Loyola University Medical Center, Maywood, IL*

STEEN HUSTED • *Department of Cardiology, Aarhus University Hospital, Aarhus, Denmark*

OMER IQBAL • *Department of Pathology, Loyola University Medical Center, Maywood, IL*

WALTER P. JESKE • *Departments of Thoracic-Cardiovascular Surgery and Pathology, Cardiovascular Institute, Loyola University Medical Center, Maywood, IL*

BRIGITTE KAISER • *Center for Vascular Biology and Medicine Erfurt, Friedrich Schiller University Jena, Erfurt, Germany*

KONSTANTINOS KONSTANTOPOULOS • *Department of Chemical and Biomolecular Engineering, Johns Hopkins University, Baltimore, MD*

JORGEN KRISTENSEN • *Tawam Hospital, Al Ain, United Arab Emirates*

ROBERT J. LEADLEY, JR. • *Cardiovascular Pharmacology, Pfizer Global Research and Development, Ann Arbor Laboratories, Ann Arbor, MI*

MAHMOUD MARASHI • *Rashid Hospital, Dubai, United Arab Emirates*

OWEN J. T. MCCARTY • *Department of Chemical and Biomolecular Engineering, Johns Hopkins University, Baltimore, MD*

SHAKER A. MOUSA • *Albany College of Pharmacy, Albany, NY*

MARGARET PRECHEL • *Department of Pathology, Cardiovascular Institute, Loyola University Medical Center, Maywood, IL*

MOHAMAD QARI • *King Abdul-Aziz University Hospital, Jeddah, Saudi Arabia*

HATEM QUTUB • *King Faisal University, Alkhobar, Saudi Arabia*

RONALD J. SHEBUSKI • *CarePoint Medical Inc., Eden Prairie, MN*

JEANINE M. WALENGA • *Departments of Thoracic-Cardiovascular Surgery and Pathology, Cardiovascular Institute, Loyola University Medical Center, Maywood, IL*

1

Highlights of Latest Advances in Antithrombotics

Shaker A. Mousa

1. Platelets, Thromboembolic Disorders, and Antiplatelets

Thrombosis is still the leading cause of morbidity and mortality, and thus, effective antithrombotic strategies remain a critical therapeutic objective. The past decade has witnessed considerable progress in the development of newer anticoagulants, antiplatelets, and thrombolytics for the prevention and treatment of various thromboembolic disorders.

The transition of coronary-artery plaque from stable to unstable with the subsequent plaque rupture at the shoulder region leads to thrombotic complications, or acute coronary syndromes (ACS), ranging from unstable angina to acute myocardial infarction (AMI). Plaque rupture results in the exposure of the thrombogenic surface, leading to platelet adhesion, platelet activation, platelet aggregation, and secretion. Platelets play a major role in health and disease.

Antiplatelet therapies have provided a distinct clinical benefit in various arterial thromboembolic disorders, including aspirin and clopidogrel. Aspirin is currently considered to be the gold-standard antiplatelet agent based on its high benefit-to-cost and benefit-to-risk ratios. Another class of antiplatelet agents includes Ticlopidine and its improved version, clopidogrel adenosine 5′ diphosphate (ADP) inhibition, which has demonstrated comparable efficacy to that of aspirin.

2. Clopidogrel: A Novel ADP Antagonist

In the CAPRIE trial, both aspirin and clopidogrel have been compared. Clopidogrel may be a valuable alternative to aspirin for those patients for whom aspirin fails to achieve therapeutic benefit. A number of preclinical studies have suggested an additive to synergistic potential in combining aspirin and clopidogrel, this was further confirmed in a randomized CURE clinical trial,

From: *Methods in Molecular Medicine, vol. 93: Anticoagulants, Antiplatelets, and Thrombolytics*
Edited by: S. A. Mousa © Humana Press Inc., Totowa, NJ

with a significant benefit-to-risk ratio for patients with various thromboembolic disorders.

Recent clinical studies have validated the benefit of the aspirin and dipyridamole combination in stroke patients. Clopidogrel (75 mg QD) demonstrated rapid oral absorption, significant platelet aggregation, and inhibition (40–60%), and bleeding time increases as much as twofold above baseline value. Clopidogrel (5.32% event rate/yr) demonstrated 8.7% overall relative risk reduction over aspirin (5.83% event rate/yr) in preventing MI, ischemic stroke, or vascular death. Clopidogrel (2.5% event rate/yr) resulted in a 19.2% relative risk reduction as compared to aspirin (3.6% event rate/yr) in reducing fatal and non-fatal MI.

The CLASSICS trial compared the efficacy and safety of clopidogrel (75 mg QD) + aspirin (325 mg QD) vs ticlopidine (250 mg QD) + aspirin (325 mg/d). The overall cardiovascular event rates were low and comparable between the clopidogrel and the ticlopidine arms. Clopidogrel + aspirin is superior to ticlopidine + aspirin in coronary stenting. Pretreatment with clopidogrel + aspirin prior to stenting was beneficial. The latest CURE trial demonstrated an additive effect on the efficacy of clopidogrel + aspirin in arterial thrombosis, with reasonable safety profiles.

3. Intravenous Platelet GPIIb/IIIa Antagonists

3.1. Abciximab

The EPIC and EPILOG trials have established the clinical benefit of Abciximab in reducing the risk of ischemic complications in patients undergoing percutaneous coronary intervention. In addition to its platelet $\alpha IIb\beta 3$ blockade, Abciximab blocks $\alpha v\beta 3$, and to some extent Mac-1 integrin. The implication of these additional effects on efficacy and safety has not yuet been determined as compared to the specific platelet $\alpha IIb\beta 3$ antagonists such as integrilin and Tirofiban.

3.2. Eptifibatide (Integrilin)

Eptifibatide is a cyclic KGD peptide that is specific for platelet $\alpha IIb\beta 3$ integrin. Eptifibatide has demonstrated clinical benefits in patients with non-ST-segment elevation and acute ischemic syndromes, and in patients undergoing PCI. Additionally, initial data and ongoing clinical trials suggest its potential value in combination with thrombolytics, stent in PCI, and in peripheral-artery diseases.

3.3. Aggrastat (Tirofiban) in ACS

Aggrastat is a non-peptide RGD mimetic that is specific for platelet $\alpha IIb\beta 3$ integrin. The clinical benefit of Aggrastat was established in various trials including prism, Restore, and prism-plus. Tirofiban demonstrated a significant reduction in refractory ischemia in unstable angina/non-Q wave MI patients as compared to heparin (prism). In the prism-plus trial, Tirofiban + heparin resulted in a significant reduction in refractory ischemia and MI as compared to heparin alone. The Restore trial, Tirofiban plus heparin reduced the incidence of adverse outcomes at 2 and 7 d after PTCA. Tirofiban as well as other GPIIb/IIIa antagonists are in clinical trials in combination with low-molecular-weight heparin (LMWH).

4. Oral Platelet GPIIb/IIIa Antagonists

4.1. Discontinued Oral Platelet GPIIb/IIIa Antagonists in Clinical Development

The clinical benefit of platelet GPIIb/IIIa blockade is well-documented with intravenous (iv) GPIIb/IIIa antagonists. Intravenous platelet GPIIb/IIIa antagonists have proven to be of clinical benefit in reducing ischemic complications following angioplasty and in unstable angina and non-Q-wave MI. Recently, clinical results with three oral GPIIb/IIIa inhibitors in large phase III trials showed lack of clinical benefit over aspirin. These trials include Excite (Xemilofiban), OPUS-TIMI 16 (Orbofiban), Symphony (Sibrafiban). In those trials with oral GPIIb/IIIa antagonists' composite end points—that is, reduction of MI events, mortality, and urgent revascularization demonstrated a lack of significant clinical benefit. However, subgroup analysis demonstrated potential benefit in the reduction of the need for revascularization post-interventional procedures. The exact reason for the failure of oral as compared to iv GPIIb/IIIa blockade suggest the critical need to achieve steady-state antiplatelet effective levels with the oral agents or the need for heparin.

4.2. Roxifiban

The latest oral GPIIb/IIIa antagonist with high affinity and specificity for both activated and resting human platelets along with a slow platelet dissociation rate. Roxifiban represents a demonstrated new generation oral platelet GPIIb/III antagonist. Because of its unique platelet-binding kinetics, it has demonstrated distinct pharmacokinetic and pharmacodynamic profiles in various preclinical and clinical studies. All clinical trials with all oral GPIIb/IIIa antagonists are being discontinued because of the failure of various GPIIb/IIIa antagonists (xemilofiban, orbifiban, lotrafiban) in various large phase III trials.

5. Highlights of the Latest Developments in Anticoagulants

The past decade has witnessed remarkable progress in the development of newer anticoagulants and anti-platelets. An understanding of the pathogenesis of thrombotic and vascular disorders has greatly facilitated these developments to target blood vessels, platelets, and the protease network involving the coagulation, thrombolytic, and the fibrinolytic systems. Improved processing from the natural sources, biotechnology, and organic chemistry strategies have played a major role in these developments. Such drugs as the LMWH, oral unfractionated heparin (UFH) synthetic heparin, and antithrombin agents. Many of the important drugs, such as the LMWH, pentasaccharide, direct antithrombin, direct antiXa agents, and biotechnology-derived therapeutic agents, are highlighted in this issue.

5.1. Low Molecular Weight Heparin (LMWH)

LMWH represents the most significant development in antithrombotic therapy. The potential advantages of these drugs as antithrombotic agents are based on high bioavailability (85–95%) after subcutaneous (sc) administration, long plasma half-life resulting in a predictable response, and less bleeding for a clinically significant antithrombotic effect as compared to UFH. LMWH preparations currently in use are produced by different techniques, have variable molecular weight distribution, and therefore are likely to have different pharmacokinetic and pharmacodynamic properties, which may have important clinical implications. Several randomized clinical trials have clearly demonstrated their efficacy and safety in preventing and treating venous and arterial thrombosis. Further expansion beyond the use of heparin in thrombosis is in progress.

5.1.1. The Use of LMWH in Pregnancy

Thromboembolism is a leading contributor to obstetric morbidity as well as mortality, occurring with an incidence between 0.1% and 0.4% during pregnancy, and the rate of recurrent thromboembolism can be as high as 12.5% among pregnant women with a history of thrombosis during previous pregnancy. LMWH do not cross the placental blood-barrier, and are associated with a better compliance, lesser risk for thrombocytopenia, bleeding complications, or osteopenia as compared to UFH. The use of LMWH in obstetric patients is controversial with respect to the time and duration of therapy, monitoring, and dose adjustment. The utility of LMWH in the obese subset of the patient population and patients with renal failure must be defined in clinical trials for each individual LMWH.

5.1.2. LMWH in ACS: MI Management

It is well-established that LMWH offer advantages in comparison with UFH in the prevention and treatment of DVT. Therefore, they are likely to offer some advantages in arterial diseases, particularly coronary-artery diseases as compared to UFH. This was demonstrated with Enoxaparin (Essence and TIMI 11B) and recently with Dalteparin (FRIX II). The potential value of other LMWH in that setting must be established.

5.1.3. LMWH and Cancer

Venous thromboembolism is an important complication in patients who are receiving treatment for cancer. LMWH may offer opportunities to improve the prevention and treatment of VTE in cancer, but further randomized trials are required in order to separate the anticancer from the anticoagulant effects. These agents may also prolong survival in patients with malignant disease, and are currently being evaluated in this indication.

6. Progress in the Development of Synthetic Pentasaccharides

Pentasaccharides are synthetic high ATIII-affinity heparinomimetics defined as being the critical structure of heparin that binds to ATIII and elicits an anti-factor Xa activity. Several pentasaccharides have been produced that vary in potency and biological half-life. The original SR 90107A/ORG and the SANORG were recently approved by the Food and Drug Administration (FDA) for venous prophylaxis indications and are in various other clinical trials.

6.1. Bivalirudin (Hirulog)

Bivalirudin is a highly specific and reversible direct thrombin inhibitor, which has been shown in clinical trials for percutaneous transluminal angioplasty to have a significant reduction in death, MI, urgent revascularization, and major hemorrhage. Current trials are evaluating its safety with concomitantly administered GPIIb/IIIa, thrombolytics, and other antiplatelet agents.

6.2. Argatroban

Argatroban is a novel direct thrombin inhibitor, which has been developed for treatment in heparin-induced thrombocytopenia (HIT) as an alternative to UFH. Two large studies have examined the effect of treatment with Argatroban in HIT compared to conventional treatment. The results of these trials have demonstrated the efficacy of Argatroban in the various presentations of HIT.

6.3. Anti-Xa Agents

High affinity and selectivity toward the Xa as compared to other serine proteases characterize newly developed anti-Xa agents. In addition to the inhibition of plasmatic coagulation processes—such as the prevention of thrombin generation and of thrombin-mediated platelet reactions, as well as the inactivation of clot-bound prothrombinase complexes—some of these agents may also interfere with receptor-mediated cellular effects of factor Xa that play an important role in the proliferation of vascular smooth-muscle cells (SMCs). Anti-Xa agents might become important drugs for the prophylaxis of various venous thromboembolic disorders as well as an adjunct therapy with other antithrombotics.

6.4. Heparin by Oral Delivery

Currently, UFH is not orally administered because UFH molecules are not absorbed from the gastrointestinal (GI) tract, presumably because of their size and ionic repulsion from negatively charged epithelial tissue. A novel carrier system is now available to accomplish GI absorption. Oral administration of heparin with this carrier molecule (SNAC) has produced significant alterations in aPTT, anti- IIa and Xa, and release of TFPI. The development of an oral liquid formulation has permitted evaluation in patients. The results of a recently completed Phase 11 trial, which evaluated the safety and tolerance of oral heparin administration as venous thromboprophylaxis in patients undergoing total hip arthroplasty, demonstrated limited oral bioavailability. The intra- and inter-subject variability may limit the potential utility of this formulation. However, a second-generation formulation might overcome these limitations. The PROTECT Trial—a Phase III trial evaluating SNAC heparin—is in progress. It is still undetermined whether this regimen would be cost-effective.

6.5. Recombinant Human Protein C

Protein C is a vitamin K-dependent plasma serine protease that plays a critical role in the regulation of hemostasis. A recombinant version of human activated protein C (rhAPC) has demonstrated significant benefits for the treatment of sepsis. The biology, structure/function relationships, and therapeutic rationale for rhAPC have demonstrated efficacy and safety in various experimental settings. Protein C appears to have clear safety advantages as compared to other anticoagulant strategies.

6.6. Antitissue Factor (TF)

Inhibition of the coagulation cascade can be accomplished by blocking the cascade at one of several points. Many of the currently available therapies have been directed at blocking the downstream portion of the process, including thrombin action and Xa. An approach that may offer some advantages over the present therapies is blockade of the coagulation cascade very early in the process at the TF/VIIa level. However, there is no evidence yet available in favor of this approach.

Suggested Readings

Fitzgerald, G. A. and Shipp, E. (1992) Antiplatelet and anticoagulant drugs in coronary vascular disease. *Ann Epidemiol.* **2(4),** 529–542.

Gresele, P. and Agnelli, G. (2002) Novel approaches to the treatment of thrombosis. *Trends Pharmacol. Sci.* **23(1),** 25–32.

Hirsh, J. (1996) New antithrombotics for the treatment of acute and chronic arterial ischemia. *Vasc. Med.* **1(1),** 72–78.

Hirsh, J. and Weitz, J. I. (1999) New antithrombotic agents. *Lancet* **353(9162),** 1431–1436.

Leadley, R. J. Jr., Chi, L., Rebello, S. S., and Gagnon, A. (2000) Contribution of in vivo models of thrombosis to the discovery and development of novel antithrombotic agents. *J. Pharmacol. Toxicol. Methods* **43(2),** 101–116.

Radziwon, P., Boczkowska-Radziwon, B., Giedrojc, J., Schenk, J., Wojtukiewicz, M. Z., Kloczko, J., et al. (1998) Effects of polysulfonate derivative (GL 522-Y-1) on coagulation in vitro and thrombosis in vivo. *Haemostasis* **28(2),** 86–92.

Verstraete, M. (1995) New developments in antiplatelet and antithrombotic therapy. *Eur. Heart J.* **16 (Suppl. L),** 16–23.

Vivekananthan, D. P. and Moliterno. D. J. (2002) Glycoprotein IIb/IIIa combination therapy in acute myocardial infarction: tailoring therapies to optimize outcome. *J. Thromb. Thrombolysis* **13(1),** 35–39.

Vivekananthan, D. P., Patel, V. B., and Moliterno, D. J. Glycoprotein IIb/IIIa antagonism and fibrinolytic therapy for acute myocardial infarction. *J. Interv. Cardiol.* **15(2),** 131–139.

Weitz, J. and Hirsh, J. (1993) New anticoagulant strategies. *J. Lab. Clin. Med.* **122(4),** 364–373.

2

Antiplatelet, Anticoagulant, and Thrombolytic Drug Interactions

Omer Iqbal and Shaker A. Mousa

1. Introduction

Despite recent major pharmacological and device advances, percutaneous coronary intervention (PCI) remains a costly procedure with significant periprocedural risk. Heparin has maintained the foundation of procedural anticoagulation, but heparin anticoagulation is unpredictable because it is an indirect thrombin inhibitor, which requires heparin cofactor II-antithrombin for its actions. Antithrombin levels vary widely in patients. In addition, the heparinantithrombin complex is too large to inhibit clot-bound or fibrin-bound thrombin. Clinical functions can alter antithrombin levels, which further reduce heparin's predictability. Heparin can also be inhibited by plasma proteins. These complexities can lead to both excessive anticoagulation with clinical bleeding and subtherapeutic heparinization with clinical coronary occlusion. Finally, heparin is associated with a 1–3% incidence of heparin-induced thrombocytopenia (HIT), which carries an increased risk for acute, subacute, and chronic thrombotic occlusion. The major pharmacological improvement in platelet efficacy has been the addition of glycoprotein IIb/IIIa inhibitors for PCIs. However, all GPIIb/IIIa inhibitors are associated with a risk of bleeding. Reduction of heparin doses has resulted in less clinical bleeding, but bleeding still occurs in a significant number of patients.

Investigations with direct thrombin inhibitors have been undertaken for both non-ST-elevation myocardial infarction (MI) and PCI. Hirudin has shown a small but definite reduction in coronary ischemia compared to heparin in acute coronary syndromes (ACS), but hirudin is associated with a statistically significant increase in the frequency of major bleeding. The modifications in the

From: *Methods in Molecular Medicine, vol. 93: Anticoagulants, Antiplatelets, and Thrombolytics*
Edited by: S. A. Mousa © Humana Press Inc., Totowa, NJ

hirudin molecule have resulted in bivalirudin, which has been tested in >4000 PCI patients compared to heparin. Bivalirudin showed a significant reduction in major bleeding (13.0% vs 9.89%, $p<0.001$) compared to heparin, indicating a trend toward fewer ischemic complications. Argatroban is smallest of the direct thrombin inhibitors, and has similar pharmacodynamics to bivalirudin (reversible, short half-life). A large body of evidence suggests that direct thrombin inhibitors (hirudin and bivalirudin) are more efficacious than heparin for treatment of ACS and that the small molecules—short half-life, reversible thrombin inhibitors (bivalirudin and argatroban)—are safer than heparin. The improved efficacy of argatroban should reduce the need for adjuvant GPIIb/IIIa inhibition, and therefore reduce bleeding as well as pharmacologic costs.

Argatroban (Novastan), a direct thrombin inhibitor, is a carboxy acid derivative that belongs to a class of peptidomimetics that also includes inogatran, efegatran, and napsagatran. Argatroban has now been approved in the United States as an alternative to heparin in patients with HIT. It binds covalently to the active site of thrombin (1). Argatroban was used in one trial of 50 patients with HIT who were undergoing plasma thromboplastin component antecedent percutaneous transluminal coronary angioplasty (PTCA) at a dose of 350 µg/kg bolus, and yielded encouraging results.

Reperfusion therapy of acute myocardial infarction (AMI) to establish reperfusion as quickly as possible is of primary importance. The use of fibrinolytics in combination with low molecular weight heparins (LMWHs) have provided encouraging results in randomized clinical trials. The encouraging results seen with LMWHs instead of unfractionated heparin (UFH) represent a definitive advancement in the field. If LMWHs are exerting their effects mainly their enhanced anti-Xa inhibition, then more specific and direct factor Xa inhibitors may be advantageous (4). The GPIIb/IIIa inhibitors can be used in combination with the thrombolytic agents in patients with AMI. Activase™ (alteplase, recombinant) in combination with GPIIb/IIIa inhibitors or TNKase in combination with GPIIb/IIIa inhibitors can be used in patients with AMI.

The thrombi in the coronary arteries that cause AMI comprise of a platelet core in a fibrin-thrombin matrix. Following successful thrombolysis, re-occlusion is caused by excessive platelet activation, which makes the thrombi difficult to lyse. In these situations, adjunctive use of thrombolytic agents with GPIIb/IIIa inhibitors will prevent platelet activation and aggregation (5). Platelets bind to the walls of the vessel by attachment at Ia or Ib receptors on the platelet surface. Platelet-platelet binding is a result of interaction between GPIIb/IIIa receptors involving the fibrinogen and vWF (6).

Gold et al. have demonstrated that the platelet Fab fragment of the murine antibody 7E3-F(ab)2 to GPIIb/IIIa binds tightly to the GPIIb/IIIa receptor and inhibits platelet aggregation (7). In the TAMI-8, a non-randomized multicenter pilot study, 60 patients with AMI were given Activase with varied abciximab dosages of 0.1, 0.15, 0.20, and 0.25 mg/kg given at 3, 6, and 15 h after a 100-mg dose of Activase administered over a period of 3 h. Despite limitations of the study being small and not blinded, the safety profile was similar in the abciximab and control groups. However, in abciximab-treated patients, fewer major bleeding events, decreased recurrent ischemic events, and better coronary-artery patency, as evaluated by angiography, were observed.

An ongoing, double-blind, randomized, placebo-controlled, crossover trial of abciximab alone or in combination with low-dose Activase is being carried out in 26 patients with AMI. Each patient presented within 6 h of symptom onset with ST-segment elevation. Patients were initially given aspirin and heparin, and then randomized to receive either abciximab 0.25 mg/kg bolus or placebo followed by an angiogram 60–90 min later. Patients were crossed over and given the opposite treatment. A second angiogram was taken 10 min later. The results of the second angiogram, in which patients received abciximab alone, showed that eight patients had thrombolysis in myocardial infarction (TIMI) grade 0 flow, five patients had TIMI grade 1 flow, five patients had TIMI grade 2 flow, and eight patients had TIMI grade 3 flow. The results of the angiogram in patients who received Activase and placebo have not yet been reported *(8)*.

Antman et al. also reported the results from the dose-finding and dose-confirmation phases of the TIMI-14 trial, which evaluated the use of thrombolytic therapy in combination with abciximab in patients with AMI *(9)*.

TNKase—a new, genetically engineered variant of t-PA—is produced by recombinant DNA technology. TNKase is fibrin-specific. This fibrin specificity decreases systemic activation of plasminogen and the resulting breakdown of the circulating fibrinogen when compared to a molecule that lacks this feature. The ASSENT-2 trial was a phase III, randomized, double-blind trial that compared TNKase with Activase. Anticoagulants such as heparin and vitamin K antagonists, acetylsalicylic acid, dipyridamole, and GPIIb/IIIa inhibitors, may increase the risk of bleeding if administered prior to, during, or after TNKase therapy.

Combination strategies of LMWH with GPIIb/IIIa inhibitor or LMWH with a thrombolytic agent or thrombolytic agent with GPIIb/IIIa inhibitors may provide better approaches in the management of thrombosis or thromboembolic complications *(10,11)*. Orally available drugs with rapid onset of action and no need for laboratory monitoring will be more suited for postsurgical prophylaxis of patients undergoing major hip or knee replacement surgeries than the LMWH or coumadin. A prodrug form of melagatran exhibits good bioavailability after oral administration, and has undergone phase II clinical evaluation for prophylaxis of thrombosis in orthopedic patients. For patients who develop venous thromboembolism (VTE) without identifiable risk factors requiring long-term oral anticoagulation, orally active drugs that target thrombin or factor Xa may show better outcomes. With the dawning of the genomic era, future drug development and drug interactions that utilize microarray technology will go hand in hand with the diagnosis of disease or drug interactions at the genetic or molecular level.

Although the development of new antithrombotic and new anticoagulant drugs has been rather impressive, optimized use of aspirin, oral anticoagulants, and heparin has added a new dimension in the management of thrombotic disorders. Polytherapeutic approaches have been used to treat thrombotic disorders. The development of synthetic pentasaccharides represents a validation of the target specificity of heparins. Additional targets will be described in the near future, and heparins will provide other drugs with biochemical and functional specificities.

Pentasaccharide has undergone various phase II and phase III trials *(12–15)*, and a recent publication has provided comparative evidence on the therapeutic effectiveness of this drug *(16)*. However, it should be emphasized that pentasaccharide contains only one of the multiple pharmacological properties of heparin. Such a selective approach may have narrower therapeutic implications; however, in combination with other drugs this new antithrombotic oligosaccharide may provide similar effects to those observed with aspirin/clopidogrel combinations. The PENTATHLON study showed a rebound effect at 6.0 mg, and the rate of thrombosis was higher than in the lowered dose of 3.0 mg/kg. Furthermore, the bleeding was higher in the 3.0-mg dose in comparison to the comparative group in which enoxaparin was used. The rebound thrombotic effect is paradoxical, and may be explained on the basis of biochemical limitations. The fact that pentasaccharide produced an increased bleeding in the 3.0-mg group as compared to the 30-mg bid groups treated with enoxaparin was also an important consideration for the relatively higher rates of bleeding. An arbitrary dose of 2.5 mg was chosen for the additional studies. This is remarkable because there was no weight adjustment in these patients and with a statistical difference between 2.5 and 3.0 mg dose in a population with a weight of 60–90 kg, it is difficult to demonstrate the physical differences. In renal compromise, the accumulation of pentasaccharide can be readily attained, and one would expect a strong bleeding outcome. In the REMBRANDT trial, pentasaccharide demonstrated no significant differences between the dosages of 7.5 and 10 mg. This may be because of the saturation of AT by pentasaccharide. Interestingly, unlike the PENTATHLON study, in this study at a 10-mg dose, no bleeding complications were observed. If the hemorrhagic threshold of pentasaccharide is so low that a reduction of 0.5-mg dosage provides different results, then it may be more useful to adjust the dosage. Careful dosage selection of pentasaccharide is warranted before it is used in any combination therapy to avoid undesirable bleeding complications.

Oral anticoagulant drugs such as warfarin also exert their therapeutic effects by multiple mechanisms. These drugs are optimized for the management of thrombotic and cardiovascular disorders using the INR and the dosage optimization approaches. Oral heparin and oral antithrombin formulations are individually developed as potential replacements for the oral anticoagulant agents. The development of oral thrombin inhibitors and oral heparin formulations as a potential replacement for oral anticoagulants are rather significant. These drugs are currently in phase III clinical trials. However, marked variations in the oral absorption, metabolic conversion, alterations in hepatic function, and the absorption indices will markedly influence their bioavailability. It is difficult to predict whether these drugs will ever achieve therapeutic potential as oral anticoagulants. Warfarin has a track record in multiple indications, with an enormous clinical database. The apparent problems associated with warfarin may also be observed with oral heparin and thrombin inhibitors. These oral heparin and thrombin formulations have different degrees of bioavailabilities. Since a specific antagonist is not available, caution should be exercised—especially when these agents are used in combination with other anticoagulants to avoid uncontrolled bleeding complications. Careful calibration of dosages is warranted before any attempt to combine these oral formulations with other anticoagulant agents.

The current trend in the reperfusion therapy for AMI involves the use of fibrinolytic therapy in combination with more effective antithrombotic therapy to enhance early coronary patency and myocardial perfusion and to prevent reocclusion (*17*). The GUSTO V, ASSENT-3, and HERO-2 trials have shown that more effective antiplatelet and/or anticoagulant therapies can reduce myocardial infarction (MI) rates by more than 20% (*18–20*). Benefits of the adjunctive use of GPIIb/IIIa and coronary intervention have been demonstrated (*21*).

2. Combination Fibrinolytic and GPIIb/IIIa Inhibitor Therapy

Inhibition of the final common pathway of platelet aggregation is important, especially when these GPIIb/IIIa inhibitors are combined with fibrinolytic therapy. Initial results of Phase II angiographic studies, with half-dose t-PA (*9*), reteplase (*22,23*), or tenecteplase (*24–26*) when combined with either abciximab (*9,23–25*), eptifibatide (*25,27*), or tirofiban (*26*) markedly improved infarct artery TIMI grade 3 flow (*9,22,27*). These results were less consistent in confirmation phases (*27*), and were found to be less evident in later studies (*23–25*). Combination fibrinolytic and GPIIb/IIIa inhibitor showed greater extent of ST-segment resolution, as observed in most of the trials (*9,24*). This demonstrates the importance of platelet involvement in microvascular occlusion after fibrinolysis (*28*) and better early ST-segment resolution and improved myocardial perfusion and survival because of combination fibrinolytic and more potent antiplatelet therapy *(29)*.

The GUSTO V trial of 16,000 patients found no significant improvement in survival with half-dose reteplase and abciximab; however, the trial did demonstrate non-inferiority to reteplase alone *(18)*. The secondary benefits of combination therapy included a lower rate of reinfarction (2.3% vs 3.5%) and less need for urgent coronary intervention. Although intracranial hemorrhages were the same at 0.6%, higher rates of ICH were observed in patients >75 yr of age. Thus, half-dose reteplase or tenecteplase combined with abciximab is an effective combination in young patients. A combination strategy of GPIIb/IIIa inhibitors with reduced-dose fibrinolytic therapy before acute angioplasty, or "facilitated angioplasty," needs to be tested. A combination strategy of half-dose reteplase and abciximab followed by early angioplasty is safe, with good clinical outcomes *(30)*. Randomized clinical trials involving the strategies of earliest combination pharmacologic reperfusion therapy combined with coronary intervention are now in progress.

3. Combination Fibrinolytic and LMWH Therapy

LMWHs in combination with fibrinolytic therapy have been evaluated in five randomized clinical trials *(24,31–34)*.

1. The HART-2 study: The strategy of enoxaparin or unfractionated heparin (UFH) with t-PA was compared, and it was found that enoxaparin was at least as effective as UFH as an adjunct to t-PA, with higher recanalization rates and less occlusion at 5–7 d *(31)*.
2. The ENTIRE study: This study compared enoxaprin to UFH, and full-dose to half-dose tenecteplase with abciximab in a factorial design *(24)*. Enoxaparin showed similar TIMI 3 flow rates, and showed an advantage over UFH in regard to the ischemic events during a period of 30 d.
3. The ASSENT-PLUS study: This study compared dalteparin to UFH with t-PA *(32)*.
4. The AMI-SK trial: This trial compared enoxaparin vs placebo with streptokinase, and demonstrated better coronary-artery patency at 8 d and reduced rates of infarction and recurrent ischemia with enoxaparin *(33)*.
5. The ASSENT-3 trial: This trial evaluated the efficacy and safety of tenecteplase in combination with enoxaparin, abciximab, or UFH in 6000 patients. Enoxaparin significantly reduced, from 15.4 to 11.4%, the primary efficacy composite end points of death, reinfarction, and recurrent ischemia.

3.1. Ongoing Trials

1. The ASSENT-3 PLUS study: Approximately 1600 patients treated with tenecteplase are being randomized to enoxaparin vs UFH in the prehospital setting.

2. The EXTRACT trial: Approximately 21,000 patients will be evaluated to compare enoxaparin vs UFH with a fibrinolytic agent of the investigator's choice to evaluate death and reinfarction in a more definitive manner.

4. Combination Fibrinolytic and Direct Thrombin Inhibitor Therapy

Over 36,000 patients with AMI treated with direct thrombin inhibitors in 11 randomized clinical trials showed a 15% relative reduction ($p = 0.001$) in the composite end points of death and MI at the end of treatment *(35)*. The first AMI trial designed to evaluate mortality with a direct thrombin inhibitor—bivalirudin compared to heparin in patients treated with streptokinase—was the HERO-2 trial, which demonstrated no effect on mortality, but one-quarter reduction in reinfarction from 2.3% to 1.6% at 4 d ($p = 0.001$), with a minor increase in the risk of bleeding complications.

5. Experimental Evidence for the Interactions Between Antiplatelets and Anticoagulant Using Thrombelastography

5.1. Thrombelastography (TEG)

TEG has been used in various hospital settings since its development by Hartert in 1948 and others. The principle of TEG is based on the measurement of the physical viscoelastic characteristics of blood clots. Clot formation is monitored at 37°C in an oscillating plastic cylindrical cuvet ("cup") and a coaxially suspended stationary piston ("pin") with a 1-mm clearance between the surfaces. The cup oscillates in either direction every 4.5 s with a 1-s mid-cycle stationary period, resulting in a frequency of 0.1 Hz. The pin is suspended by a torsion wire that acts as a torque transducer. During clot formation, fibrin fibrils physically link the cup to the pin, and the rotation of the cup is transmitted to the pin via the viscoelasticity of the clot, is displayed on-line using an IBM-compatible personal computer and customized software (Haemoscope Corp., Skokie, IL). The torque experienced by the pin is plotted as a function of time, as shown by the different TEG clot parameters.

The following TEG parameters were monitored:

r: The period of time of latency from the time that the blood was placed in the TEG® until the initial fibrin formation. R-time is prolonged by anticoagulants and is shortened by hypercoagulable states.

K: K-time is a measure of the speed needed to reach a certain level (20 mm) of clot strength. K and α both measure similar information, and both are affected by the availability of fibrinogen, which determines the rate of clot buildup; in the presence of factor XIII, which enables crosslinking of fibrin to form a stable clot; and to a lesser extent, by platelets.

α: Measures the rapidity (kinetics) of fibrin buildup and crosslinking, that is the speed of clot strengthening. α is decreased by anticoagulants that affect fibrinogen and platelet function.

MA (maximum amplitude): A direct function of the maximum dynamic properties of fibrin and platelet bonding, which represents the ultimate strength of the platelet/fibrin clot. *Maximum Amplitude* (MA, in mm), is the peak rigidity manifested by the clot at 45–90 min.

5.2. Blood Sampling

Whole blood can be collected into siliconized Vacutainer tubes (Becton-Dickinson, Rutherford, NJ) containing 3.2% trisodium citrate, so that a ratio of citrate to whole blood of 1 : 9 (v/v) is maintained. TEG was performed within 3 h of blood collection on a slow-speed rocker.

Two different conditions can be used for blood collection and induction of clot formation. These include the following: i) Calcium was added back at an average of 2.25 mM concentration followed by the addition of tissue factor (TF) (25 ng/cup) for the in vitro studies. This $CaCl_2$ concentration showed only a minimal effect on clot formation and clot strength. ii) Recalcification by adding 10 mM calcium resulted in a similar peak MA. The in vitro effects of GPIIb/IIIa antagonists, anticoagulants such as heparin or LMWH, or a combination of both at sub-effective levels on platelet/fibrin clot dynamics were examined.

LMWHs are shown to act at multiple sites, including inhibition of factor Xa, inhibition of thrombin, and via the increase in cellular release of tissue-factor pathway inhibitor (TFPI). Platelet GPIIb/IIIa blockade represents the common pathway for platelet aggregation. The present study was undertaken to determine the interactions between the LMWH tinzaparin and various platelet GPIIb/IIIa antagonists, including abciximab, integrilin, tirofiban, or roxifiban, on TF-induced platelet fibrin-clot strength (PFCS). Computerized thrombelastography (TEG) was used to determine the ability of platelets and fibrin to augment human blood clot formation and strength under conditions of maximal platelet activation accelerated by TF in human blood. The effect of sub-effective concentrations of tinzaparin (20–30% PFCS inhibition) on the dose-response of the GPIIb/IIIa antagonists and vice versa was examined. Additionally, studies in dogs given sub-effective subcutaneous (sc) doses of roxifiban (0.1 mg/kg), tinzaparin (100 IU/kg), or combinations of both on ex vivo clot retraction induced by TF using TEG were determined. Under these conditions, platelets significantly enhance clot strength eightfold relative to platelet-free fibrin clots. Abciximab and roxifiban effectively inhibited this enhancement of clot strength. In contrast, integrilin or tirofiban were much less effective. The combination of sub-effective tinzaparin and roxifiban or abciximab resulted in distinct synergy in improving the antiplatelet and anticoagulant effect mediated

Table 1
Effect of Tinzaparin and Integrilin on Inhibition of Platelet/Fibrin Clot

Antithrombotics	Conc	% Inhibition of platelet/fibrin clot
Tinzaparin	0.1 µg/mL	5 ± 2
Tinzaparin	0.2 µg/mL	12 ± 4
Integrilin	0.3 µ*M*	0
Integrilin + tinzaparin	0.3 µ*M* + 0.1 µg/mL	80 ± 9
Integrilin + tinzaparin	0.3 µ*M* + 0.2 µg/mL	100 ± 0

Data represent mean ± SD, $n = 5$.

by TF. Similar synergistic interactions were demonstrated after sc administration of roxifiban and tinzaparin at reduced doses in dogs. The in vitro dose-response relationship of PFCS using TF-TEG at reduced levels of tinzaparin with clinically achievable levels of tirofiban or integrilin significantly inhibited PFCS. These data suggest the potential of low-dose tinzaparin with either low-dose GPIIb/IIIa antagonists (abciximab or roxifiban) or with full-dose GPIIb/IIIa antagonists (integrilin or tirofiban) in the prevention and treatment of various thromboembolic disorders. The effect of tinzaparin on inhibition of platelet/fibrin clot are given in Table 1.

5.3. Need for Heparin

Results from PRISM, PRISM-PLUS, and PURSUIT suggest an important role for concomitant heparin in trials with intravenous (iv) GPIIb/IIIa inhibitors. Greater clinical benefit was shown in the patients who received the IIb/IIIa inhibitor plus heparin as compared to the IIb/IIIa inhibitor alone. These data suggested the potential benefit of heparin. Recent studies from our laboratory demonstrated a synergistic effect of heparin with class II GPIIb/IIIa antagonists in inhibiting platelet/fibrin clot dynamics. Additionally, heparin plus class I demonstrated additive effects in inhibiting clot dynamics.

Similar synergistic interactions were demonstrated between GPIIb/IIIa antagonists and thrombolytics, based on this in vitro model and based on experimental in vivo models of thrombosis as well as clinical investigations.

References

1. Fitzgerald, D. and Murphy, N. (1996) Argatroban: a synthetic thrombin inhibitor of low relative molecular mass. *Coron. Artery Dis.* **7,** 455–458.
2. Lewis, B., Matthas, W., Grassman, J. D., et al. (1997) Results of phase 2/3 trial of argatroban anticoagulation during PTCA of patients with heparin-induced thrombocytopenia (HIT). *Circulation* **96,** 1–217 (abstract).

3. Lewis, B. E., Wallis, D. E., Berkowitz, S. D., et al. (2001) Argatroban anticoagulant therapy in patients with heparin-induced thrombocytopenia. *Circulation* **103,** 1838–1843.

4. Coussement, P. K., Bassand, J. P., Convens, C., et al. (2001) A synthetic factor-Xa inhibitor (ORG31540/SR9017A) as an adjunct to fibrinolysis in acute myocardial infarction. The PENTALYSE study. *Eur. Heart J.* **22,** 1716–1724.

5. Topol, E. (1998) Toward a new frontier in myocardial reperfusion therapy: emerging platelet pre-eminence. *Circulation* **97,** 221–218.

6. Coller, B. S. (1990) Platelet and thrombolytic therapy. *N. Engl. J. Med.* **322,** 33–42.

7. Gold, H., Coller, B., Yasuda, T., et al. (1988) Rapid and sustained coronary artery recanalization with combined bolus injection of recombinant tissue type plasminogen activator and monoclonal antiplatelet GPIIb/IIIa antibody in a canine preparation. *Circulation* **77,** 670–677.

8. Gold, H., Keriakes, D., Dinsmore, R., et al. (1997) A randomized, placebo-controlled crossover trial of ReoPro alone or combined with low dose plasminogen activator for coronary reperfusion in patients with acute myocardial infarction: preliminary results. *Circulation* **96,** 1–474.

9. Antman, E., Giugliano, R., Bibson, M., et al. (1999) Abciximab facilitates the rate and extent of thrombolysis: results of the Thrombolysis in Myocardial Infarction (TIMI) 14 trial. *Circulation* **99,** 2720–2732.

10. Iqbal, O., Messmore, H., Hoppensteadt, D., Fareed, J., and Wehrmacher, W. (2000) Thrombolytic drugs in acute myocardial infarction. *Clin. Applied Thromb./ Haemost.* **6(1),** 1–13.

11. Iqbal, O., Walenga, J. M., Lewis, B. E., and Bakhos, M. (2000) Bleeding complications with glycoprotein IIb/IIIa inhibitors. *Drugs Today* **36(8),** 503–514.

12. Turpie, G. (2000) The PENTATHLON 2000 study: comparison of the first synthetic factor Xa inhibitor with low molecular weight heparin in the prevention of venous thromboembolism (VTE) after elective hip replacement surgery. *Blood* **96(11),** Abstract #2112.

13. Lassen, M. R. (2000) The EPHESUS study: comparison of the first synthetic factor Xa inhibitor with low molecular weight heparin (LMWH). The prevention of venous thromboembolism (VTE) after elective hip replacement surgery. *Blood* **96(11),** Abstract #2109.

14. Erickson, B. (2000) The PENTHIFRA study: comparison of the first synthetic Factor Xa inhibitor with low molecular weight heparin (LMWH). The prevention of venous thromboembolism (VTE) after hip fracture surgery. *Blood* **96(11),** Abstract #2110.

15. Bauer, K. (2000) The PENTAMAKS study: comparison of the first synthetic Factor Xa inhibitor with low molecular weight heparin. The prevention of venous thromboembolism (VTE) after elective major knee surgery. *Blood* **96(11),** Abstract #2111.

16. Turpie, A. G. G., Gallus, A. S., and Hoek, J. A. (2001) For the pentasaccharide investigators: a synthetic pentasaccharide for the prevention of deep vein thrombosis after total hip replacement. *N. Engl. J. Med.* **344(9),** 619–625.

17. Granger, C. B. (2002) Reperfusion therapy for Acute Myocardial Infarction, in *Textbook of Cardiovascular Medicine*, Vol. 5, No. 2, Lippincott, Philadelphia, PA, pp. 1–14.

18. Topol, E. J. (2001) The GUSTO V Investigators. Reperfusion therapy for acute myocardial infarction with fibrinolytic therapy or combination reduced fibrinolytic therapy and platelet glycoprotein IIb/IIIa inhibition: the GUSTO V randomized trial. *Lancet* **357,** 1905–1914.

19. Efficacy and safety of tenecteplase in combination with enoxaparin, abciximab, or unfractionated heparin: the ASSENT-3 randomized trial in acute myocardial infarction. The assessment of safety and efficacy of a new thrombolytic regimen (ASSENT)-3 investigators. *Lancet* **358,** 605–613.

20. White, H. and the HERO-2 Investigators (2001) Thrombin-specific anticoagulation with bivalirudin versus heparin in patients receiving fibrinolytic therapy for acute myocardial infarction: the HERO-2 randomized trial. *Lancet* **358,** 1855–1863.

21. Stoen, G. W., Grines, C. L., Cox, D. A., et al. (2002) Comparison of angioplasty with stenting, with or without abciximab, in acute myocardial infarction. *N. Engl. J. Med.* **346,** 957–966.

22. The SPEED Group (Strategies for the Patency Enhancement in the Emergency Department) (2001) Randomized trial of abciximab with and without low-dose reteplase for acute myocardial infarction. *Circulation* **101,** 2788–2794.

23. Antman, E. M., Gibson, C. M., de Lemos, J. A., et al. (2000) Combination reperfusion therapy with abciximab and reduced dose reteplase: results from TIMI 14. the Thrombolysis in Myocardial Infarction (TIMI)14 Investigators. *Eur. Heart J.* **21,** 1944–1953.

24. Antman, E. M., Louwerenburg, H. W., Baars, H. F., et al. (2002) Enoxaparin as adjunctive antithrombin therapy for ST-elevation myocardial infarction: results of the ENTIRE-Thrombolysis in Myocardial Infarction (TIMI) 23 Trial. *Circulation* **105,** 1642–1649.

25. Giugliano, R. P., Roe, M. T., Zeymer, U., et al. (2001) Restoration of epicardial and myocardial perfusion in acute ST-elevation myocardial infarction with combination eptifibatide and reduced dose tenecteplase: dose finding results from the INTEGRITI Trial (abstract). *Circulation* **104,** II–538, 2001.

26. Llevadot, J., Giugliano, R. P., and Antman, E. M. (2001) Bolus fibrinolytic therapy in acute myocardial infarction. *JAMA* **286,** 442–449.

27. Brener, S. J., Zeymer, U., Adgey, A. A., et al. (2002) Eptifibatide and low dose tissue plasminogen activator in acute myocardial infarction: the integrelin and low dose thrombolysis in acute myocardial infarction (INTRO-AMI) Trial. *J. Am. Coll. Cardiol.* **39,** 377–386.

28. Topol, E. J. and Yadav, J. S. (2000) Recognition of the importance of embolization in atherosclerotic vascular disease. *Circulation* **101,** 570–580.

29. Roe, M. T., Ohman, E. M., Maas, A. C., et al. (2001) Shifting the open-artery hypothesis downstream: the quest for optimal reperfusion. *J. Am. Coll. Cardiol.* **37,** 9–18.

30. Herrmann, H. C., Moliterno, D. J., Ohman, E. M., et al. Facilitation of early per-
    cutaneous coronary intervention after reteplase with or without abciximab in acute
    myocardial infarction: results from the SPEED (GUSTO-4 Pilot) Trial. *J. Am.
    Coll. Cardiol.* **36,** 1489–1496.
31. Ross, A. M., Molhoek, P., Lundergan, C., et al. (2001) Randomized comparison
    of enoxaparin, a low molecular weight heparin, with unfractionated heparin adjunc-
    tive to recombinant tissue plasminogen activator thrombolysis and aspirin: second
    trial of Heparin and Aspirin Reperfusion therapy (HART II). *Circulation* **104,**
    648–652.
32. Wallentin, L., Dellborg, D. M., Lindahl, B., Nilsson, T., Pehrsson, K., and Swahn,
    E. (2001) The low-molecular-weight-heparin dalteparin as adjuvant therapy in
    acute myocardial infarction: the ASSENT PLUS Study. *Clin. Cardiol.* **24 (3
    Suppl.),** L112–L114.
33. Alonso, A, for the AMI-SK Investigators. Preliminary results of the AMI-SK trial.
    Am. Coll. Cardiol. 50th Scientific Session, March 2001, Orlando, Florida.
34. Baird, S. H., Menown, I. B. A., McBride, S. J., Trouton, T. G., and Wilson, C. (2002)
    Randomized comparison of enoxaparin with unfractionated heparin following fib-
    rinolytic therapy for acute myocardial infarction. *Eur. Heart J.* **23,** 627–632.
35. Direct Thrombin Inhibitor Collaboration Investigators (2002) Direct thrombin
    inhibitors in acute coronary syndromes: principal results of a meta-analysis based
    on individual patient's data. *Lancet* **359,** 294–302.

3

Evaluation of Platelet Antagonists in In Vitro Flow Models of Thrombosis

Owen J. T. McCarty, James P. Abulencia, Shaker A. Mousa, and Konstantinos Konstantopoulos

1. Introduction

Intravascular thrombosis is one of the most frequent pathological events that affects mankind, and a major cause of morbidity and mortality in developed countries. There is abundant evidence suggesting that platelets play a pivotal role in the pathogenesis of arterial thrombotic disorders, including unstable angina (UA), myocardial infarction (MI), and stroke *(1–3)*. The underlying pathophysiological mechanism of these processes has been recognized as the disruption or erosion of a vulnerable atherosclerotic plaque, leading to local platelet adhesion and subsequent formation of partially or completely occlusive platelet thrombi.

The specific platelet-surface receptors that support these initial adhesive interactions are determined by the local fluid dynamic conditions of the vasculature and the extracellular matrix (ECM) constituents exposed at the sites of vascular injury *(4)*. Under high shear conditions, the adhesion of platelets to exposed subendothelial surfaces of atherosclerotic or injured vessels presenting collagen and von Willebrand's factor is primarily mediated by the platelet glycoprotein (GP)Ib/IX/V complex *(4,5)*. This primary adhesion to the matrix activates platelets, ultimately leading to platelet aggregation-mediated predominantly by the binding of adhesive proteins such as fibrinogen and vWF to GPIIb/IIIa *(4,5)*. In addition, direct platelet aggregation in the bulk phase under conditions of abnormally elevated fluid shear stresses, analogous to those occurring in atherosclerotic or constricted arterial vessels *(6)*, may be important. Shear-induced platelet aggregation is dependent upon the availability of vWF

From: *Methods in Molecular Medicine, vol. 93: Anticoagulants, Antiplatelets, and Thrombolytics*
Edited by: S. A. Mousa © Humana Press Inc., Totowa, NJ

and the presence of both GPIb/IX and GPIIb/IIIa on the platelet membrane. It has been postulated that at high shear stress conditions, the interaction of vWF with the GPIb/IX complex is the initial event that triggers platelet activation, as well as the binding of vWF to GPIIb/IIIa to induce platelet aggregate formation *(4)*.

Several studies have identified the pivotal role of GPIIb/IIIa in arterial thrombosis. Thus, this platelet integrin receptor has emerged as a rational therapeutic target in the management of acute coronary syndromes (ACS). The first platelet GPIIb/IIIa antagonist developed was abciximab, a chimeric Fab fragment of the monoclonal antibody (mAb) 7E3 *(7)*. Various large-scale clinical trials have demonstrated the efficacy of abciximab against major ischemic events in patients undergoing percutaneous coronary interventions (reviewed in *8*). Additionally, studies with the small-molecule GPIIb/IIIa antagonists eptifibatide and tirofiban have illustrated the clinical benefits of intravenous (iv) use of specific GPIIb/IIIa inhibitors in patients with ACS *(8)*. However, clinical development programs with orally active, rapidly reversible GPIIb/IIIa antagonists including xemilofiban (EXCITE), orbofiban (OPUS) and sibrafiban (SYMPHONY) were halted because of lack of efficacy, and perhaps increased thrombotic events *(9)*. The lack of clinical benefit for the oral agents is puzzling, and may be partially attributed to under-dosing. GPIIb/IIIa antagonists, when administered at suboptimal levels, may transiently bind to the platelet receptor and induce conformational changes, which then allow fibrinogen binding to occur after the drug dissociates from the receptor *(10)*. Along these lines, it was recently shown that oral administration of orbofiban enhanced platelet reactivity, as determined by increased fibrinogen binding to the platelet surface and elevated P-selectin expression levels *(11)*. Therefore, ex vivo monitoring must reflect the actual in vivo antiplatelet efficacy in order to optimize therapeutic dose regimens, and thus achieve clinical benefit.

A variety of methods have been utilized to evaluate the ex vivo and/or in vitro efficacy of platelet antagonists, including photometric aggregometry, whole blood electrical aggregometry, and particle counter methods. In photometric aggregometry, a sample is placed in a stirred cuvet in the optical light path between a light source and a light detector. Aggregate formation is monitored by a decrease in turbidity, and the extent of aggregation is measured as a percentage of maximal light transmission. The major disadvantage of this technique is that it cannot be applied in whole blood, since the presence of erythrocytes interferes with the optical responses. Furthermore, it is insensitive to the formation of small aggregates *(12)*. Particle counters are used to quantitate the size and the number of particles suspended in an electrolyte solution by monitoring the electrical current between two electrodes immersed in the solution. Aggregation in this system is quantitated by counting the platelets before and after stimulation, and is usually expressed as a percentage of the initial count *(13,14)*. However, the disadvantage of this technique is that it cannot distinguish platelets and platelet aggregates from other blood cells of the same size. Thus, one is limited to counting only a fraction of single platelets, as well as aggregates that are much larger than erythrocytes and leukocytes *(14)*. The technique of electrical aggregometry allows the detection of platelet aggregates as they attach to electrodes that are immersed in a stirred cuvet of whole blood or platelet suspensions. Such an attachment results in a decrease in conductance between the two electrodes that can be quantitated in units of electrical resistance. However, one disadvantage of this method is that it is not sensitive in the detection of small aggregates *(15)*.

This chapter discusses two complementary in vitro flow models of thrombosis that can be used to accurately quantify platelet aggregation in anticoagulated whole blood specimens, and to evaluate the inhibitory efficacy of platelet antagonists. i) A viscometric-flow cytometric assay to measure direct shear-induced platelet aggregation in the bulk phase *(16–19)*; and ii) a parallel-plate perfusion chamber coupled with a computerized videomicroscopy system to quantify the adhesion and subsequent aggregation of human platelets in anticoagulated whole blood flowing over an immobilized substrate (e.g., collagen I) *(19–21)*. Furthermore, a third in vitro flow assay is described in which surface-anchored platelets are pre-incubated with a GPIIb/IIIa antagonist, and unbound drug is washed away prior to the perfusion of THP-1 monocytic cells, thereby enabling us to distinguish agents with markedly distinct affinities and receptor-bound lifetimes *(19,21)*.

2. Materials

1. Anticoagulant solution (sodium citrate, porcine heparin, PPACK).
2. Fluorescently labeled platelet-specific antibody.
3. Dulbecco's phosphate-buffered saline (D-PBS) (with and without Ca^{2+}/Mg^{2+}).
4. Formaldehyde.
5. Type I collagen, from bovine Achille's tendon.
6. 0.5 mol/L glacial acetic acid in water.
7. Glass cover slips (24 × 50 mm; Corning; Corning, NY).
8. Silicone sheeting (gasket) (0.005-in or 0.010-in thickness; Specialty Manufacturing Inc., Saginaw, MI).
9. Quinacrine dihydrochloride.
10. Prostaglandin E_1 (PGE1) and EGTA.
11. Thrombin.
12. Bovine serum albumin (BSA).
13. *N*-2-hydroxyethylpiperazine *N'*2-ethane sulfonic acid (HEPES)-Tyrode buffer (129 m*M* NaCl, 9.9 m*M* $NaHCO_3$, 2.8 m*M* KCl, 0.8 m*M* K_2PO_4, 0.8 $MgCl_2 \cdot 6H_2O$, 1 m*M* $CaCl_2$, 10 m*M* HEPES, 5.6 m*M* dextrose).

14. 3-aminopropyltriethoxysilane (APES).
15. Acetone.
16. 70% nitric acid in water.
17. THP-1 monocytic cells.
18. Platelet antagonists such as abciximab.

3. Methods

The methods described here outline three dynamic adhesion/aggregation assays used to evaluate the in vitro and/or ex vivo efficacy of platelet antagonists: (i) a viscometric-flow cytometric assay to measure shear-induced platelet-platelet aggregation in the bulk phase, (ii) a perfusion chamber coupled with a computerized videomicroscopy system to visualize in real time and quantify (iia) the adhesion and subsequent aggregation of platelets flowing over an immobilized substrate (e.g., extracellular matrix [ECM] protein) and (iib) free-flowing monocytic cell adhesion to immobilized platelets.

3.1. Isolation of Human Platelets

The steps described in **Subheading 3.1.1.–3.1.3.** outline the procedure for isolation and purification of platelets from whole blood obtained by venipuncture from human volunteers.

3.1.1. Venous Blood Collection

Obtain blood sample by venipuncture from an antecubital vein into polypropylene syringes containing either sodium citrate (0.38% final concentration) or heparin (10 U/mL final concentration) *(19)*.

3.1.2. Preparation of Platelet-Rich Plasma

Centrifuge anticoagulated whole blood at 160g for 15 min to prepare platelet-rich plasma (PRP) (*see* **Note 1**).

3.1.3. Isolation of Washed Platelets

1. PRP specimens are subjected to a further centrifugation (1,100g for 15 min) in the presence of 2 μM PGE$_1$ *(22)*.
2. The platelet pellet is resuspended in HEPES-Tyrode buffer containing 5 mM EGTA and 2 μM PGE$_1$ *(22)*.
3. Platelets are then were washed via centrifugation (1,100g for 10 min) and resuspended at 2 × 10^8/mL in HEPES-Tyrode buffer *(22)*, and kept at room temperature for no longer than 4 h before use in aggregation/adhesion assays.

3.2. Viscometric-Flow Cytometric Methodology

The cone-and-plate viscometer is an in vitro flow model used to investigate the effects of bulk fluid shear stress on suspended cells. Anticoagulated whole blood specimens (or isolated cell suspensions) are placed between the two platens (both of stainless steel) of the viscometer. Rotation of the upper conical platen causes a well-defined and uniform shearing stress to be applied to the entire fluid medium *(4)*. The shear rate (γ) in this system can be readily calculated from the cone angle and the speed of the cone using the formula:

$$\gamma = \left(\frac{2\,\pi\omega}{60\theta_{cp}}\right) \tag{1}$$

where γ is the shear rate in s^{-1}, ω is the cone rotational rate in revolutions per min (rev/min) and θ_{cp} is the cone angle in radians. The latter is typically in the range of 0.3 to 1.0°. The shear stress, τ, is proportional to shear rate, γ, as shown by: $\tau = \mu \times \gamma$, where μ is the viscosity of the cell suspension (the viscosity of anticoagulated whole blood is ~0.04 cp at 37°C). This type of rotational viscometer is capable of generating shear stresses from ~2 dyn/cm^2 (venous level) to greater than 200 dyn/cm^2 (stenotic arteries) *(see* **Note 2***)*.

Single platelets and platelet aggregates generated upon shear exposure of blood specimens are differentiated from other blood cells on the basis of their characteristic forward-scatter and fluorescence (by the use of fluorophore-conjugated platelet specific-antibodies) profiles by flow cytometry *(17,18)*. This technique requires no washing or centrifugation steps that may induce artefactual platelet activation, and allows the study of platelet function in the presence of other blood elements. The steps described in this section outline the procedure used to quantify platelet aggregation induced by shear stress in the bulk phase as well as the inhibitory effects of platelet antagonists *(16,19)*.

1. Incubate anticoagulated whole blood with platelet antagonist or vehicle (control) at 37°C for 10 min.
2. Place a blood specimen (typically ~500 µL) on the stationary platen of a cone-and-plate viscometer maintained at 37°C.
3. Take a small aliquot (~3 µL) from the pre-sheared blood sample (*see* **Note 3**), fix it with 1% formaldehyde in D-PBS (~30 µL), and process it as outlined in **steps 6–8**.
4. Expose the blood specimen, in the presence or absence of a platelet antagonist, to well-defined shear levels (typically 4000 s^{-1} to induce significant platelet aggregation in the absence of a platelet antagonist) for prescribed periods of time (typically 30–60 s).
5. Take a small aliquot (3 µL) from the sheared blood specimen, and immediately fix it with 1% formaldehyde in D-PBS (~30 µL).
6. Incubate the fixed blood samples with a saturating concentration of a flucrescently labeled platelet-specific antibody, such as anti-GPIb(6D1)-fluorescein isothiocyanate (FITC), for 30 min in the dark.
7. Dilute specimens with 2 mL of 1% formaldehyde, and analyze them by flow cytometry.

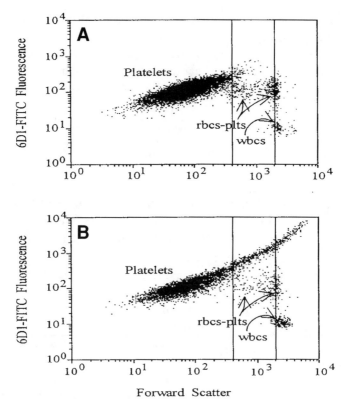

Fig. 1. Quantification of shear-induced platelet aggregation by flow cytometry. (**A**) corresponds to an unsheared blood specimen. (**B**) corresponds to a blood specimen that has been subjected to a pathologically high level of shear stress for 30 s. As can be seen in the Figure, there are three distinct cell populations. The upper population consists of platelets and platelet aggregates. The "rbcs-plts" population corresponds to platelets associated with erythrocytes and leukocytes (*see* **Note 4**). The "wbcs" population consists of some leukocytes that have elevated levels of FITC autofluorescence. The left vertical line separates single platelets (≤4.5 μm in diameter) from platelet aggregates, whereas the right vertical line separates "small" from "large" platelet aggregates. The latter were defined to be larger than 10 μm in equivalent sphere diameter. Reproduced from *Thrombosis and Haemostasis* (1995) **74(5),** 1329–1334, by copyright permission of the Schattauer GmbH *(17)*.

8. Flow-cytometric analysis is used to distinguish platelets from other blood cells on the basis of their characteristic forward scatter and fluorescence profiles, as shown in **Fig. 1**. Data acquisition is then carried out on each sample for a set period (usually 100 s), thereby allowing equal volumes for both the pre-sheared and

sheared specimens to be achieved. As a result, the percent platelet aggregation can be determined by the disappearance of single platelets into the platelet aggregate region using the formula:

$$\% \text{ platelet aggregation} = (1 - Ns/Nc) \times 100 \qquad (2)$$

where Ns represents the single-platelet population of the sheared specimen and Nc represents the single-platelet population of the pre-sheared specimen. By comparing the extents of platelet aggregation in the presence and absence of a platelet antagonist, its antiplatelet efficacy can be readily determined.

3.3. Platelet Adhesion and Subsequent Aggregation onto Collagen I Under Dynamic Flow Conditions

The steps described in **Subheadings 3.3.1.** and **3.3.2.** outline an in vitro flow model of platelet thrombus formation that can be used to evaluate the ex vivo and/or in vitro efficacy of platelet antagonists. In vivo, thrombus formation may be initiated by platelet adhesion from rapidly flowing blood onto exposed subendothelial surfaces of injured vessels containing collagen and vWF, with subsequent platelet activation and aggregation. The use of a parallel-plate flow chamber provides a controlled and well-defined flow environment based on the chamber geometry and the flow rate through the chamber *(4)*. The wall shear stress, τ_w, assuming a Newtonian and incompressible fluid, can be calculated using the formula:

$$\tau_w = \frac{6\,\mu Q}{wh^2} \qquad (3)$$

where Q is the volumetric flow rate, μ is the viscosity of the flowing fluid, h is the channel height, and b is the channel width. A flow chamber typically consists of a transparent polycarbonate block, a gasket whose thickness determines the channel depth, and a glass cover slip coated with an ECM protein such as type I fibrillar collagen. The apparatus is held together by vacuum. Shear stress is generated by flowing fluid (e.g., anticoagulated whole blood or isolated cell suspensions) through the chamber over the immobilized substrate under controlled kinematic conditions using a syringe pump. Combining the parallel-plate flow chamber with a computerized epifluorescence videomicroscopy system enables us to visualize in real time and separately quantify the adhesion and subsequent aggregation of human platelets in anticoagulated whole blood (or isolated platelet suspensions) flowing over an immobilized substrate *(19–21)*.

3.3.1. Preparation of Collagen-Coated Surfaces

1. Dissolve 500 mg collagen type I from bovine Achille's tendon into 200 mL of 0.5 mol/L acetic acid in water, pH 2.8.

2. Homogenize for 3 h.
3. Centrifuge the homogenate at 200g for 10 min, collect supernatant, and measure collagen concentration by a modified Lowry analysis *(23)*.
4. Coat glass cover slips with 200 µL of fibrillar collagen I suspension on all but first 10 mm of the slide length (coated area = 12.7 × 23), and place in a humid environment at 37°C for 45 min.
5. Rinse excess collagen with 10 mL of D-PBS maintained at 37°C before assembly into the flow chamber (*see* **Note 5**).

3.3.2. Platelet Perfusion Studies

1. Add the fluorescent dye quinacrine dihydrochloride to anticoagulated whole blood samples at a final concentration of 10 µ*M* immediately after blood collection.
2. Prior to the perfusion experiment, incubate blood with either a platelet antagonist or vehicle (control) at 37°C for 10 min.
3. Perfuse anticoagulated whole blood through the flow chamber for 1 min at wall shear rates ranging from 100 s^{-1} (typical of venous circulation) to 1500 s^{-1} (mimicking partially constricted arteries) for prescribed periods of time (e.g., 1 min). Platelet-substrate interactions are monitored in real time using an inverted microscope equipped with an epifluorescent illumination attachment and silicon-intensified target video camera, and recorded on videotape (*see* **Note 6**). The microscope stage and flow chamber are maintained at 37°C by an incubator heating module and incubator enclosure during the experiment.
4. Videotaped images are digitized and computer-analyzed at 5, 15, and 60 s for each perfusion experiment. The number of adherent individual platelets in the microscopic field of view during the initial 15 s of flow is determined by image processing and used as the measurement of platelet adhesion that initiates platelet thrombus formation. The number of platelets in each individual thrombus is calculated as the total thrombus intensity (area × fluorescence intensity) divided by the average intensity of single platelets determined in the 5-s images (*see* **Note 7**). By comparing the extents of platelet aggregation in the presence and absence of a platelet antagonist, its antiplatelet efficacy can be determined (**Fig. 2**). Along these lines, any potential inhibitory effects of a platelet antagonist on platelet adhesion can be readily evaluated.

3.4. Cell Adhesion to Immobilized Platelets Using a Parallel-Plate Flow Chamber

The steps described in **Subheadings 3.4.1.–3.4.3.** outline an in vitro flow assay to distinguish agents with markedly distinct affinities and off-rates. In this assay, immobilized platelets are pretreated with a GPIIb/IIIa antagonist, and any unbound drug is washed away before the perfusion of monocytic THP-1 cells. We have demonstrated that agents with slow platelet off-rates such as XV454 ($\tau_{1/2}$ of dissociation = 110 min; K$_d$ = 1 nm) and abciximab ($\tau_{1/2}$ of dissociation = 40 min; K$_d$ = 9.0 nm) *(19)* that are distributed predominantly as receptor-

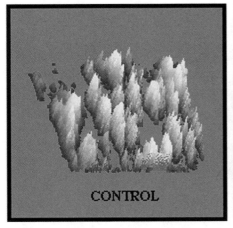 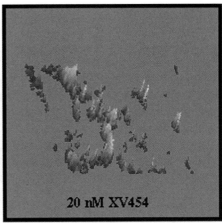

Fig. 2. Three-dimensional computer-generated representation of platelet adhesion and subsequent aggregation on collagen I/von Willebrand factor from normal heparinized blood perfused in the absence (control) or presence of a GPIIb/IIIa antagonist (XV454) at 37°C for 1 min at 1,500 s^{-1}. Reproduced from *Arterioscl. Thromb. B. Vasc. Biol.* (2001) **21,** 149–156 by copyright permission of Lippincott, Williams, & Wilkins *(19)*.

bound entities with little unbound in the plasma, can effectively block these heterotypic interactions *(19,21)*. In contrast, agents with relatively fast platelet dissociation rates such as orbofiban ($\tau_{1/2}$ of dissociation = 0.2 min; Kd >110 nm), whose antiplatelet efficacy depends on the plasma concentration of the active drug, do not exhibit any inhibitory effects *(19,21)*.

3.4.1. Preparation of 3-Aminopropyltriethoxysilane Treated Glass Slides

1. Soak glass cover slips overnight in 70% nitric acid.
2. Wash cover slips with tap water for 4 h.
3. Dry cover slips by washing once with acetone, followed by immersion in a 4% solution of APES in acetone for 2 min.
4. Repeat **step 3**, followed by a final rinse of the glass coverslips with acetone.
5. Wash cover slips 3× with water, and allow them to dry overnight.

3.4.2. Immobilization of Platelets on 3-Aminopropyltriethoxysilane Treated Glass Slides

1. Layer washed platelets or PRP (2×10^8 cells/mL) on the surface of a cover slip at 30 µL/cm^2.
2. Allow platelets to bind to APES-treated cover slip in a humid environment at 37°C for 30 min.

3.4.3. Monocytic THP-1 Cell-Platelet Adhesion Assay

1. Assemble the platelet-coated cover slip on a parallel-plate flow chamber that is then mounted on the stage of an inverted microscope equipped with a CCD camera connected to a VCR and TV monitor.
2. Perfuse the antiplatelet antagonist at the desirable concentration or vehicle (control) over surface-bound platelets, and incubate for 10 min. The extent of platelet activation can be further modulated by the presence of chemical agonists such as thrombin (0.02–2 U/mL) during the 10-min incubation. The microscope stage and flow chamber are maintained at 37°C by an incubator heating module and incubator enclosure during the experiment.
3. In some experiments, unbound platelet antagonist is removed by a brief washing step (4 min) prior to the perfusion of the cells of interest over the platelet layer. In others, the desirable concentration of the platelet antagonist is continuously maintained in the perfusion buffer during the entire course of the experiment.
4. Perfuse cells (e.g., THP-1 monocytic cells, leukocytes, tumor cells, protein-coated beads, etc.) over surface-bound platelets, either in the presence or absence of a platelet antagonist at the desirable flow rate for prescribed periods of time. THP-1 cell binding to immobilized platelets is monitored in real time, and recorded on videotape **(Fig. 3)**.
5. Determine the extent of THP-1 cell tethering, rolling, and stationary adhesion to immobilized platelets as well as the average velocity of rolling THP-1 cells (*see* **Note 8**). By comparing the corresponding extents of THP-1 cell tethering, rolling, and stationary adhesion to immobilized platelets in the presence and absence of a platelet antagonist, its antiplatelet efficacy can be determined *(19,21)*.

4. Notes

1. Low-speed centrifugation results in the separation of platelets (top layer) from larger and more dense cells such as leukocytes and erythrocytes (bottom layer). To minimize leukocyte contamination in PRP specimens, slowly aspirate the uppermost two-thirds of the platelet layer. Furthermore, certain rare platelet disorders, such as Bernard-Soulier syndrome (BSS), are characterized by larger than normal platelets that must therefore be isolated by allowing whole blood to gravity separate for 2 h post-venipuncture.
2. The mechanical force most relevant to platelet-mediated thrombosis is shear stress. The normal time-averaged levels of venous and arterial shear stresses range between 1 and 5 dyn/cm^2 and 6–40 dyn/cm^2, respectively. However, fluid shear stress may reach levels well over 200 dyn/cm^2 in small arteries and arterioles partially obstructed by atherosclerosis or vascular spasm. The cone-and-plate viscometer and parallel-plate flow chamber are two of the most common devices used to simulate fluid mechanical shearing stress conditions in blood vessels *(4)*.
3. Because of the large concentration of platelets and erythrocytes in whole blood, small aliquots (~3 µL) of pre-sheared and post-sheared specimens must be obtained and processed prior to the flow cytometric analysis. This will minimize

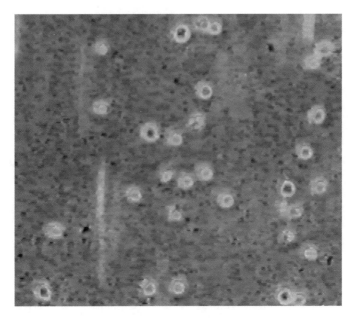

Fig. 3. Phase-contrast photomicrograph of THP-1 cells (phase bright objects) attached to a layer of thrombin-treated platelets (phase dark objects) after THP-1 cell perfusion for 3 min at a shear stress level of 1.5 dyn/cm^2.

an artifact produced as a platelet and an erythrocyte pass through the light beam of a flow cytometer at the same time *(18)*.

4. The "rbcs-plts" population represents 3–5% of the displayed cells. A small fraction (~5%) of this population seems to be leukocyte-platelet aggregates as evidenced by the use of an anti-CD45 monoclonal antibody *(18)*. The remaining events correspond to erythrocytes associated with platelets. However, it appears that the majority of the latter population is an artifact generated by the simultaneous passage of a platelet and an erythrocyte through the beam of a flow cytometer. This concept is corroborated by the fact that further dilution of pre-sheared and sheared blood specimens and/or reduction of the sample flow rate during the flow cytometric analysis results in a dramatic relative decrease of the "rbcs-plts" population *(18)*.

5. The collagen density remaining on glass cover slips after D-PBS rinsing can be measured by the difference in weight of 20 clean uncoated slides vs 20 collagen-treated slides *(24)*.

6. Experiments are optimally monitored ~100–200 μm downstream from the collagen/glass interface using a 60X FLUOR objective and 1X projection lens, which gives a 3.2×10^4 μm^2 field of view *(19,21)*. A field of view closer to the interface may lead to non-reproducible results because of variations in the collagen layering in

that region. In contrast, positions farther downstream are avoided in order to minimize the effects of upstream platelet adhesion, and subsequent aggregation on both the fluid dynamic environment as well as bulk platelet concentration.

7. The digitization of a background image (at the onset of perfusion prior to platelet adhesion to the collagen I surface) and its subtraction from a subsequent image acquired 5-s after an initial platelet adhesion event allows the determination of the fluorescence intensity emitted by a single platelet. The intensity level of each single platelet is measured as a mean gray level between 0 (black) and 255 (white) through the use of an image-processing software (e.g., OPTIMAS; Agris-Schoen Vision Systems, Alexandria, VA), and is multiplied by its corresponding area (total number of pixels covered by each single platelet). The aforementioned products are then averaged for all single-platelet events detected at the 5-s timepoint, thus enabling us to calculate the average intensity of single platelets.

8. A single field of view (10X; 0.55 mm^2) is monitored during the 3-min period of the experiment, and at the end five additional fields of view (0.55 mm^2) are monitored for 15 s each *(21)*. The following parameters can be quantified: i) the number of total interacting cells per mm^2 during the entire 3-min perfusion experiment; ii) the number of stationary interacting cells per mm^2 after 3 min of shear flow; iii) the percentage of total interacting cells that are stationary after 3 min of shear flow; and iv) the average rolling velocity (μm/s) of interacting cells. The number of interacting cells per mm^2 is determined manually by reviewing the videotapes. Stationary interacting cells per mm^2 are considered as those that move <1-cell radius within 10 s at the end of the 3-min attachment assay. To quantify their number, images can be digitized from a videotape recorder using an imaging software package (e.g., OPTIMAS). Rolling velocities can be computed as the distance traveled by the centroid of the rolling THP-1 cell divided by the time interval using image processing.

Acknowledgments

This work was supported by a Mid-Atlantic American Heart Association Grant-in-Aid and a DuPont Young Professor Grant.

References

1. Antiplatelet Trialist Collaboration. (1994) Collaborative overview of randomized trials of antiplatelet therapy-I: prevention of death myocardial infarction and stroke by prolonged antiplatelet therapy in various categories of patients. *Br. Med. J.* **308,** 81–106.

2. Fitzgerald, D. J., Roy, L., Catella, F., and Fitzgerald, G. A. (1986) Platelet activation in unstable coronary disease. *N. Eng. J. Med.* **315,** 983–989.

3. Fuster, V. (1994) Mechanisms leading to myocardial infarction: insights from studies of vascular biology. *Circulation* **90,** 2126–2146.

4. Konstantopoulos, K., Kukreti, S., and McIntire, L. V. (1998) Biomechanics of cell interactions in shear fields. *Adv. Drug Delivery Rev.* **33,** 141–164.

5. Alevriadou, B. R., Moake, J. L., Turner, N. A., Ruggeri, Z. M., Folie, B. J., Phillips, M. D., et al. (1993) Real-time analysis of shear dependent thrombus formation and its blockade by inhibitors of von Willebrand factor binding to platelets. *Blood* **81,** 1263–1276.
6. Turitto, V. T. (1982) Blood viscosity, mass transport, and thrombogenesis. *Prog. Hemostasis Thromb.* **6,** 139–177.
7. The EPIC Investigators (1994) Use of a monoclonal antibody directed against the glycoprotein IIb/IIIa receptor in high-risk coronary angioplasty. *N. Engl. J. Med.* **330,** 956–961.
8. Konstantopoulos, K. and Mousa, S. A. (2001) Antiplatelet therapies: platelet GPIIb/IIIa antagonists and beyond. *Current Opinion in Investigational Drugs* **2,** 1086–1092.
9. Mousa, S. A. (1999) Antiplatelet therapies: recent advances in the development of platelet GPIIb/IIIa antagonists, in *Current Interventional Cardiology Reports,* Vol. 1. (Holmes, D. R., ed.), Current Science, Philadelphia, PA, pp. 243–252.
10. Peter, K., Schwarz, M., Ylanne, J., Kohler, B., Moser, M., Nordt, T., et al. (1998) Induction of fibrinogen binding and platelet aggregation as a potential intrinsic property of various glycoprotein IIb/IIIa inhibitors. *Blood* **92,** 3240–3249.
11. Holmes, M. B., Sobel, B. E., Cannon, C. P., and Schneider, D. J. (2000) Increased platelet reactivity in patients given orbofiban after an acute coronary syndrome. An OPUS-TIMI 16 substudy. *Am. J. Cardiol.* **85,** 491–493.
12. Gear, A. R. L. and Lambrecht, J. K. (1981) Reduction in single platelets during primary and secondary aggregation. *Thromb. Haemostasis* **45,** 298.
13. Peterson, D. M., Stathopoulos, N. A., Giorgio, T. D, Hellums, J. D., and Moake, J. L. (1987) Shear-induced platelet aggregation requires von Willebrand factor and platelet membrane glycoproteins Ib and IIb-IIIa. *Blood* **69,** 625–628.
14. Jen, C. J. and McIntire, L. V. (1984) Characteristics of shear-induced aggregation in whole blood. *J. Lab. Clin. Med.* **103,** 115–124.
15. Sweeney, J. D., Labuzzetta, J. W., Michielson, C. E., and Fitzpatrick, J. E. (1989) Whole blood aggregation using impedance and particle counter methods. *Am. J. Clin. Pathol.* **92,** 794–797.
16. Konstantopoulos, K., Kamat, S. G., Schafer, A. I., Bañez, E. I., Jordan, R., Kleiman, N. S., et al. (1995) Shear-Induced Platelet Aggregation is inhibited by in vivo infusion of an anti-glycoprotein IIb/IIIa antibody fragment, c7E3 Fab, in patients undergoing coronary angioplasty. *Circulation* **91,** 1427–1431.
17. Konstantopoulos, K., Grotta, J. C., Sills, C., Wu, K. K., and Hellums, J. D. (1995) Shear-induced platelet aggregation in normal subjects and stroke patients. *Thromb. Haemostasis* **74,** 1329–1334.
18. Konstantopoulos, K., Wu, K. K., Udden, M. M., Bañez, E. I., Shattil, S. J., and Hellums, J. D. (1995) Flow cytometric studies of platelet responses to shear stress in whole blood. *Biorheology* **32,** 73–93.
19. Abulencia, J. P., Tien, N., McCarty, O. J. T., Plymire, D., Mousa, S. A., and Konstantopoulos, K. (2001) Comparative antiplatelet efficacy of a novel, nonpep-

tide GPIIb/IIIa antagonist (XV454) and Abciximab (c7E3) in Flow Models of Thrombosis. *Arterioscler. Thromb. Vasc. Biol.* **21,** 149–156.

20. Turner, N. A., Moake, J. A., Kamat, S. G., Schafer, A. I., Kleiman, N. S., and McIntire, L. V. (1995) Comparative real-time effects on platelet adhesion and aggregation under flowing conditions of in vivo aspirin, heparin, and monoclonal antibody fragment against glycoprotein IIb-IIIa. *Circulation* **91,** 1354–1362.

21. Mousa, S. A., Abulencia, J. P., McCarty, O. J. T., Turner, N. A., and Konstantopoulos, K. (2002) Comparative efficacy between the glycoprotein IIb/IIIa antagonists roxifiban and orbofiban in inhibiting platelet responses in flow models of thrombosis. *J. Cardiovasc. Pharmacol.* **39,** 552–560.

22. Evangelista, V., Manarini, S., Rotondo, S., Martelli, N., Polischuk, R., McGregor, J. L., et al. (1996) Platelet/polymorphonuclear leukocyte interaction in dynamic conditions: evidence of adhesion cascade and cross talk between P-selectin and the beta 2 integrin CD11b/CD18. *Blood* **88,** 4183–4194.

23. Folie, B. J., McIntire, L. V., and Lasslo, A. (1988) Effects of a novel antiplatelet agent in mural thrombogenesis on collagen-coated glass. *Blood* **72,** 1393–1400.

24. Ross, J. M., McIntire, L. V., Moake, J. L., and Rand, J. H. (1995) Platelet adhesion and aggregation on human type VI collagen surfaces under physiological flow conditions. *Blood* **85,** 1826–1835.

4

Heparin and Low Molecular Weight Heparin in Thrombosis, Cancer, and Inflammatory Diseases

Shaker A. Mousa

1. Introduction

Despite the research and development efforts in newer anticoagulants, unfractionated heparin (UFH) and low molecular weight heparin (LMWH) will continue to play a pivotal role in the management of thrombotic disorders. Although bleeding and heparin-induced thrombocytopenia (HIT) represent major side effects of this drug, it has remained the anticoagulant of choice for the prophylaxis and treatment of arterial and venous thrombotic disorders, surgical anticoagulation, and interventional usage. It is the understanding of the structure of heparin that led to the development of LMWHs, synthetic heparinomimetics, antithrombin (AT), and anti-Xa agents.

In recent years, clinical data and studies have clarified both the potential and the shortcomings of anticoagulant therapy in the prevention and treatment of thromboembolic disorders. The discovery and introduction of heparin derivatives such as LMWHs have enhanced the clinical options for the management of thromboembolic disorders while enhancing the safety of therapy. In the United States LMWHs are currently approved for the prophylaxis and treatment of deep venous thrombosis (DVT). LMWH uses are also being expanded for additional indications for the management of unstable angina and non Q-wave myocardial infarction (MI) *(1–4)*. In addition to the approved uses, LMWHs are currently being tested for several newer indications. Because they are polypharmacological agents, these drugs are expected to find uses in several other clinical indications such as inflammatory diseases and cancer. Additional pharmacological studies and well-designed clinical trials in which various pharmacokinetic and pharmacodynamic parameters are studied will provide addi-

From: *Methods in Molecular Medicine, vol. 93: Anticoagulants, Antiplatelets, and Thrombolytics*
Edited by: S. A. Mousa © Humana Press Inc., Totowa, NJ

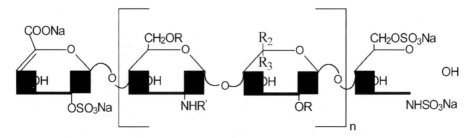

Fig. 1. Example of a structure of representative LMWH: Tinzaparin. $n = 1–25$, R = H or SO_3Na, R′ = H or SO_3Na or $COCH_3$; R_2 = H and R_3 = COONa or R_2 = COONa and R_3 = H.

tional evidence on the clinical individuality of each of this class of novel agents *(1–4)*. The key reason for the success of heparin in thrombosis and beyond is its polypharmacological site of actions for the prevention and treatment of mutifactorial diseases that will only benefit slightly with single pharmacological mechanism-based agents. Thromboembolic disorders are driven by hypercoaguable, hyperactive platelet, pro-inflammatory, endothelial dysfunction, and pro-angiogenesis states. Heparin can effectively modulate all of those mutifactorial components as well as the interface among those components.

As heparin was discovered more than half a century ago, our knowledge of the chemical structure and molecular interactions of this fascinating polycomponent was limited at the early stages of its development. Through the efforts of a major multidisciplinary group of researchers and clinicians, it is now well-recognized that heparin has multiple sites of actions and can be used in multiple indications. It is not too distant in the future to witness the impact of these drugs on the management of various diseases.

Tinzaparin sodium **(Fig. 1)** is a LMWH produced by controlled enzymatic depolymerization of conventional, unfractionated porcine heparin *(3,5)*. Tinzaparin is a potent anticoagulant as compared to other known LMWH *(6)*. Tinzaparin is more effective than UFH as treatment for DVT, is effective in the treatment of pulmonary embolism (PE), and the prevention of DVT in abdominal surgery patients, and is superior to warfarin as thromboembolism prophylaxis in subjects who are undergoing orthopedic joint (hip or knee) replacement surgery *(7–10)*. It is also an effective anticoagulant for hemodialysis extracorporeal circuits *(11)*. Tinzaparin has been marketed for more than 10 yr in Europe, 6 yr in Canada, and more recently, has been FDA-approved in the United States and worldwide under the trade name Innohep (Leo Pharmaceutical Products). Indications approved in countries outside the United States include treatment of DVT, treatment of PE, prevention of DVT following hip or knee replacement surgery, prevention of DVT following general surgery, and anticoagulation of extracorporeal circuits during hemodialysis.

Anti-Xa activity has served as the primary biomarker for evaluating the exposure of Tinzaparin and other LMWHs. It is used to define in vitro potency and to monitor therapeutic response *(12)*. Because LMWHs are polycomponent moieties with multiple biological actions each with distinct time-courses, the true pharmacokinetic behavior of these agents cannot be evaluated with assays developed for a single pharmacological activity. The absolute bioavailability is approx 90% based on anti-Xa activity *(12,13)* and 93% based on plasma tissue-factor pathway inhibitor (TFPI).

Recent clinical trials in which LMWHs with different anti-Xa to anti-IIa ratios were tested in DVT patients following hip replacement found no difference in efficacy or safety measures as compared to UFH *(13,14)*, despite distinct differences in biomarker activity profiles. However, anti-Xa activity is sensitive as an indicator of molecular weight distribution differences with various heparin fractions *(3,5,15)*. LMWHs vary in their affinity for ATIII, presumably because of production method *(16)*. Such differences have been cited as a partial explanation for the differences in LMWH pharmacodynamics as evaluated by anti-Xa activity, and one reason why they cannot be used interchangeably. In contrast, TFPI, a vascular endothelial biomarker, might represent a greater potential for the role of LMWH in various diseases *(17,18)*.

2. Pharmacology of Heparin and LMWH

UFH is a highly negatively charged glycosaminoglycan (GAG) that binds freely and nonspecifically to various proteins, and effectively binds to antithrombin III (ATIII). Since plasma protein levels of ATIII are variable, constant monitoring of the UFH dose is required. UFH is currently indicated for the prevention of DVT in low-risk patients (<40 yr of age; undergoing uncomplicated surgery; no risk for thromboembolism) and high-risk patients (>40 yr of age, undergoing major or orthopedic surgery, with previous DVT) *(19–21)*. The UFH dose should be monitored to keep the activated partial thromboplastin time (APTT) at 1.5 to provide adequate prophylaxis. Under these circumstances, an increased risk for postoperative bleeding accompanies the use of UFH *(20,22)*. UFH is also indicated for the treatment of DVT, given as a continuous intravenous (iv) administration concomitant with warfarin (started on d 1 or d 2 after the qualifying event, for 3 mo). Additional indications for UFH include treatment of acute PE, myocardial infarction (MI), unstable angina, embolism in patients with atrial fibrillation (AF), and in acute peripheral arterial occlusion *(23–28)*.

Longterm UFH administration has been shown to increase osteoclastic activity and bone resorption, which may be related to the dosage rather than duration of exposure to UFH *(20,29)*. Hypersensitivity to UFH preparations may cause necrosis of skin overlying the injection site, which is believed to be the result of the formation of antigen-antibody complexes, with or without deposition of platelets. UFH injections have also been associated with metabolic changes, such as a marked increase in both lipolytic activity and plasma levels of free fatty acids, which may cause complications in patients with type II hyperlipidemia *(29)*.

LMWHs have a lower reactivity to platelets, which correlates inversely with the anticoagulant activity in normal platelet-rich plasma (PRP). However, LMWH fractions with low and high antithrombotic activity reacted equally with platelets in PRP depleted of AT, suggesting the formation of heparin-AT complexes that protect platelets from aggregation *(30)*. LMWHs are less affected than UFH by platelet factor 4 (PF4), a protein that effectively neutralizes heparin molecules *(31,32)*.

In contrast to UFH, LMWHs have a lower affinity to bind to plasma proteins, endothelial cells, and macrophages. This difference in binding profile explains the pharmacokinetic differences observed between LMWHs and UFH. The binding of UFH to plasma proteins reduces its anticoagulant activity, which combined with the variations in plasma concentrations of heparin-binding proteins, is reflected in its unpredictable anticoagulant response **(Table 1)**.

LMWHs exhibit improved subcutaneous (sc) bioavailability; lower protein binding; longer half-life; variable number of ATIII binding sites; variable GAG contents; variable antiserine protease activities (anti-Xa, anti-IIa, anti-Xa/anti-IIa ratio, and other anticoagulation factors); variable potency in releasing TPFPI; variable levels of vascular endothelial-cell-binding kinetics *(15–18)*. For these reasons, during the last decade LMWHs have increasingly replaced UFH in the prevention and treatment of venous thromboembolic disorders such as venous thromboembolism (VTE). Randomized clinical trials have demonstrated that individual LMWHs used at optimized dosages are at least as effective and probably safer than UFH. The convenient once- or twice daily sc dosing regimen without the need for monitoring has encouraged the wide use of LMWHs. It is well-established that different LMWHs vary in their physical and chemical properties because of the differences in their methods of manufacturing. These differences translate into differences in their pharmacodynamic and pharmacokinetic characteristics *(16)*. The World Health Organization (WHO) and United States Food and Drug Administration (FDA) regard LMWHs as individual drugs that cannot be used interchangeably *(16,33)*.

Bioavailability of LMWHs after iv or sc administration is greater than for UFH, and was determined to be between ~87% and 98%. By contrast, UHF has a bioavailability of 15–25% after sc administration. LMWHs have a biological half-life (based on anti-Xa clearance) nearly double that of UFH. The half-life

Table 1
UFH vs LMWH

UFH	LMWH
Continuous, iv infusion	BID or QD sc injection
Primarily administered in hospital	Administered in hospital, office, or home
Usually administered by healthcare professionals	Administered by patient, caregiver, or professional
Monitoring and dosing adjustments	No monitoring, fixed, or weight-based dosing
Frequent dosing errors	More precise dosing
Risk of thrombocytopenia and osteoporosis	Decreased risk of adverse events
Cheap, but not cost-effective	Demonstrated pharmacoeconomic benefits
Requires 5–7 d in the hospital	Requires 0–2 d in the hospital

of LMWHs enoxaparin, deltaparin, tinzaparin, and others has been documented to be between ~100 and 360 min, depending on whether the administration of LMWH was iv or sc. The anti-Xa activity persists longer than AT activity, which reflects the faster clearance of longer heparin chains *(34)*.

LMWH, in doses based on patient weight, needs no monitoring, possibly because of the better bioavailability, longer plasma half-life, and more predictable anticoagulant response of LMWHs compared with UFH, when administered subcutaneously. Although LMWHs are more expensive than UFH, a pilot study in pediatric patients found that sc LMWH administration reduced the number of necessary laboratory assays, nursing hours, and phlebotomy time *(35)*.

LMWHs are expected to continue to diminish UFH use, through development programs for new indications and increased clinician comfort with use of the drugs. In addition, as both patients and healthcare providers recognize the relative simplicity of administration with a sc injection, together with real cost savings and quality-of-life benefits by reducing hospital stays, the trend toward outpatient use will continue.

3. LMWH Differentiation: Structure–Function Differences

The variations in molecular composition and pharmacological properties of LMWHs are reflected in clinical trials that have reported differences in clinical efficacy and safety. Therefore, each LMWH should be considered a unique substance. The main differences between LMWHs are variations in the amount of pharmacologically active product, varying chemical and physical compositions resulting in different biologic actions, and differences in results from clinical trials performed at optimized doses for each agent. The FDA considers each LMWH to be a distinct drug that cannot be interchanged with another LMWH.

LMWHs have different physiochemical characteristics because of their diverse methods of preparation, which make them non-interchangeable. The anticoagulant potency of heparin is measured as USP U/mg. This method is only applicable to LMWHs at high doses, when their anticoagulant properties are apparent. Anti-Xa activity has not enabled standardization of the biologic actions of LMWHs, since it does not address the ATIII-independent actions of LMWHs. The European Pharmacopoeia Commission has nevertheless adopted anti-Xa activity as a measure of LMWH potency. Since other markers of pharmacological activity also differ among LWMHs, their anti-IIa activity may prove useful in determining the biologic activity of each LMWH.

3.1. Method of Manufacturing

All of the commercially available LMWHs are manufactured by depolymerization of porcine mucosal heparin preparations. Bovine heparins are not used in their production because of viral contamination. LMWHs are prepared either by chemical or enzymatic digestion methods *(5)*. Most LMWHs exhibit approximately one-third of the molecular weight of regular heparin. Initially, the clinical batches of LMWHs were prepared by ethanolic fractionation of heparin. However, because of cost and limited availability of heparin for the sizeable isolation of these agents, chemical and enzymatic depolymerization procedures have been developed. Physical methods such as irradiation and the ultrasonification process have also been employed in the preparation of these agents. All of the currently available LMWHs are currently manufactured by chemical or enzymatic depolymerization of porcine mucosal heparin *(3,15,16)*. Controlled depolymerization processes have been widely used to produce products with similar molecular weights; however, marked differences in the chemical composition of each of these products were noted during the depolymerization process. Tinzaparin is the only known LMWH that is prepared by enzymatic hydrolysis with heparinase *(3,5,15,16)*.

Although the depolymerization process results in lower molecular weight heparin products (MW 4–8 *Kd*), these products exhibit differences in both of their molecular structural and functional properties *(15,16)*. Optimized methods are currently employed to prepare LMWHs, which exhibit a similar molecular profile. However, because of the significant differences in the chemical or enzymatic procedures, structural variations are found in all of these agents. Therefore, these differences exert significant influence on the biologic action of these products *(6)*. Safety and efficacy comparison of these agents in well-designed clinical trials to demonstrate clinical differences in each of the individual products have only recently become available. Initial attempts to standardize LMWHs because of their biologic actions, such as anti-Xa potency, have failed. A potency designation because of the anti-Xa actions represents only one of the several properties of these agents. Furthermore, this assay only measures the AT-III affinity-based actions of some of the components of these agents. Many of the pharmacological actions of LMWHs are based on the non-ATIII affinity components of the drugs. These include the release of TFPI, t-PA, inhibition of adhesion molecule release, decrease in the circulating von Willebrand's Factor, and modulation of blood flow. Most of these effects are not measurable through the conventional methods to assay heparin such as the anti-Xa, anti-IIa, and global anticoagulant tests.

Because a wide range of GAGs of varying chain length and molecular weight typifies UFH, treatment and response are difficult to standardize and predict. LMWHs are depolymerized heparin preparations, derived by chemical or enzymatic methods. The method of production of LMWHs influences their pharmacokinetic properties and anticoagulant activities. The differing methods of LMWH preparation result in considerable molecular heterogeneity, which are apparent in the demonstrated differences among LMWHs in anti-IIa and anti-Xa activities, platelet interactions, and protamine and PF4 neutralization activities. The LMWHs are bioequivalent (anti-Xa, USP), and their biologic effects also vary according to the route of administration. Significantly different bleeding profiles were noted for each of the LMWHs, depending on whether they were administered intravenously or subcutaneously.

3.2. Molecular Weight Distribution

The resulting molecules have a mean molecular mass of 4–8 *Kd*. More than 60% of the polysaccharides have molecular masses between 2 and 8 *Kd*, resulting in a reduction in thrombin-neutralizing capacity (anti-IIa activity). The anticoagulant properties of heparins depend on the presence of specific pentasaccharide sequences with a high affinity to ATIII *(5,15,16)*. The depolymerization methods result in modified ATIII-binding sites on the heparins and reduced activity of specific LMWHs. LMWHs have different properties and characteristics, a direct result of their method of synthesis and the resulting molecular weight distribution *(5,15,16)*.

3.3. Degree of Sulfation

Chemical modifications of the end groups and internal structure, degree of sulfation, and charge density vary from product to product, and affect the characteristics of the products. Depending on the method of preparation, the LMWHs are different mixtures of various polysaccharides, antifactor X (anti-Xa), anti-IIa activities, endothelial TFPI release, and different biologic actions *(6,16)*.

4. Plasmatic Effects

Heparin affects the coagulation cascade at multiple sites. Heparin-mediated effects could be classified as either AT-dependent or AT-independent. Individual LMWHs have predictable pharmacological actions, increased bioavailability, prolonged half-life ($t_{1/2}$), and sustained activity compared to UFH, making it possible to provide adequate anticoagulation for DVT prophylaxis with one sc administration per 24 h in the case of some LMWHs (3).

The anti-IIa-to-anti-Xa ratio for UFH is approximately one. By convention, the anti-Xa effect of LMWHs is identical, although the anti-IIa increases as the heparin molecular weight increases. US pharmacopoeia amidolytic measurements of the various LMWHs have demonstrated differences in anti-Xa activities for each LMWH (33). However, since anti-IIa and anti-Xa activities of each LMWH do not represent the total antithrombotic and antihemorrhagic effects of the respective agents, the International Society on Thrombosis and Haemostasis recommends that vial labeling should be based on weight. Labeling should also include specific anti-IIa and anti-Xa activity as evaluated against the International Standard and the recommended therapeutic dose (20).

Pharmacokinetic studies have shown that LMWHs have a relatively high bioavailability after sc injection as compared to UFH, and demonstrated a longer half-life of their anticoagulant anti-Xa activity than UFH, LMWHs have been demonstrated to be highly effective in the prevention of venous thrombosis in surgery patients (22,24,36), and in patients undergoing hip surgery (9). Initial reports of a high incidence of bleeding have been reevaluated. When used in lower, more appropriate doses for preventing thrombosis, LMWHs have not been associated with an increased risk of perioperative bleeding. Other side effects such as thrombocytopenia and skin necrosis also occur with LMWHs, but the occurrence rate appears to be much lower than with UFH (37).

5. Vascular Effects

The vascular vs plasmatic effects of LMWH is currently gaining tremendous interest in explaining the actions of LMWH in various settings. The role of TFPI as the heparin vascular component in the prevention of thrombosis was originally reported to be limited. Subsequent studies have challenged this view. TFPI interferes with enzyme-substrate interactions, resulting in a complex of four proteins: TFPI, TF, Xa, and IIa. This interaction can occur at the endothelial surface, and TFPI may thus be involved in maintaining a nonthrombotic state in the endothelium. TFPI also interacts with several mechanisms, including elastase, protease generation, low-density lipoproteins, and tissue factor (TF) mediation of platelet and macrophage activation. TFPI is released into the bloodstream after administration of UFH or LMWHs, and prophylactic LMWH administration can increase TFPI plasma-concentrations *(17,38)*. TFPI has demonstrated synergism with heparin in clotting assays, and may contribute to the antithrombotic effects of heparin *(6)*. High cellular distribution has been shown in endothelial cells with limited distribution in platelets, monocytes, or other cells.

In vitro studies of tinzaparin have demonstrated a time-dependent and saturable binding profile on endothelial cells, with both low and high affinity for binding *(39)*. Heparin is shown to increase endothelial TFPI release in an ATIII-independent mechanism. The release of endothelial TFPI is directly dependent on the molecular weight and the degree of sulfation. There is no release of TFPI with the pentasaccharide, but as the MW increases above 2000–3000 Daltons and up to 8000 Daltons, a significant increase in TFPI release *(17)* has been demonstrated. The degree of sulfation also contributes significantly to the endothelial TFPI release *(17)* at the same molecular weight. Different LMWHs demonstrated different capacities in releasing endothelial TFPI.

A fivefold increase in the plasma level of TFPI after administration of tinzaparin at the DVT treatment dose and by threefold above basal after administration at the prophylaxis dose were documented. Heparin-released TFPI in itself has potent anticoagulant properties in inhibiting platelet/fibrin clot formation, strength, and dynamics. A synergistic interaction was found between tinzaparin and TFPI in clotting assays. The combination of LWMH and TFPI is far more potent in clotting assays than either one alone *(40)*.

Another non-ATIII-mediated action of LMWHs is the promotion of fibrinolysis *(31)*. Tinzaparin was shown to affect fibrinolysis; prophylactic use of tinzaparin for DVT increased levels of tissue plasminogen activator (t-PA) and fibrin and fibrinogen degradation products and enhanced α_2-antiplasmin activity. Levels of t-PA antigen were significantly elevated in patients undergoing total hip replacement who were receiving tinzaparin for up to 7 d for DVT prophylaxis.

6. Clinical Experiences in VTE

The commercial use of LMWHs began in the mid-1980s for hemodialysis and the prophylaxis of DVT in general surgery. The initial clinical development of LMWHs remained sequestered in the European continent during the initial years. Later, these drugs were introduced in North America. In the initial stages of the development of these drugs, only Nadroparin, Dalteparin, and Enoxaparin were used. Subsequently, several other LMWHs such as ardeparin, tinzaparin, reviparin, and parnaparin were introduced. These LMWHs constitute a group of important medications, with total sales reaching nearly 2.5 billion dollars and expanded treatment plans reaching far beyond the initial indications for the prophylaxis of postsurgical DVT.

Efficacy and safety comparisons of LMWHs vs UFH have demonstrated that LMWHs were at least as effective as UFH in reducing mortality rates after acute DVT. LMWHs were also shown to be as safe as UFH with respect to major bleeding complications, and as effective as UFH in preventing thromboembolic recurrences. Meta-analyses of trials evaluating enoxaparin, tinzaparin, dalteparin, and others in the treatment of DVT showed that LMWHs were likely to be more effective than UFH in the prevention of recurrent venous thromboembolism. LMWHs were also associated with a lower incidence of major bleeding and lower mortality rate in this clinical setting, particularly in patients with cancer. Trials of fixed doses of SC LMWHs, adjusted for body wt, and no monitoring, showed that LMWHs were safer and more effective than adjusted-dose UFH. The authors of this analysis cautioned that the conclusions were based on trials with only two LMWHs (fraxiparin and tinzaparin). LMWHs are not interchangeable; therefore, the conclusions on efficacy and safety of tinzaparin and fraxiparin cannot be extrapolated to other LMWHs.

The largest trial comparing a LMWH with UFH evaluated fixed-dose sc tinzaparin vs adjusted-dose continuous iv heparin in 432 patients for the initial treatment of proximal-vein thrombosis, using objective documentation of clinical outcomes. Warfarin sodium was administered on d 2 of therapy, and continued for 3 mo. The incidence of new thromboembolism was higher in the UFH group ($p < 0.7$). The risk of major bleeding was reduced by 95% for patients in the tinzaparin treatment regimen ($p < 0.06$). Risk reduction for death was 51% in favor of the LMWH regimen ($p = 0.49$), which was particularly striking in patients with cancer. The long-term use of tinzaparin may have a greater effect on the incidence of death, bleeding, and recurrent thromboembolism in patients with metastatic carcinomas *(9)*.

Initial sc therapy with tinzaparin was concluded to be as safe and effective as iv UFH in patients with acute pulmonary embolism (PE). The benefit and ease of administration of LMWH in patients with DVT may be extended to patients with acute symptomatic PE and stable hemodynamics *(41)*. A study of SC LMWH in patients with proximal DVT vs iv UFH evaluated the clinical outcomes, cost, and cost-effectiveness of both methods. The American-Canadian Thrombosis Study randomized 432 patients and found sc tinzaparin sodium to be at least as clinically effective and safe as iv UFH, and also less expensive. The cost-effectiveness of the LMWH administration could have been even greater if outpatient therapy had been implemented *(36)*. Once again, the results of this study could not be extrapolated to other LMWHs, since their molecular composition and pharmacokinetic profiles differ and their costs may therefore vary considerably *(36)*.

Table 2
Comparison Between LMWH and Pentasaccharide

LMWH	Pentasaccharide
Inhibits Xa and IIa	Strong anti-Xa effect, no IIa effect
Prophylaxis: ⇓ in recurrent VTE of 2.8%	⇓ In recurrent VTE (2.4%) reported with dalteparin as comparitor)
⇑ TFPI activities vs other agents	Does not affect plasma TFPI levels
Apparent mortality benefit in cancer and IBD patients.	Nothing is available, and it is unlikely to have an impact
Competitive pricing	Anticipate high pricing
Indicated for QD dosing	QD dosing
Low HIT rate (~1%)	No HIT (0%)
Pharmacoeconomic outcomes data-supportive	No pharmacoeconomic data
Antidote: protamine sulfate or heparinase	No antidote
VTE treatment well-documented	Not available yet

LMWHs have an efficacy profile equivalent to or better than UFH, and the safety profile includes fewer complications than UFH. Nevertheless, several side effects have been documented. Although initially believed to be absent with LMWHs, HIT has been reported in a few LMWH-treated patients. However, the frequency with which this side effect occurs is far smaller than with UFH. Because LMWHs are considered to be less immunogenic because of their lower molecular weights, LMWH anticoagulation therapy may be possible in patients who have HIT *(37)*.

6.1. LMWH vs Pentasaccharide

Advantages for LMWH as compared to the pentasaccharide are shown in **Table 2**, which illustrates a polypharmacological effects for LMWH at various levels beyond anti-Xa.

References

1. Weitz, J. I. (1997) Low-molecular-weight heparin. *N. Engl. J. Med.* **337,** 688–698.
2. Mousa, S. A. and Fareed, J. W. (2001) Advances in anticoagulant, antithrombotic and thrombolytic drugs. *Exp. Opin. Invest. Drugs* **10(1),** 157–162.
3. Fegan, C. D. (1998) Tinzaparin as an antithrombotic: an overview. *Hosp. Med.* **149,** 1285–1288.

4. Aguilar, D. and Goldhaber, S. Z. (1999) Clinical uses of low molecular weight heparin. *Chest* **115(5),** 1418–1423.

5. Linhardt, R. J. and Gunay, N. S. (1999) Production and chemical processing of low molecular weight heparins. *Semin. Thromb. Hemost.* **25(3),** 5–16.

*6. Mousa, S. A. (2000) Comparative efficacy among different low molecular weight heparin (LMWHs) & drug interaction: implications in the management of vascular disorders. *Thromb. Haemostasis* **26(1)(Suppl. 1),** 39–46.

7. Hull, R. D., Raskob, G. E., Pineo, G. F., Green, D., Towbridge, A. A., Elliott, C. G., et al. (1992) Subcutaneous low-molecular weight heparin compared with continuous intravenous heparin in the treatment of proximal-vein thrombosis. *N. Engl. J. Med.* **326, 975–982.

8. Simonneau, G., Sors, H., Charbonnier, B., Page, Y., Laaban, J.-P., Bosson, J.-L., et al. (1997) A comparison of low-molecular-weight heparin with unfractionated heparin for acute pulmonary embolism. *N. Engl. J. Med.* **337,** 663–669.

9. Hull, R. D., Raskob, G. E., Pineo, G. F., Rosenbloom, D., Evans, W., Mallory, T., et al. (1993) A comparison of subcutaneous low-molecular weight heparin with warfarin sodium for prophylaxis against deep-vein thrombosis after hip or knee implantation. *N. Engl. J. Med.* **329,** 1370–1376.

10. Leizorovicz, A., Picolet, H., Peyrieux, J. C., Boissel, J. P., and the HBPM research group. (1991) Prevention of perioperative deep vein thrombosis in general surgery: a multicenter double blind study comparing two doses of logiparin and standard heparin. *Br. J. Surg.* **78,** 412–416.

11. Ryan, K. E., Lane, D. A., Flynn, A., Shepperd, J., Ireland, H. A., and Curtis, J. R. (1991) Dose finding study of a low molecular weight heparin, tinzaparin, in haemodialysis. *Thromb. Haemostasis* **66(3),** 277–282.

12. Pedersen, P. C., Østergaard, P. B., Hedner, U., Bergqvist, D., and Mätzsch, T. (1991) Pharmacokinetics of low molecular weight heparin, logiparin, after intravenous and subcutaneous administration to healthy volunteers. *Thromb. Res.* **61,** 477–487.

13. Mätzsch, T., Bergqvist, D., Hedner, U., and Østergaard, P. B. (1987) Effects of an enzymatically depolymerized heparin as compared with conventional heparin in healthy volunteers. *Thromb. Haemostasis* **57(1),** 97–101.

14. Mousa, S. A., Bozarth, J., Hainer, J., et al. (2001) Pharmacodynamic of tinzaparin following 175 IU/Kg SC administration in healthy volunteers on plasma TFPI. *Thromb. Haemostasis* P2299.

---

*This study provides a comparative total anticoagulant efficacy among different LMWH showing dependency on the molecular weight and degree of sulfation.

**This is a key double-blind clinical trial comparing the efficacy and safety of LMWH to UFH in-patients with VTE.

15. Emmanuele, R. M. and Fareed, J. (1987) The effect of molecular weight on the bioavailability of heparin. *Thromb. Res.* **48,** 591–596.
16. Brieger, D. and Dawes, J. (1997) Production method affects the pharmacokinetic and *ex vivo* biological properties of low molecular weight heparins. *Thromb. Haemostasis* **77(2),** 317–322.
17. Mousa, S. A., Bozarth, J., Larnkjaer, A., and Johanson, K. (2000) Vascular effects of heparin molecular weight fractions and LMWH on the release of TFPI from human endothelial cells. *Blood* **16(11),** 59, 3928.
18. Kaiser, B., Hoppensteadt, D., and Fareed, J. (2000) Tissue factor pathway inhibitor for cardiovascular disorders. *Emerging Drugs* **5(1),** 73–87.
19. Verstraete, M. (1990) Pharmacotherapeutic aspects of unfractionated and low molecular weight heparins. *Drugs* **40,** 498–530.
20. Lindblad, B. (1988) Prophylaxis of postoperative thromboembolism with low dose heparin alone or in combination with dihydroergotamine. A review. *Acta Chir. Scand. Suppl.* **543,** 31–42.
21. Hull, R., Delmore, T., Carter, C., Hirsh, J., Genton, E., Gent, M., et al. (1982) Adjusted subcutaneous heparin versus warfarin sodium in the long-term treatment of venous thrombosis. *N. Engl. J. Med.* **306,** 189–194.
22. Hull, R. D., Raskob, G. E., Hirsh, J., Jay, R. M., Leclerc, J. R., Geerts, W. H., et al. (1986) Continuous intravenous heparin compared with intermittent subcutaneous heparin in the initial treatment of proximal-vein thrombosis. *N. Engl. J. Med.* **315,** 1109–1114.
23. Cruickshank, M. K., Levine, M. N., Hirsh, J., Roberts, R., and Siguenza, M. (1991) A standard heparin nomogram for the management of heparin therapy [see comments]. *Arch. Intern. Med.* **151,** 333–337.
24. Hull, R. D., Raskob, G. E., Rosenbloom, D., Lemaire, J., Pineo, G. F., Baylis, B., et al. (1992) Optimal therapeutic level of heparin therapy in patients with venous thrombosis. *Arch. Intern. Med.* **152,** 1589–1595.
25. Goldhaber, S. Z. (1996) Thrombolytic therapy for venous thromboembolism, in *Disorders of Thrombosis* (Hull, R. and Pineo, G. F., eds.), W.B. Saunders Co, pp. 321–328.
26. Gueret, P., Dubourg, O., Ferrier, A., Farcot, J. C., Rigaud, M., and Bourdarias, J. P. (1986) Effects of full-dose heparin anticoagulation on the development of left ventricular thrombosis in acute transmural myocardial infarction. *J. Am. Coll. Cardiol.* **8,** 419–426.
27. Neri Serneri, G. G., Gensini, G. F., Poggesi, L., Trotta, F., Modesti, P. A., Boddi, M., et al. (1990) Effect of heparin, aspirin, or alteplase in reduction of myocardial ischaemia in refractory unstable angina (published erratum appears in Lancet 1990 Apr 7;335[8693]:868). *Lancet* **335,** 615–618.
28. Bounameaux, H., Verhaeghe, R., and Verstraete, M. (1986) Thromboembolism and antithrombotic therapy in peripheral arterial disease. *J. Am. Coll. Cardiol.* **8,** 98B–103B.

29. Matzsch, T., Bergqvist, D., Hedner, U., Nilsson, B., and Ostergaard, P. (1986) Heparin-induced osteoporosis in rats. *Thromb. Haemostasis* **56,** 293–294.

30. Salzman, E. W., Rosenberg, R. D., Smith, M. H., Lindon, J. N., and Favreau, L. (1980) Effect of heparin and heparin fractions on platelet aggregation. *J. Clin. Invest.* **65,** 64–73.

31. Friedel, H. A. and Balfour, J. A. (1994) Tinzaparin. A review of its pharmacology and clinical potential in the prevention and treatment of thromboembolic disorders. *Drugs* **48,** 638–660.

32. Padilla, A., Gray, E., Pepper, D. S., and Barrowcliffe, T. W. (1992) Inhibition of thrombin generation by heparin and low molecular weight (LMW) heparins in the absence and presence of platelet factor 4 (PF4). *Br. J. Haematol.* **82,** 406–413.

33. Fareed, J., Jeske, W., Hoppensteadt, D., Clarizio, R., and Walenga, J. M. (1998) Low-molecular-weight heparins: pharmacological profile and product differentiation. *Am. J. Cardiol.* **82,** 3L–10L.

34. Boneu, B., Caranobe, C., Cadroy, Y., Dol, F., Gabaig, A. M., Dupouy, D., et al. (1988) Pharmacokinetic studies of standard unfractionated heparin, and low molecular weight heparins in the rabbit. *Semin. Thromb. Hemost.* **14,** 18–27.

35. Sutor, A. H., Massicotte, P., Leaker, M., Andrew, M. (1997) Heparin therapy in pediatric patients. *Semin. Thromb. Hemost.* **23,** 303–319.

36. Freedman, M. D. (1996) Low molecular weight heparins: an emerging new class of glycosaminoglycan antithrombotic. *J. Clin. Pharmacol.* **31,** 298–306. *Circulation* **93,** 2212–2245.

37. Fareed, J., Walenga, J. M., Hoppensteadt, D., Huan, X., and Nonn, R. (1989) Biochemical and pharmacological in-equivalence of low molecular weight heparins. *Ann. NY Acad. Sci.* **556,** 333–353.

38. Lindahl, A. K., Abildgaard, U., and Stokke, G. (1990) Release of extrinsic pathway inhibitor after heparin injection: increased response in cancer patients. *Thromb. Res.* **59,** 651–656.

39. Larnkjaer, A., Ostergaard, P. B., and Flodgaard, H. J. (1994) Binding of low molecular weight heparin (Tinzaparin sodium) to bovine endothelial cells in vitro. *Thromb. Res.* **75,** 185–194.

40. Ostergaard, P., Nordfang, O., Petersen, L. C. , Valentin, S., and Kristensen, H. (1993) Is tissue factor pathway inhibitor involved in the antithrombotic effect of heparins? Biochemical considerations. *Haemostasis* **23 (Suppl. 1),** 107–111.

41. Hull, R. D., Raskob, G. E., Rosenbloom, D., Pineo, G., Lerner, R. G., Gafni, A., et al. (1997) Treatment of proximal vein thrombosis with subcutaneous low-molecular-weight heparin vs. intravenous heparin. *Arch. Intern. Med.* **157,** 289–294.

5

Are Low Molecular Weight Heparins the Same?

Shaker A. Mousa

1. Introduction

Low molecular weight heparins (LMWHs) are glycosaminoglycans (GAGs) of different chain length, molecular weight distribution, and different physiochemical characteristics that result from their diverse methods of preparation, which make them non-interchangeable. The anticoagulant potency of heparin is measured as USP U/mg. This method is only applicable to LMWHs at high doses, when their anticoagulant properties are apparent. Anti-Xa activity has not enabled standardization of the biologic actions of LMWHs, since it does not address the ATIII-independent actions of LMWHs. Yet the European Pharmacopoeia Commission has adopted anti-Xa activity as a measure of LMWH potency. Since other markers of pharmacological activity also differ among LMWHs, their anti-IIa activity, tissue-factor pathway inhibitor (TFPI) releasing capacity, anti-inflammatory, and other cellular effects should be useful biomarkers in determining the biologic activity of each LMWH.

2. LMWH Differentiation: Structure–Function Differences

The variations in molecular composition and pharmacological properties of LMWHs are reflected in clinical trials that reported differences in clinical efficacy and safety. Therefore, each LMWH should be considered to be a unique substance. The main differences between LMWHs are variations in the amount of pharmacologically active product, varying chemical and physical compositions resulting in different biologic actions, and differences in results from clinical trials performed at optimized doses for each agent. The Food and Drug Administration (FDA), World Health Organization (WHO), and other national organizations consider each LMWH to be a distinct drug that cannot be interchanged with another LMWH.

From: *Methods in Molecular Medicine, vol. 93: Anticoagulants, Antiplatelets, and Thrombolytics*
Edited by: S. A. Mousa © Humana Press Inc., Totowa, NJ

Table 1
Low Molecular Weight Heparins (LMWHs)
and Their Chemical Characteristics

LMWHs	Characteristics
Nadroparin	Presence of 2,5-anhydro-D-mannose at reducing terminus
Enoxaparin	Presence of 4,5 unsaturated uronic acid at nonreducing terminus
Dalteparin	Presence of 2,5-anhydro-D-mannose at reducing terminus
Certoparin	Presence of 2,5-anhydro-D-mannose at reducing terminus
Tinzaparin	Presence of 4,5-unsaturated uronic acid at nonreducing terminus
Reviparin	Presence of 2,5-anhydro-D-mannose at reducing terminus
Ardeparin	Labile glycosidic bonds

2.1. Method of Manufacturing

All of the commercially available LMWHs are manufactured by depoly-merization of porcine mucosal heparin preparations *(1)*. LMWHs are prepared by either chemical or enzymatic digestion methods (**Table 1**). Most LMWHs exhibit approximately one-third of the molecular weight of regular heparin. Initially, the clinical batches of LMWHs were prepared by ethanolic fraction-ation of heparin. However, because of cost and limited availability of heparin for the sizeable isolation of these agents, chemical and enzymatic depolymer-ization procedures were developed. All of the currently available LMWHs are currently manufactured by chemical or enzymatic depolymerization of porcine mucosal heparin (**Table 1**). Controlled depolymerization processes were widely used to produce products with similar molecular weights; however, marked dif-ferences in the chemical composition of each of these products were imposed during the depolymerization process. Tinzaparin is the only LMWH known that is prepared by enzymatic hydrolysis with heparinase. A distinct improvement in the pharmacokinetic and pharmacodynamic properties of the class of LMWH over the parent-unfractionated heparin (UFH) has been clearly demonstrated (**Table 2**).

Although the depolymerization process results in lower molecular weight heparin products (MW 4–8 *Kd*), these products exhibit differences in both their molecular structural and functional properties. Optimized methods are cur-rently used to prepare LMWHs, which exhibit a similar molecular profile. However, because of the significant differences in the chemical or enzymatic procedures, structural variations are found in all of these agents. Therefore, these differences exert a significant influence on the biologic action of these products *(2)*. Safety and efficacy comparison of these agents in well-designed

Table 2
UFH vs LMWH

UFH	LMWH
Continuous iv infusion	BID or QD subcutaneous injection
Primarily administered in hospital	Administered in hospital, office, or home
Usually administered by healthcare professionals	Administered by patient, caregiver, or professional
Monitoring and dosing adjustments	No monitoring, fixed or weight-based dosing
Frequent dosing errors	More precise dosing
Risk of thrombocytopenia and osteoporosis	Decreased risk of adverse events
Cheap, but not cost-effective	Demonstrated pharmacoeconomic benefits
Requires 5–7 d in the hospital	Requires 0–2 d in the hospital

clinical trials to demonstrate clinical differences in each of the individual products are not available at this point. Initial attempts to standardize LMWHs on the basis of their biologic actions, such as anti-Xa potency, have failed. A potency designation on the basis of the anti-Xa actions represents only one of the various properties of these agents. Many of the pharmacological actions of LMWHs are based on the non-ATIII affinity components *(3–7)*. These include the release of TFPI, t-PA, inhibition of adhesion molecules, decrease in the circulating von Willebrand's Factor, and modulation of blood flow **(Table 3)**. Most of these effects are not measurable with the conventional methods such as the anti-Xa, anti-IIa, or global anticoagulant methods.

The method of production of LMWHs influences their pharmacokinetic and pharmacodynamic properties as well as their anticoagulant and antithrombotic activities *(1–3)*. The various methods of LMWH preparation result in considerable molecular heterogeneity, which are apparent in the demonstrated differences among LMWHs in anti-IIa and anti-Xa activities, platelet interactions, protamine, and PF4 neutralization activities *(8)*.

2.2. Molecular Weight Distribution (Fig. 1)

The resulting molecules have a mean molecular mass of 4–8 *Kd*. More than 60% of the polysaccharides have molecular masses between 2 and 8 *Kd*, resulting in a reduction in thrombin-neutralizing capacity (anti-IIa activity). The plasmatic anticoagulant properties of heparins depend on the presence of specific Pentasaccharide sequences with a high affinity to ATIII/factor Xa. The

Table 3
Variable Poly-Components and Poly-Pharmacological Effects of LMWHs as a Function of Their Structural Heterogenicity

Site of Actions	Pharmacological Effects
ATIII-dependent plasmatic effects	Anti-Xa, Anti-IIa, and other coagulation factors
ATIII-independent vascular effects	TFPI, nitric oxide, vWF
Cell adhesion molecule modulation	Selectins (P, L, and E-Selectins) and immunoglobulins (soluble ICAM-1 andVCAM-1)
Fibrinolytic system	t-PA and PAI-1
Inflammatory mediators	TNF-α, IL-6, etc.

depolymerization methods result in modified ATIII-binding sites on the heparins and in reduced activity of specific LMWHs. LMWHs have different characteristics, a direct result of their method of synthesis and the resulting molecular weight distribution *(8–11)*.

2.3. Degree of Sulfation

Chemical modifications of the end groups and internal structure, degree of sulfation, and charge density vary from product to product and affect the characteristics of the end products. Depending on the method of preparation, the LMWHs are different mixtures of various polysaccharides, different anti-Factor X (anti-Xa), anti-IIa activities, endothelial TFPI release, and different biologic actions *(4,6)*.

2.4. Pharmcokinetics, Pharmacodynamics, and Elimination

Tinzaparin (Logiparin,® Innohep®), a LMWH with an average molecular weight of 6.5 *Kd*, is synthesized through depolymerization of heparin by heparinase, an enzyme isolated from *Flavobacterium heparinum (12)*. This allows for the production of a LMWH with intact structure and highest level of sulfation. The bioavailability of the tinzaparin fraction with anti-Xa activity is higher than the fraction with anti-IIa activity. The absorption half-life for anti-Xa is ~200 min. The difference may indicate that bioavailability is dependent on molecular weight. Longer chain lengths are necessary for anti-IIa activity rather than for anti-Xa activity. Anti-Xa bioavailability is ~90%, as measured in healthy volunteers. Based on a one-compartment model, the elimination half-life was calculated to be 82 min *(12)*. The elimination half-life was found to be dose-dependent. The half-life after intravenous (iv) administration of 5000 IU a-Xa

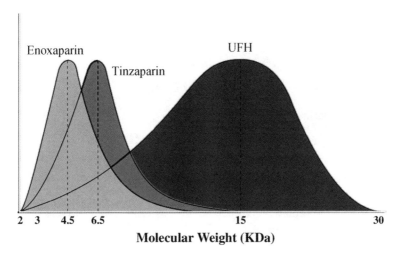

Fig. 1. Molecular weight distribution of two different LMWH as compared to UFH.

was determined to be ~112 min, compared with 61 min for the same dose of UFH. Tinzaparin is distributed mainly into two compartments, plasmatic and vascular. This feature allows for initial and delayed renal elimination of tinzaparin. Because of tinzaparin's high vascular distribution, it does not accumulate in patients with renal failure. Thus, there is no need for dose adjustment with tinzaparin in contrast to UFH or other LMWH.

The elimination route of UFH, tinzaparin, or other LMWH is predominantly via renal excretion, with about 90% of the administered dose detectable in the urine (over a period of 7 d). The majority of renal excreted material is recovered during the first 24 h post-administration. A minimal amount is excreted in three feces *(12)*. The renal excreted LMWH fraction is characterized by lower molecular mass that has no anti-Xa activity.

In contrast to UFH, tinzaparin does not exhibit significant accumulation in patients with renal failure *(13)*. This is because of the differences in the compartments for distribution. Tinzaparin exhibits a strong vascular distribution, with a relatively long residence time (sulfation) in addition to its plasmatic distribution. UFH is distributed into the plasma protein pool and free plasma pool, and with limited vascular distribution. In general, the lower the molecular weight distribution, the greater the plasmatic distribution and the lesser the vascular distribution. The pentasaccharide is 100% plasmatic distribution and 0% vascular distribution. In patients with renal failure, pentasacchride would have the highest accumulation with a greater incidence of bleeding if doses are not adjusted, as with other LMWH with relatively low molecular weight distribution and relatively low sulfate/carboxylate ratios.

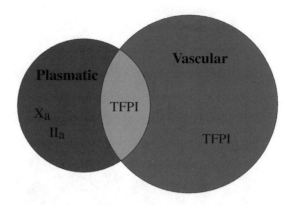

Fig. 2. Vascular vs plasmatic effects of heparin and LMWH.

3. Anticoagulation: Plasmatic vs Vascular-Mediated Effects (Fig. 2)

3.1. Plasmatic Effects at Different Steps in the Coagulation Cascade

Heparin affects the coagulation cascade at multiple sites. Heparin-mediated effects could be classified as either AT-dependent or AT-independent. Individual LMWHs have predictable pharmacological actions, increased bioavailability, prolonged half-life, and sustained activity compared with UFH, making it possible to provide adequate anticoagulation for DVT prophylaxis and treatment with once-a-day subcutaneous (sc) administration in the case of some LMWHs such as tinzaparin *(13)*.

The anti-IIa-to-anti-Xa ratio for UFH is approximately one. By convention, the anti-Xa effect of LMWHs is identical, although the anti-IIa decreases as the heparin molecular weight decreases. US Pharmacopoeia amidolytic measurements of the various LMWHs have demonstrated differences in anti-Xa activities for each LMWH *(8)*. However, since anti-IIa and anti-Xa activities of each LMWH do not represent the total antithrombotic and anti-hemorrhagic effects of the respective agents, the International Society on Thrombosis and Haemostasis recommends that vial labeling should be based on weight. Labeling should also include specific anti-IIa and anti-Xa activity as evaluated against the International Standard and the recommended therapeutic dose. The antithrombotic potency and potential bleeding effects of one product cannot be extrapolated to another on the basis of weights in mg of anti-Xa or anti-IIa activity.

Pharmacokinetic studies have shown that LMWHs have a relatively high bioavailability after sc injection as compared to UFH, and demonstrate a longer half-life of their anticoagulant anti-Xa activity than UFH. LMWHs have been demonstrated to be highly effective in the prevention of venous thrombosis in surgery patients *(14–16)*, and in patients undergoing hip surgery *(17)*. Initial reports of a high incidence of bleeding have been reevaluated. When used in lower, more appropriate doses for preventing thrombosis, LMWHs have not been associated with an increased risk of perioperative bleeding. Other side effects such as thrombocytopenia and skin necrosis also occur with LMWHs, but the occurrence rate appears to be much lower than with UFH *(10)*.

3.2. Vascular Effects in the Endothelium

The vascular vs plasmatic effects of LMWH are a topic of increasing interest as a way to explain the actions of LMWH in various settings. The role of TFPI as the heparin vascular component in the prevention of thrombosis was originally reported to be limited. Subsequent studies have challenged this view. TFPI interferes with enzyme-substrate interactions, resulting in a complex of four proteins: TFPI, TF, Xa, and VIIa. This interaction can occur at the endothelial surface, and TFPI may therefore be involved in maintaining a non-thrombotic state in the endothelium. TFPI also interacts with several mechanisms, including elastase, protease generation, low-density lipoproteins, and TF mediation of platelet and macrophage activation. TFPI is released into the bloodstream after administration of UFH or LMWHs; prophylactic LMWH administration can increase TFPI plasma-concentrations *(4,5,18,19)*. TFPI has demonstrated synergism with heparin in clotting assays, and may contribute to the antithrombotic effects of heparin *(3)*. High cellular distribution is shown in endothelial cells with limited distribution in platelets, monocytes, or other cells.

3.2.1. Effects of LMWH on Endothelial TFPI

In vitro studies of tinzaparin have demonstrated a time-dependent and saturable binding profile on endothelial cells, with both low and high affinity for binding *(6)*. Heparin is shown to increase endothelial TFPI release in an ATIII-independent mechanism. The release of endothelial TFPI is directly dependent on the molecular weight (**Fig. 3**) and the degree of sulfation (**Fig. 4**). There is no release of TFPI with the pentasaccharide, but as the molecular weight increases above 2000–3000 Dalton and up to 8000 Dalton, a significant increase in TFPI release has been demonstrated *(4)*. The degree of sulfation also contributes significantly to the endothelial TFPI release at the same molecular weight (**Fig. 4**). Thus, different LMWHs demonstrate different capacity in releasing endothelial TFPI *(4)*.

Anti-Xa activity has served as the primary biomarker for evaluating the exposure of LMWHs. It is used to define the in vitro potency and to monitor therapeutic response. Because LMWHs are poly-component moieties with multiple biological actions, each with distinct time-courses, the true pharmacoki-

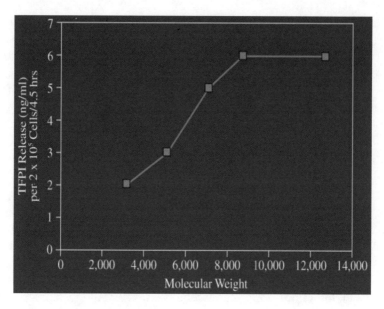

Fig. 3. In vitro effect of molecular weight distribution on the release of TFPI from human endothelial cells.

netic behavior of these agents cannot be evaluated with assays developed for a single pharmacological activity. Heparin has multiple effects beyond anti-Xa and anti-IIa, ranging from the inhibition of tissue factor (TF) activity to the enhancement of TFPI levels and resulting in a shift in the TF-to-TFPI ratio, a more important upstream as compared to the Xa/IIa ratio *(20,21)*.

Clinical trials in which LMWHs with distinct in vitro potency (anti-Xa: anti-IIa ratio) and ex vivo anti-Xa and anti-IIa activities were tested in deep venous thrombosis (DVT) patients following hip replacement found no difference in efficacy or safety measures, despite distinct differences in biomarker activity profiles *(22,23)*. LMWHs vary in their affinity for ATIII, presumably because of production method of the GAGs and their molecular weight distributions *(22,23)*. In contrast, TFPI, an ATIII-independent vascular-endothelial biomarker, might represent a greater potential for the role of LMWH in various diseases and in differentiating LMWHs.

Based on current methods, plasma levels of TFPI increase rapidly following the sc injection of tinzaparin sodium, reaching maximum and sustained levels for up to 5 h. The absolute bioavailability is approx 90%, based on anti-Xa activity *(24)*, and 95% based on TFPI *(18)*.

The effect of molecular weight on the bioavailability of heparin has been well-appreciated and anti-Xa activity is accepted as a sensitive biomarker for

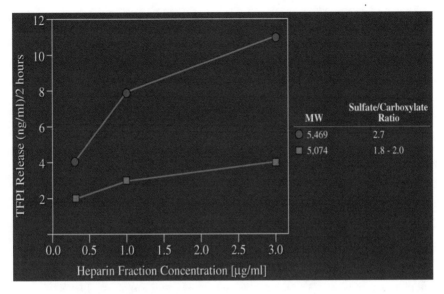

Fig. 4. Effect of different sulfate/carboxylate ratio at fixed molecular weight on TFPI release from human endothelial cells.

the various heparin molecular weight fractions. Whether or not these fractions have any pharmacological activity has been a topic of much debate.

Comparisons among agents are less straightforward, and the biomarker response from one such agent may not be transmittable to another with respect to outcomes that these markers may contribute to but certainly do not predict. A composite of several markers may be required to make such comparisons. Continued exploration of mechanistic determinants of activity to better quantify the effects of these important medicines is warranted.

References

1. Linhardt, R. J. and Gunay, N. S. (1999) Production and chemical processing of low molecular weight heparins. *Semin. Thromb. Hemost.* **25(3),** 5–16.
2. Brieger, D. and Dawes, J. (1997) Production method affects the pharmacokinetic and *ex vivo* biological properties of low molecular weight heparins. *Thromb. Haemostasis* **77(2),** 317–322.
*3. Mousa, S. A. (2000) Comparative efficacy among different low molecular weight heparin (LMWHs) & drug interaction: implications in the management of vascular disorders. *Thromb. Haemostasis* **26(1)(Suppl. 1),** 39–46.

---

*This study provides a comparative total anticoagulant efficacy among different LMWH showing dependency on the molecular weight and degree of sulfation.

4. Mousa, S. A., Bozarth, J., Larnkjaer, A., and Johanson, K. (2000) Vascular effects of heparin molecular weight fractions and LMWH on the release of TFPI from human endothelial cells. *Blood* **16(11),** 59, 3928.

5. Lindahl, A. K., Abildgaard, U., and Stokke, G. (1990) Release of extrinsic pathway inhibitor after heparin injection: increased response in cancer patients. *Thromb. Res.* **59,** 651–656.

6. Larnkjaer, A., Ostergaard, P. B., and Flodgaard, H. J. (1994) Binding of low molecular weight heparin (Tinzaparin sodium) to bovine endothelial cells in vitro. *Thromb. Res.* **75,** 185–194.

7. Ostergaard, P., Nordfang, O., Petersen, L. C., Valentin, S., and Kristensen, H. (1993) Is tissue factor pathway inhibitor involved in the antithrombotic effect of heparins? Biochemical considerations. *Haemostasis* **23 (Suppl. 1),** 107–111.

8. Fareed, J., Jeske, W., Hoppensteadt, D., Clarizio, R., and Walenga, J. M. (1998) Low-molecular-weight heparins: pharmacological profile and product differentiation. *Am. J. Cardiol.* **82,** 3L–10L.

9. Boneu, B., Caranobe, C., Cadroy, Y., Dol, F., Gabaig, A. M., Dupouy, D., et al. (1988) Pharmacokinetic studies of standard unfractionated heparin, and low molecular weight heparins in the rabbit. *Semin. Thromb. Haemost.* **14,** 18–27.

10. Freedman, M. D. (1991) Low molecular weight heparins: an emerging new class of glycosaminoglycan antithrombotic. *J. Clin. Pharmacol.* **31,** 298–306. *Circulation* (1996) **93,** 2212–2245.

11. Fareed, J., Walenga, J. M., Hoppensteadt, D., Huan, X., and Nonn, R. (1989) Biochemical and pharmacological in-equivalence of low molecular weight heparins. *Ann. NY Acad. Sci.* **556,** 333–353.

12. Friedel, H. A. and Balfour, J. A. (1994) Tinzaparin. A review of its pharmacology and clinical potential in the prevention and treatment of thromboembolic disorders. *Drugs* **48,** 638–660.

13. Hull, R. D., Raskob, G. E., Rosenbloom, D., Pineo, G., Lerner, R. G., Gafni, A., et al. (1997) Treatment of proximal vein thrombosis with subcutaneous low-molecular-weight heparin vs. intravenous heparin. *Arch. Intern. Med.* **157,** 289–294.

14. Simonneau, G., Sors, H., Charbonnier, B., Page, Y., Laaban, J.-P., Bosson, J.-L., et al. (1997) A comparison of low-molecular-weight heparin with unfractionated heparin for acute pulmonary embolism. *N. Engl. J. Med.* **337,** 663–669.

15. Hull, R. D., Raskob, G. E., Hirsh, J., Jay, R. M., Leclerc, J. R., Geerts, W. H., et al. (1986) Continuous intravenous heparin compared with intermittent subcutaneous heparin in the initial treatment of proximal-vein thrombosis. *N. Engl. J. Med.* **315,** 1109–1114.

16. Hull, R. D., Raskob, G. E., Rosenbloom, D., Lemaire, J., Pineo, G. F., Baylis, B., et al. (1992) Optimal therapeutic level of heparin therapy in patients with venous thrombosis. *Arch. Intern. Med.* **152,** 1589–1595.

17. Hull, R. D., Raskob, G. E., Pineo, G. F., Rosenbloom, D., Evans, W., Mallory, T., et al. (1993) A comparison of subcutaneous low-molecular weight heparin with

Warfarin sodium for prophylaxis against deep-vein thrombosis after hip or knee implantation. *N. Engl. J. Med.* **329,** 1370–1376.

18. Mousa, S. A., Bozarth, J., Hainer, J., Sprogel, P., Johansen, K., and Barrett, J. (2001) Pharmacodynamic of tinzaparin following 175 iu/kg subcutaneous administration in healthy volunteers on plasma tissue factor pathway inhibitor (TFPI). *Thromb. Haemostasis* P2299.

19. Kaiser, B., Hoppensteadt, D., and Fareed, J. (2000) Tissue factor pathway inhibitor for cardiovascular disorders. *Emerging Drugs* **5(1),** 73–87.

20. Mousa, S. A., Bozarth, J. M., Wilson, M., Cohen, M., Khalil-and Ibrahim, M. (2001) Effects of heparin on plasma tissue factor (TF) and tissue factor pathway inhibitor (TFPI) in patients with acute myocardial infarction (AMI). *J. Am. Coll. Cardiol.* **37(2, Suppl. A),** 354A, 1217.

21. Gori, A. M., Pepe, G., Attanasio, M., Falciani, M., Abbate, R., Prisco, D., et al. (1999) Tissue factor reduction and tissue factor pathway inhibitor release after heparin administration. *Thromb. Haemostasis* **81,** 589–593.

22. Bara, L., Planes, A., and Samama, M.-M. (1999) Occurrence of thrombosis and haemorrhage, relationship with anti-Xa, anti-IIa activities, and D-dimer plasma levels in patients receiving low molecular weight heparin, enoxaparin or tinzaparin, to prevent deep vein thrombosis after hip surgery. *Br. J. Haematol.* **104,** 230–240.

23. Brieger, D. and Dawes, J. (1997) Production method affects the pharmacokinetic and ex vivo biological properties of low molecular weight heparins. *Thromb. Haemostasis* **77(2),** 317–322.

24. Pedersen, P. C., Østergaard, P. B., Hedner, U., Bergqvist, D., and Mätzsch, T. (1991) Pharmacokinetics of low molecular weight heparin, logiparin, after intravenous and subcutaneous administration to healthy volunteers. *Thromb. Res.* **61,** 477–487.

6

Antithrombotic Drugs for the Treatment of Heparin-Induced Thrombocytopenia

Walter P. Jeske and Jeanine M. Walenga

1. Introduction

Heparin remains the anticoagulant of choice in the therapy of thromboembolic events. Heparin is effective in the prevention and treatment of venous thromboembolism (VTE), as a surgical anticoagulant, and in interventional cardiology *(1)*. Heparin is also used in the treatment of unstable angina and acute myocardial infarction (AMI), and in some patients with disseminated intravascular coagulation. Although the clinical effects of heparin are meritorious, side effects do occur. Bleeding is the primary undesirable effect of heparin. Heparin-induced thrombocytopenia (HIT), the most frequent of drug-induced allergies, necessitates the use of alternative agents to treat or prevent thrombus formation.

2. Clinical Manifestations of HIT

The diagnosis of HIT should be based on clinical criteria and platelet count, and not solely on HIT laboratory tests. Most authors define thrombocytopenia in HIT as a platelet count below 100,000–150,000/μL or a 30–50% decrease in platelet count from baseline *(2)*. Although HIT is typically associated with a platelet count of 38,000–60,000/μL, there is no platelet count at which a diagnosis of HIT can be made, or excluded, with certainty. Thrombocytopenia may be relative, but not absolute.

If no previous heparin exposure can be determined and the decrease in platelet count immediately after heparin administration is only moderate, a transient HIT that is not immune-mediated should be suspected *(3)*. This form of HIT is known as HIT type I **(Table 1)**. Laboratory testing is an important consideration in such patients. The diagnosis of HIT type I is supported by nega-

From: *Methods in Molecular Medicine, vol. 93: Anticoagulants, Antiplatelets, and Thrombolytics*
Edited by: S. A. Mousa © Humana Press Inc., Totowa, NJ

Table 1
Types of HIT

Type I HIT
- Nonimmune-mediated
- Benign
- Mild thrombocytopenia
- Thrombocytopenia corrects despite continuation of heparin

Type II HIT
- Immune-mediated
- Thrombocytopenia, which follows heparin exposure with a reduction in platelet count to less than 100,000/µL or a 30% decrease in platelet count from baseline
- Heparin exposure which precedes the thrombocytopenia by at least 5 d (at the current period or any time earlier)
- Reasonable exclusion of other clinical causes of thrombocytopenia—e.g., a degree of thrombocytopenia following cardiac surgery is expected
- May be associated with thrombosis—onset of new thrombotic event or extension of previous thrombosis

tive laboratory tests. Patients with this benign form of HIT can continue with heparin treatment without consequence.

HIT type II is a more serious form of HIT, which is immune-mediated and can result in serious thrombotic complications. The diagnosis of HIT type II depends on clinical criteria with confirmation by specific laboratory tests. Functional assays, such as platelet aggregometry or the serotonin-release assays, detect HIT antibodies by their ability to activate platelets. Enzyme-linked immunosorbent assays (ELISA) to identify these antiheparin-PF4 antibodies are also available. Unexplained thrombocytopenia or unexplained thromboembolism in a patient who is receiving heparin is sufficient reason to suspect a diagnosis of HIT *(3,4)*. A link must be established between heparin and thrombocytopenia; other causes of thrombocytopenia must be excluded.

An early diagnosis of HIT in cardiac surgery patients can be difficult to make, as most patients have platelet counts between 100,000/µL and 150,000/µL during the early postoperative period *(2)*. Ongoing studies by the authors suggest that HIT may be associated with an immediate postoperative platelet count decrease >50% from the pre-operative count without a trend of increasing platelet count during the following postoperative days. It is important to exclude postoperative platelet-consumptive processes such as unrecognized hematoma formation or hemorrhage *(2)*.

The time required to develop HIT antibody from the initial heparin exposure is typically 5 d, but can be longer or shorter if an anamnestic response is produced *(5,6)*. The dose of heparin and route of administration do not seem to make any difference in the frequency of HIT. Like other antibody responses, the HIT antibody response varies in an individual patient. This can be seen from the varying titers of antibody to the heparin-platelet factor (PF) 4 complex *(7,8)*. The duration of antibody production in individual patients is also variable. The antibody response in most patients ranges from a period of weeks to months; but patients have remained HIT antibody-positive for more than 1 yr. One may observe a delay in platelet rise in some HIT patients with a negative lab assay after heparin removal, and a positive lab assay may be observed in the face of rising platelet counts after heparin removal *(3)* Both cases are HIT.

Failure to monitor platelet counts and to evaluate the patient for manifestations of thromboembolism or hemorrhage may result in a delay in diagnosis. Rechallenge with heparin after resolution of the thrombocytopenia to confirm the diagnosis of HIT is dangerous, and should not be performed.

HIT occurs in approx 1–2% of all individuals exposed to heparin *(9,10)*. The majority of cases are found in medically and surgically treated adults, but can also be observed during pregnancy and in the newborn *(11–13)*. The most dramatic clinical expression of HIT is HIT antibody-driven thrombosis. Thrombosis can occur anywhere throughout the venous or the arterial circulation *(3,10,13,14)*. HIT in patients with thrombosis (HITTS) is most often associated with deep venous thrombosis (DVT) and pulmonary embolism (PE), but unusual thromboses, including mesenteric ischemia, spinal-artery thrombosis, visceral infarctions, cerebral infarction, and myocardial infarction (MI) are not uncommon *(2,13)*. Thrombi are probably also formed in many HIT patients in locations that do not result in clinically expressed adverse events, and can develop when platelet counts are normal.

Studies suggest that the diagnosis of HIT predicts future clinically significant thrombotic events *(2,3,13,15)*. Patients with clinically diagnosed HIT have a 35% probability of developing a clinically significant thrombosis during their hospitalization *(13)*. Patients with HIT or HITTS carry a reported mortality of 25–30% and amputation rates of up to 25% *(13)*. The apparent paradox of a fall in platelet count with thrombotic rather than hemorrhagic complications is analogous to the syndrome of thrombotic thrombocytopenic purpura (TTP) *(3)*. Therefore, these patients require careful monitoring and aggressive treatment, possibly including prophylactic anticoagulant therapy.

3. Pathophysiology of HIT

HIT type II is an immune reaction triggered by the generation of antibodies that bind to a complex of heparin coupled with a peptide or protein on the platelet or endothelial cell-surface *(16–23)*. The currently accepted mechanism of the pathophysiology of HIT is based on the development of an IgG antibody targeted toward the heparin-PF4 complex *(16,21)*. This antibody causes platelet activation, aggregation, and subsequent platelet and endothelial-cell destruction *(17,19,24–27)*. The antibody is not heparin specific, and has been shown to react with highly sulfated materials including dextran sulfate, pentosan polysulfate, but not dextran, dermatan sulfate or de-sulfated heparin *(20,28)*.

The Fab region of the antibodies recognize the heparin-PF4 complex, and the Fc portion of the antibody binds to the FcγRIIa receptors on the platelet *(16–18,21,22,29)*. Complexes of heparin-PF4-IgG accumulate on the platelet surface and stimulate platelets, which releases additional PF4, creating a positive feedback cycle. In addition, heparin sulfate on the endothelial-cell surface can also bind PF4. The antibody to the heparin-PF4 complex binds to the cell-bound complex, resulting in endothelial-cell damage *(19,23,25–27)*. The damaged endothelial cells act as a starting point for the thrombotic event, potentially through exposure of tissue factor (TF), which is enhanced by the recruitment of monocytes and further TF release from these cells *(30)*. The release of platelet microparticles *(24,31)* that are rich in phospholipid and adhesion molecules further contributes to platelet aggregation, endothelial-cell change, and thrombosis.

Platelet activation plays a central role in HIT; however, platelet activation does not occur as an isolated physiological response. Leukocyte activation, leukocyte binding to platelets, leukocyte binding to endothelial cells, and the activation of the inflammatory state also occur in the presence of heparin-dependent antibodies *(25,26,32–35)*.

Studies with cultured endothelial cells have demonstrated that there is an increase in the expression of adhesion molecules (ICAM-1, VCAM, E-Selectin), inflammatory cytokines (IL-1β, IL-6) and prothrombotic substances (TF, PAI-1) upon incubation with anti-heparin-PF4 antibodies *(26,34)*. From these studies, it is clear that endothelial-cell behavior is related to the vascular bed from which they are derived. Although human bone-marrow endothelial cells could be activated by isolated HIT IgG and PF4 alone, the activation response with human umbilical vein endothelial cells (HUVEC) was dependent on the presence of platelets or prestimulation with TNFα. HIT patients have been shown to have elevated circulating levels of TF, thrombomodulin, soluble P-selectin, and PAI-1 compared to normal individuals, suggesting endothelial injury and/or activation in patients with HIT *(25,35)*.

Platelet activation induced by anti-heparin-PF4 antibodies results in enhanced binding of platelets to monocytes and neutrophils *(32)*. Such interactions can lead to alterations in the functions of both the platelets and leukocytes. Measured as increased CD11b expression, neutrophils are activated upon incubated with HIT serum *(33)*. Studies suggest that this activation response is dependent on platelets. Another study has shown that isolated monocytes express TF following incubation with purified HIT IgG *(30)*. Thus, it appears that there is also an inflammatory component to the HIT response.

The wide spectrum of clinical manifestations described in patients who develop HIT may be explained by the heterogeneity of the components that comprise its mechanism. HIT antibodies are usually of the IgG_2 isotype, although other IgG isotypes as well as IgA and IgM antibodies have been identified in these patients *(16,21,22,36)*. The heparin-PF4 antibody titer does not correlate with the severity of clinical manifestations of HIT *(7,8)*, suggesting that there are other still unknown components or mechanisms. Both functional and non-functional antibodies, in terms of their ability to activate platelets, have been identified in patients with HIT *(36,37)*. Such antibodies may arise from different epitopes on the heparin-PF4 complex. Whether these non-functional antibodies are truly benign is unknown. However, there is evidence of an increased prevalence of MI, recurrent angina, urgent revascularization, and stroke within the year following detection of antibodies *(38)*. There is a range of affinities of antibodies to the heparin-PF4 complex, and only the highest-affinity antibodies appear to cause platelet activation, as demonstrated by the serotonin-release assay *(39,40)*. Other studies have also shown that antibodies from some patients with HIT can cause platelet activation independent of heparin *(36)*.

The platelet FcγRIIA-receptor genotype imparts a degree of risk on patients for developing HIT, but this does not seem to be a major factor *(41)*. Heparin itself is heterogeneous in amino acid and protein content and degree of sulfation from lot to lot and from manufacturer to manufacturer. These add other levels of heterogeneity to the spectrum of HIT.

4. Anticoagulant Options for Patients With HIT

Despite the devastating consequences of the heparin antibody, the diagnosis of the immune form of HIT is not made promptly in many hospital units. The clinical management of patients who are believed to have HIT demands a meticulous search for heparin exposure, including vascular line flushes and heparin-coated catheters. All heparin should be immediately discontinued. Early discontinuation of heparin alone does not appear to significantly affect the thrombotic event rate, although early recognition may improve mortality *(13)*. In one study, one-third of all HIT patients in whom heparin was stopped as soon as the diagnosis was made developed a new thrombosis *(13)*. Thus, prophylaxis against thrombosis may be beneficial. Although the discontinuation of heparin removes the stimulus for HIT antibody production, it also eliminates the usual treatment for thrombosis. Untreated thrombus will continue to propagate, and will become a clinically significant thrombotic event. Therefore, alternatives to heparin are needed in this patient population for the prophylaxis and treatment of thrombotic events and for use in interventional and surgical procedures.

4.1. Traditional Management Options

Most of the early anticoagulation treatment alternatives for patients with HIT have been less than optimal because of high bleeding risk, slow onset of activity, long half-life, poor efficacy, and lack of an antidote. The conventional anticoagulants aspirin and dextran are of limited value in the treatment of patients with HIT-associated thrombosis (2). Dextran interferes with platelet aggregation and fibrin polymerization, thus delaying the onset of aggregation and the overall degree of aggregation. However, tachyphylaxis or anaphylaxis to dextran can occur. Aspirin has been used with some success, but often has no effect in HIT patients (42). Aspirin is usually initiated only after thrombocytopenia has resolved to a level of at least 100,000/µL platelets.

4.2. Low Molecular Weight Heparins

Considered to be less antigenic than heparin because of their smaller size, low molecular weight heparins (LMWHs) were believed to play a role as alternative anticoagulants in patients with HIT. Based on a review of clinical trials carried out in the 1990s, there was a lower risk of immune sensitization and lower risk of developing HIT with LMWH treatment (0.3% vs 2.8%) (43). The molecular weight of heparin may contribute to its ability to generate functional antibodies. Fractions of heparin with mean molecular weights less than 5000 Daltons do not activate platelets in the presence of antibody (44). This may be a key factor in the lower incidence of HIT in patients treated with LMWH; however, data for all LMWHs and for both prophylactic and therapeutic doses is not available.

Nonetheless, it is clear that in a patient with established HIT, the use of LMWHs would be associated with a high risk of continuation of the disease process. In vitro results unequivocally demonstrate that LMWHs will produce platelet aggregation in the presence of heparin antibody. Although the response is less than that for heparin (80% vs 100% positive reactors), it remains significant (28,45). There have been limited reports on the successful use of LMWHs in HIT-positive patients (46–49). However, some authors caution that evidence for reducing the thrombus extension was not documented in all patients (49–51). If in vitro platelet aggregation with LMWH is positive, treatment must be avoided or stopped (47) The current American College of Chest Physicians (ACCP) recommendation is that LMWH should not be given to patients with HIT, as the potential for cross-reactivity with the heparin antibody is high (1).

4.3. Warfarin

For patients with mechanical prosthetic valves, atrial fibrillation (AF), and an underlying hypercoagulable state, the ideal management strategy is to keep the patients prophylactically anticoagulated with oral anticoagulants (2,4).

However, warfarin should not be used as the sole treatment for HIT-associated thrombosis. With warfarin, the required loading period of 48–72 h leaves patients without anticoagulant protection during that period. This can be prevented by overlapping use of a direct thrombin inhibitor during initial warfarin dosing. Warfarin also inhibits protein C, potentially resulting in a prothrombotic state that can lead to tissue necrosis. To avoid skin necrosis, full anticoagulation with warfarin should be delayed until the patient is out of the acute phase of HIT and platelet counts exceed 100,000/μL *(52)*. Once the international normalized ratio (INR) for warfarin is stable in the therapeutic range, the intravenous (iv) thrombin inhibitor can be tapered off. An important point to consider when using a combination of direct thrombin inhibitor and oral anticoagulant is that the PT/INR is also affected by direct thrombin inhibitors *(53–55)*. Higher than expected INR values will be obtained for patients on a combination of direct thrombin inhibitors and warfarin, but without the same relationship between INR and bleeding risk. A nomogram is available that can be used to help direct dosing. A practical recommendation is to co-administer warfarin and the thrombin inhibitor until an INR of 3–4 is achieved. The thrombin inhibitor can then be withdrawn, and the INR can be reassessed. Low-dose aspirin can be added to the regimen once warfarin is therapeutic.

4.4. Ancrod

The defibrinating agent ancrod (Arvin®; Knoll; Whippany, NJ) is a purified fraction of venom from the Malaysian pit viper *Agkistrodon rhodostroma*. Theoretically, it is useful in patients with HIT because of its mechanism of action, which differs from that of heparin. Ancrod acts on the fibrinogen molecule enzymatically, cleaving off the fibrinopeptides A but not the fibrinopeptides B. Soluble fibrin is formed, to which tissue plasminogen activator (tPA) and plasminogen bind. Generated plasmin degrades the fibrin. Fibrin deposition and clot formation are prevented by endogenous fibrinolysis. Thrombosis can occur if the endogenous fibrinolytic system is not optimal, or if the infusion of ancrod is rapid enough that the rate of fibrin formation is greater than the rate of fibrin degradation. Ancrod has been used in cardiac surgery for anticoagulation of the cardiac surgery pump in patients with HIT, with treatment performed 24–48 h prior to surgery. This treatment is no longer recommended because it carries an inherent risk of bleeding, thrombosis, and treatment failure *(56)*. This agent is no longer available for clinical use.

4.5. Direct Thrombin Inhibitors

The recommended treatment for patients with HIT antibody is to anticoagulate with a direct thrombin inhibitor *(1)*. The FDA has approved hirudin (lepirudin, Refludan® [Berlex; Wayne, NJ]) and argatroban (Acova®

Table 2
Differences Between the Two Direct Thrombin Inhibitors

Argatroban	Hirudin
Shorter half-life	Longer half-life
Anticoagulant response rapidly reversed	Anticoagulant response slowly reversed
No antibody formation	Antibodies are generated that delay its elimination; antibodies are generated that decrease its anticoagulant activity
May have less bleeding side effect	May have more bleeding side effect
Metabolized in the liver	Cleared via the kidney
Requires dose adjustment in liver disease patients	Requires dose adjustment in renal diseasepatients
Effectively monitored by aPTT and ACT	Monitored by aPTT and ACT, but response times are different from argatroban

[GlaxoSmithKline; Philadelphia, PA]) for the treatment of HIT-associated thrombosis. Pharmacologic characteristics of these agents are compared in **Table 2**. Argatroban has also been approved for prophylaxis of HIT-associated thrombosis. These drugs have no structural similarity to heparin, and thus do not crossreact with the HIT antibody *(2,28,57,58)*. The level of anticoagulation can be monitored with standard aPTT testing for both drugs.

4.5.1. Argatroban: Prophylaxis and Treatment of Thrombosis

A multicenter study conducted to evaluate the safety and efficacy of arga-troban in patients with HIT used continuous iv argatroban at 2 µg/kg/min for an average of 6 d (14 d maximum) in 160 HIT patients and 144 HITTS patients *(59)*. Dosage was adjusted to maintain the activated partial thromboplastin time (aPTT) between 1.5 and 3.0× baseline. Outcomes assessed during and for a period of 30 d following therapy were compared with those from 147 HIT and 46 HITTS historical control patients.

The primary efficacy composite end points of new thrombosis, all-cause amputation, or all-cause death were significantly reduced in argatroban-treated patients vs controls with HIT (25.6% vs 38.8%, $p = 0.014$). In patients with HITTS the composite incidence in argatroban-treated patients was 43.8% vs 56.5%, $p = 0.13$. Significant between group differences by time-to-event analysis of the composite end point favored argatroban treatment in HIT ($p = 0.01$) and HITTS ($p = 0.014$) patients. Argatroban therapy, relative to controls, also significantly reduced new thrombosis and death due to thrombosis ($p < 0.05$).

No difference was detected in the incidence of major bleeding vs controls (HIT: 3.1% vs 6.5%, $p = 0.20$; HITTS: 10.4% vs 9.2%, $p = 0.74$), although minor bleeding was increased (HIT: 40% vs 12%, $p < 0.001$; HITTS: 42% vs 17%, $p < 0.001$), primarily at procedural sites. Argatroban-treated patients achieved therapeutic aPTTs generally within 4–5 h of starting therapy, and, compared to controls, had a significantly more rapid rise in platelet count ($p = 0.0001$).

4.5.2. Argatroban: Interventional Cardiology

Frequently, patients with HIT require coronary interventional procedures. The feasibility of using argatroban in this patient population was investigated several years ago *(60–62)*. Subsequently, two trials (ARG216 and ARG310/311) evaluated the safety and efficacy of argatroban as anticoagulant therapy for percutaneous coronary interventional (PCI) procedures, including percutaneous transluminal coronary angioplasty, stent implantation and rotational atherectomy, in HIT patients *(63)*. Patients ($n = 91$; 112 PCIs) were treated with a 350 µg/kg bolus argatroban followed by a 25 µg/kg/min infusion. Efficacy of anticoagulation in argatroban-treated PCI HIT patients was measured in comparison to the Cleveland Clinic PCI angioplasty registry of heparin-treated non-HIT patients during the concordant time of patient enrollment. Safety of argatroban in PCI was evaluated by comparing the bleeding rate with argatroban to the heparin-only arm of the EPILOG trial, which was also conducted during the same period as patient enrollment in the argatroban PCI trials.

The 94.5% acute procedural success rate in patients who were undergoing their initial PCI with argatroban compared favorably with the 94.0% procedural success rate with heparin. No unsatisfactory outcomes occurred during repeat PCIs with argatroban ($n = 21$). Only one patient experienced major periprocedural bleeding. The safety of argatroban during PCI was at least equivalent to the safety of heparin during PCI (1.1% major bleeding rate with argatroban vs 3.1% with heparin).

Adequate anticoagulation as measured by the activated clotting time (ACT) was achieved in 97.8% of argatroban-treated patients after the initial argatroban bolus. The target ACT for PCI of 300–450 s was achieved within 10 min of initiation of argatroban *(61)*. An ACT of >300 s was maintained throughout the interventional procedure in more than 80% of the argatroban-treated patients. A repeat argatroban bolus of 150 µg/kg generally re-established a therapeutic ACT. An ACT of 200–250 s was recommended when argatroban is used in conjunction with a GPIIb/IIIa inhibitor.

Although the data is promising for the use of argatroban in PCI in HIT and non-HIT patients, the registry-style control data collection used in some of these studies could have introduced observational bias as a result of the non-blinded nature of the study design. A recent pilot study has shown that the use of argatroban in combination with glycoprotein IIb/IIIa inhibition is safe and effective in non-HIT patients undergoing percutaneous coronary intervention *(63a)*. In this study of 101 prospectively enrolled patients, a 250 µg/kg bolus + 15 µg/kg/min infusion of argatroban was observed to provide adequate anticoagulation with an acceptable bleeding risk. Further refinement of argatroban dosing is ongoing.

4.5.3. Lepirudin: Treatment of Thrombosis

Lepirudin was evaluated for safety and efficacy in the heparin-associated thrombocytopenia (HAT) study in patients with HIT confirmed by lab testing. Patients were administered one of four iv regimens: A1, HITTS patients ($n = 51$), 0.4 mg/kg bolus followed by 0.15 mg/kg/h; A2, HITTS patients receiving thrombolysis ($n = 5$), 0.2 mg/kg bolus followed by 0.1 mg/kg/h; B, HIT patients ($n = 18$), 0.1 mg/kg/h; C, during cardiopulmonary bypass surgery ($n = 8$), 0.25 mg/kg bolus and 5 mg boluses as needed *(64)*. Outcomes of 71 patients were compared to a historical control group of 120 patients. The incidence of the combined end point (death, amputation, new thromboembolic complications) was significantly reduced in lepirudin-treated patients ($p = 0.014$). Platelet counts increased rapidly in 88.7% of treated patients, and bleeding rates were similar in both groups.

In the HAT-2 study, patients with HIT confirmed by lab testing received treatment by one of three dosing regimens for 2–10 d or longer: A1, treatment, 0.4 mg/kg bolus followed by 0.15 mg/kg/h ($n = 65$); A2, in conjunction with thrombolytic therapy, 0.2 mg/kg followed by 0.1 mg/kg/h ($n = 4$); B, prophylaxis, 0.01 mg/kg/h ($n = 43$) *(65)*. Outcomes of 95 patients compared with those of 120 historical control patients showed aPTT >1.5× baseline and platelet count normalization by d 10 in 69% of treated patients. Within 35 d after HIT confirmation fewer lepirudin-treated patients than historical control patients experienced outcome events ($p = 0.12$). Bleeding events in the lepirudin group were more frequent (44.6 vs 27.2%; $p = 0.0001$).

These studies showed that anticoagulation with argatroban or hirudin significantly reduces the risk of thrombosis and thromboembolic complications (new thrombosis, amputation, or death) associated with HIT. This benefit was achieved with an acceptable safety profile.

4.5.4. Lepirudin: Cardiac Surgery

Perhaps the greatest obstacle to overcome in the management of patients with HIT antibody is anticoagulation during surgical coronary revascularization. Standard heparin protocols, restricted to the surgery itself, can be employed after antibody titers are allowed to decrease *(3,66)*. Additionally, performing surgery with a combination of heparin and an antiplatelet agent such as tirofiban or iloprost may prove to be a useful option *(67,68)*. Postoperative or long-term use of heparin should be replaced with a direct thrombin inhibitor and/or warfarin.

The use of hirudin as an anticoagulant during cardiopulmonary bypass surgery (coronary-artery grafting, aortic-valve replacement) in patients with HIT has been described in a number of small studies and case reports *(69–77)*. Although large-scale trials to identify the optimal dosage of hirudin have not been performed, it appears that clotting can be avoided at hirudin concentrations of approx 3–5 µg/mL *(71,74)*. It may be possible to monitor such levels of hirudin using the ecarin clotting time. However, this assay has not been standardized, and is not widely available. As in patients without HIT, the risk of bleeding is increased when hirudin-treated HIT patients have impaired renal function.

4.5.5. Other Uses of Thrombin Inhibitors in HIT Patients

Several case reports describe the successful use of argatroban anticoagulation in HIT patients requiring renal or carotid stent placement *(77a,b)*. Doses of argatroban were similar to those that are used for coronary interventions. The use of both argatroban and lepirudin for anticoagulation in HIT patients requiring hemodialysis has been described *(77c–77g)*. Lepirudin has been shown in a limited number of patients to provide safe and effective anticoagulation for performing percutaneous coronary interventions in patients with HIT *(77h,77i)*.

4.5.6. Danaparoid

The low molecular weight heparinoid danaparoid (Orgaran®; Organon; Oss, The Netherlands) was introduced about 12 yr ago, and was soon used as an alternative anticoagulant in patients with HIT, as no other viable drug existed at this time. Danaparoid is a mixture of non-heparin polysulfated glycosaminoglycans (GAGs) (heparin sulfate, dermatan sulfate, chondroitin sulfate) and LMWH. Although related to heparin in structure, danaparoid differs from heparin in the degree of sulfation and molecular weight. In vitro studies using HIT-positive sera have shown a decreased incidence of platelet aggregation to danaparoid compared to heparin—e.g., 18% positive reactors vs 100% for heparin *(28,78)*. As a result, there have been reported treatment failures *(79)*.

Danaparoid has been successfully used in a considerable number of patients with HIT in numerous clinical situations such as hemodialysis, plasmapheresis, treatment of pulmonary emboli, treatment of venous or arterial thrombosis, and unstable angina, and during therapy with the intra-aortic balloon pump *(80,81)*. Danaparoid has been the drug of choice for treatment of HIT patients over the last several years prior to the availability of direct thrombin inhibitors.

Typical dosing ranges from 0.5–0.8 anti-Xa U/ml for treatment of thrombosis. Although useful in many clinical cases, limitations do exist with danaparoid, including dosing guidelines that are not well-established, lack of an antagonist, and monitoring assays that are usually unavailable. In addition, because of its long half-life (about 25 h), significant postoperative bleeding can occur with danaparoid. While danaparoid has been withdrawn from the US market by its manufacturer, it remains a useful alternative for the prophylactic and therapeutic anticoagulation of HIT patients in Europe.

4.6. Thrombolytic Agents

Patients who have limb-threatening or life-threatening thrombosis that is not corrected with thrombin-inhibitor treatment can be treated with selective thrombolytic infusion *(2,4)*. Lower doses for postoperative patients (urokinase 30,000–60,000 U/h) and higher doses (urokinase 50,000–200,000 U/h) for non-postoperative patients are recommended *(4,82–84)*. Fibrinogen levels are monitored every 8 h to maintain levels at 200 mg/dL. Thrombolytic infusions are discontinued or decreased if significant clinical bleeding is observed, and are continued until angiographic evidence of complete resolution of thrombus is found. Selective thrombolytic infusion has been more successful than surgical thrombectomy. The endothelial damage that occurs with thrombectomy, combined with the involvement of endothelial cells observed with HIT antibody, may explain the limited success with thrombectomy. However, surgical thrombectomy remains a reasonable therapy in patients who have dire clinical circumstances and cannot afford the time required for selective thrombolytic infusions.

5. Future Anticoagulants

5.1. Bivalirudin

Bivalirudin (Angiomax®, The Medicines Company; Parsippany, NJ) is a synthetic, direct thrombin inhibitor with a lower molecular weight than hirudin. Its structure is based on two small peptide sequences that bind directly to the active site of thrombin, and to the exosite of thrombin. Bivalirudin is a reversible inhibitor of thrombin, which can be used in both renally and hepatically impaired patients. Bivalirudin is currently approved in the US for use in non-HIT patients undergoing PTCA. In addition, the drug is in phase II/III development for use as an anticoagulant for off-pump coronary surgery. Limited data suggests that the use of bivalirudin provide adequate anticoagulation for off-pump surgery without increasing the propensity for bleeding relative to the use of heparin/protamine. Limited clinical experience shows that bivalirudin can be used successfully to prevent thrombosis in patients with HIT *(57a,b)*.

5.2. Factor Xa Inhibitors

Factor Xa inhibitors are another focus of new drug development. The synthetic heparin pentasaccharide (fondaparinux, Arixtra®; Sanofi-Synthélabo Organon; Paris, France) is one example. Factor Xa inhibitors have shown no platelet aggregation response at any concentration with numerous HIT positive sera that have been evaluated *(28)*. These agents would not be expected to produce a platelet activation/aggregation response to the known HIT antibody, since they do not interact with PF4 and do not release PF4 from activated platelets, as does heparin. In clinical trials to date, fondaparinux treatment has been associated with thrombocytopenia at half the frequency as that observed with LMWH treatment. There has been no known development of HIT because of fondaparinux treatment in these trials. However, it is not known if these drugs are potent enough to counteract the high level of thrombin generation that produces the hypercoagulable state in HIT.

5.3. Antiplatelet Agents

Despite the potent anticoagulant effect of direct thrombin inhibitors demonstrated in the clinical trials, an unacceptable level of thrombosis-related morbidity and mortality remains in HIT patients. The glycoprotein (GP) IIb/IIIa platelet-receptor inhibitors (abciximab, ReoPro®; Lilly; Indianapolis IN; eptifibatide, Integrilin®; Millenium Pharmaceuticals, Cambridge, MA; tirofiban, Aggrastat®; Merck, West Point, PA) and the ADP platelet receptor inhibitor (clopidogrel, Plavix®; Sanofi; Paris, France) have been shown to inhibit in vitro platelet activation/aggregation responses induced by HIT serum and heparin *(24,85)*. This includes inhibition of the formation of platelet microparticles. The thrombin inhibitors were not effective in suppressing this platelet activation *(85)*.

Limited clinical experience suggests that GPIIb/IIIa inhibitors are effective at reducing thrombus that is resistant to thrombin inhibitor treatment *(58)*. In these patients, a standard dose of a GPIIb/IIIa inhibitor was administered with a reduced dose of the direct thrombin inhibitor. There was no incidence of overt bleeding that required intervention, and all patients exhibited clinical improvement or full recovery. Although promising, optimal dosing regimens have not yet been established.

6. Conclusion

Because patients with HIT have an extremely high probability of developing thrombosis, treatment options other than heparin are essential (**Table 3**; *2,4*). Prophylaxis against thrombosis should also be considered *(2,4)*. The current ACCP guidelines for the treatment of acute HITTS include the use of

Table 3
Anticoagulant Options for the HIT Patient

Drug	Comment
Current recommendations	
Argatroban	Drug of choice; approved for prophylaxis and treatment of HIT-associated thrombosis.
Lepirudin	Drug of choice; approved for the treatment of HIT-associated thrombosis.
Danaparoid	Useful in many cases; but inconvenient monitoring, longer half-life than thrombin inhibitors, potential cross-reactivity with HIT antibodies.
Warfarin	Should not be used as sole therapy in acute phase of HIT; can be given in conjunction with thrombin inhibitors during the acute phase, or its use delayed until platelet counts begin to normalize.
Other options	
Thrombolytics	Useful only to resolve life-threatening thromboses.
Dextran	Limited value; may be associated with anaphylactic or tachyphylactic responses.
Aspirin	Not effective in most patients; lacks potent anticoagulant effect needed in HIT type II.
Ancrod	Slow onset of action; high bleeding risk; no antidote.
Contraindicated agents	
LMW heparins	Not recommended due to a high degree of in vitro cross-reactivity and the potential for in vivo cross-reactivity.
Under investigation	
Bivalrudin	Direct thrombin inhibitor with properties similar to argatroban and lepirudin; limited experience in HIT patients.
Antifactor Xa agents	Do not interact with HIT antibody; may lack potent anticoagulant activity needed in HIT type II.
Antiplatelet agents	GP IIb/IIIa antagonists and ADP-receptor blockers; effective in in vitro studies; limited data in vivo; may be useful in combination with thrombin inhibitors.

danaparoid, lepirudin, or argatroban alone or in combination with warfarin. For documented clinical thrombosis associated with HIT, patients should be treated with a direct thrombin inhibitor at therapeutic aPTT levels for 7–10 d. Warfarin should not be used during the acute phase of HIT, unless a thrombin inhibitor is being used simultaneously. Conversion to warfarin can be done when the acute phase of HIT has passed. Because of the high likelihood of cross-reactivity, the use of LMWHs in patients with HIT is not recommended.

For prophylactic treatment of HIT patients despite a lack of other indications for anticoagulation, a direct thrombin inhibitor can be initiated with low levels of anticoagulation until the thrombocytopenia resolves. This regimen is continued until laboratory evidence is provided that the HIT antibody is no longer detectable. In addition to needing anticoagulation to treat thrombosis, HIT patients can require anticoagulation for non-HIT-related events such as treatment of MI and unstable angina or long-term anticoagulation for heart valves or AF. For these situations, the use of a direct thrombin inhibitor if immediate anticoagulation is needed with switchover to warfarin is a useful option. However, optimal dosing regimens have not been established in all cases.

References

1. Hirsh, J., Warkentin, T. E., Shaughnessy, S. G., Anand, S. S., Halperin, J. L., Raschke, R., et al. (2001) Heparin and low-molecular-weight heparin: Mechanisms of action, pharmacokinetics, dosing, monitoring, efficacy and safety. *Chest* **119**, 64S–94S.
2. Lewis, B. E., Walenga, J. M., and Wallis, D. E. (1997) Anticoagulation with Novastan® (argatroban) in patients with heparin-induced thrombocytopenia and heparin-induced thrombocytopenia and thrombosis syndrome. *Semin. Thromb. Hemost.* **23(2)**, 197.
3. Messmore, H. L., Upadhyay, G., Farid, S., Parachuri, R., Wehrmacher, W., and Godwin, J. (1993) Heparin-induced thrombocytopenia and thrombosis in cardiovascular surgery, in *New Anticoagulants for the Cardiovascular Patient* (Pifarré, R., ed.), Philadelphia, Hanley & Belfus, Inc., p. 83.
4. Walenga, J. M., Lewis, B. E., Hoppensteadt, D. A., Fareed, J., and Bakhos, M. (1997) Management of heparin-induced thrombocytopenia and heparin-induced thrombocytopenia and thrombosis syndrome. *Clin. Appl. Thromb. Hemost.* **3 (Suppl. 1)**, S53–S63.
5. Warkentin, T. E. and Kelton, J. G. (2001) Temporal aspects of heparin-induced thrombocytopenia. *N. Engl. J. Med.* **344(17)**, 1286–1292.
6. Warkentin, T. E. and Kelton, J. G. (2001) Delayed onset of heparin-induced thrombocytopenia. *Ann. Intern. Med.* **135(7)**, 502–506.
7. Walenga, J. M., Jeske, W. P., Wood, J. J., Ahmad, S., Lewis, B. E., and Bakhos, M. (1999) Laboratory tests for heparin-induced thrombocytopenia: a multicenter study. *Semin. Hematol.* **36 (Suppl. 1)**, 22–28.

8. Walenga, J. M., Jeske, W. P., Fasanella, A. R., Wood, J. J., Ahmad, S., and Bakhos, M. (1999) Laboratory diagnosis of heparin-induced thrombocytopenia. *Clin. Appl. Thromb. Hemost.* **5 (Suppl. 1),** S21–S27.
9. Warkentin, T. E., Hayward, C. P., Boshkov, C. K., et al. (1994) Sera from patients with heparin-induced thrombocytopenia generate platelet derived microparticles with procoagulant activity: an explanation for the thrombotic complications of heparin induced thrombocytopenia. *Blood* **84,** 3691.
*10. Warkentin, T. E. and Kelton, J. G. (1996) A 14-year study of heparin-induced thrombocytopenia. *Am. J. Med.* **101,** 502–507.
11. Greinacher, A., Eckhardt, T., Mussman, J., et al. (1993) Pregnancy complicated by heparin associated thrombocytopenia management by a prospective *in vitro* selected heparinoid (ORG 10172). *Thromb. Res.* **71,** 123.
12. Stewart, M. W., Etches, W. S., Boshkov, L. K., et al. (1995) Heparin-induced thrombocytopenia: an improved method of detection based on lumi-aggregometry. *Br. J. Haematol.* **91,** 173.
13. Wallis, D. E., Workman, D. L., Lewis, B. E., Steen, L., Pifarré, R., and Moran, J. F. (1999) Failure of early heparin cessation as treatment for heparin-induced thrombocytopenia. *Am. J. Med.* **106(6), 629–635.
14. Moberg, P., Geary, V., and Sheikh, M. (1990) Heparin-induced thrombocytopenia: a possible complication of heparin-coated pulmonary artery catheters. *J. Cardiothorac. Anesth.* **4,** 266.
15. Weismann, R. E. and Tobin, R. W. (1958) Arterial embolism occurring with systemic heparin therapy. *AMA Arch. Surg.* **76,** 219.
16. Amiral, J., Bridey, F., Dreyfus, M., et al. (1992) Platelet factor 4 complexed to heparin is the target for antibodies generated in heparin-induced thrombocytopenia. *Thromb. Haemostasis* **68(1),** 95.
17. Aster, R. H. (1995) Heparin-induced thrombocytopenia and thrombosis. *N. Engl. J. Med.* **332,** 1374.
18. Brandt, J. T., Isenhart, C. E., Osborne, J. M., et al. (1995) On the role of platelet Fc(RIIA phenotype in heparin induced thrombocytopenia. *Thromb. Haemostasis* **74,** 1564.
19. Cines, D. B., Tomaski, A., and Tannenbaum, S. (1987) Immune endothelial-cell injury in heparin associated thrombocytopenia. *N. Engl. J. Med.* **316,** 581.
20. Greinacher, A., Michels, I., Liebenhoff, U., et al. (1993) Heparin-associated thrombocytopenia: Immune complexes are attached to the platelet membrane by the negative charge of highly sulphated oligosaccharides. *Br. J. Haematol.* **84,** 711.

---

*The authors document the high occurrence of venous thrombosis in patients with HIT and the high 30-d risk of developing thrombosis in patients initially recognized with isolated thrombocytopenia.

**Retrospective study of 113 patients with HIT demonstrating that early cessation of heparin did not reduce the morbidity associated with HIT.

21. Greinacher, A., Pötzsch, B., Amiral, J., et al. (1994) Heparin-associated thrombocytopenia: isolation of the antibody and characterization of a multi-molecular PF-4 heparin complex as the major antigen. *Thromb. Haemostasis* **71**, 247.

22. Kelton, J. G., Smith, J. W., Warkentin, T. E., et al. (1994) Immunoglobulin G from patients with heparin-induced thrombocytopenia binds to a complex of heparin and platelet factor 4. *Blood* **83**, 3232.

23. Visentin, G. P., Ford, S. E., Scott, J. P., et al. (1995) Antibodies from patients with heparin-induced thrombocytopenia/thrombosis are specific for platelet factor 4 complexed with heparin or bound to endothelial cells. *J. Clin. Invest.* **93**, 81.

24. Jeske, W. P., Walenga, J. M., Szatkowski, E., Ero, M., Herbert, J. M., Haas, S., et al. (1997) Effect of glycoprotein IIb/IIIa antagonists on the HIT serum induced activation of platelets. *Thromb. Res.* **88**, 271–281.

25. Walenga, J. M., Michal, K., Hoppensteadt, D., Wood, J. J., Bick, R. L., and Robinson, J. A. (1999) Vascular damage correlates between heparin-induced thrombocytopenia and the antiphospholipid syndrome. *Clin. Appl. Thromb. Hemost.* **5 (Suppl. 1)**, S76–S84.

26. Herbert, J. M., Savi, P., Jeske, W. P., and Walenga, J. M. (1998) Effect of SR121566A, a potent GPIIb/IIIa antagonist, on the HIT serum/heparin-induced platelet mediated activation of human endothelial cells. *Thromb. Haemostasis* **80**, 326–331.

27. Chong, B. H. (1995) Heparin-induced thrombocytopenia (Review). *Br. J. Haematol.* **89**, 431–439.

28. Walenga, J. M., Koza, M. J., Lewis, B. E., and Pifarré, R. (1996) Relative heparin induced thrombocytopenic potential of low molecular weight heparins and new antithrombotic agents. *Clin. Appl. Thromb. Hemost.* **2 (Suppl. 1)**, S21.

29. Newman, P. M. and Chong, B. H. (2000) Heparin-induced thrombocytopenia: New evidence for the dynamic binding of purified anti-PF4-heparin antibodies to platelets and the resultant platelet activation. *Blood* **96**, 182–187.

30. Pouplard, C., Lochmann, S., Renard, B., Herault, O., Colombat, P., Amiral, J., and Gruel, Y. (2001) Induction of monocyte tissue factor expression by antibodies to heparin-platelet factor 4 complexes developed in heparin-induced thrombocytopenia. *Blood* **97(10)**, 3300–3302.

31. Hughes, M., Hayward, C. P. M., Warkentin, T. E., Horsewood, P., Chorneyko, K. A., and Keltonm, J. G. (2000) Morphological analysis of microparticle generation in heparin-induced thrombocytopenia. *Blood* **96**, 188–194.

32. Jeske, W. P., Schlenker, R., Bakhos, M., and Walenga, J. M. (2000) Are leukocytes important for platelet activation in heparin-induced thrombocytopenia? *Ann. Hematol.* **79 (Suppl. I)**, A46.

33. Jeske, W. P., Vasaiwala, S., Schlenker, R., Wallis, E., and Walenga, J. M. (2000) Leukocyte activation in heparin-induced thrombocytopenia. *Blood* **96(11)**, 29b.

34. Blank, M., Shoenfeld, Y., Tavor, S., Praprotnik, S., Boffa, M. C., Weksler, B. B., et al. (2002) Anti-PF4/heparin antibodies from patients with heparin-induced thrombocytopenia provoke direct activation of microvascular endothelial cells. *Int. Immunol.* **14(2)**, 121–129.

35. Baugh, M. J., Prechel, M., Hoppensteadt, D., Wallis, E. R., Bick, R. L., and Walenga, J. M. (2000) The role of CD40-ligand and anti-annexin V antibodies in the pathophysiology of the APS and HIT. *Blood* **96(11),** 272a.

36. Ahmad, S., Walenga, J. M., Jeske, W. P., Cella, G., and Fareed, J. (1999) Functional heterogeneity of anti-heparin-platelet factor 4 antibodies: implications in the pathogenesis of the HIT syndrome. *Clin. Appl. Thromb. Hemost.* **5 (Suppl. 1),** S32–S37.

37. Ahmad, S., Walenga, J. M., Jeske, W. P., Hoppensteadt, D. A., Khan, E., Cella, G., et al. (1999) Lack of thrombocytopenic responses after low molecular weight heparin usage is due to the generation of non-functional anti-heparin-PF4 antibodies. *Blood* **94(10),** 624a.

*38. Mattioli, A. V., Bonetti, L., Sternieri, S., and Mattioli, G. (2000) Heparin-induced thrombocytopenia in patients treated with unfractionated heparin: prevalence of thrombosis in a 1 year follow-up. *Ital. Heart. J.* **1(1),** 39–42.

39. Amiral, J., Pouplard, C., Vissac, A. M., Walenga, J. M., Jeske, W., and Gruel, Y. (2000) Affinity purification of heparin-dependent antibodies to platelet factor 4 developed in heparin-induced thrombocytopenia: Biological characteristics and effects on platelet activation. *Br. J. Haematol.* **109(2),** 336–341.

40. Pouplard, C. A., Amiral, J., Vissac, A. M., Walenga, J. M., Jeske, W. P., and Gruel, Y. J. (1999) Affinity purification of different heparin-dependent antibodies to PF4 developed in HIT. Biological characteristics and effects on platelet activation. *Blood* **94(10),** 16a.

41. Carlsson, L. E., Santoso, S., Baurichter, G., Kroll, H., Papenberg, S., Eichler, P., et al. (1998) Heparin-induced thrombocytopenia: new insights into the impact of the Fc(RIIa-R-H131 polymorphism. *Blood* **92(5),** 1526–1531.

42. Kappa, J. R., Fisher, C. A., Berkowitz, H. D., Cottrell, E. D., and Addonizio, V. P. (1987) Heparin-induced platelet activation in sixteen surgical patients: Diagnosis and management. *J. Thorac. Cardiovasc. Surg.* **5,** 101.

43. Warkentin, T. E., Levine, M. N., Hirsh, J., et al. (1995) Heparin-induced thrombocytopenia in patients treated with low-molecular-weight heparin or unfractionated heparin. *N. Engl. J. Med.* **332,** 1330.

44. Ahmad, S., Walenga, J. M., Jeske, W. P., Hoppensteadt, D. A., and Bakhos, M. (2001) Molecular weight and charge dependence of heparin on the pathogenic responses of anti-heparin platelet factor 4 antibodies. *Thromb. Haemostasis* **(July Suppl.),** CD-ROM, P2729.

45. Greinacher, A., Feigl, M., and Mueller-Eckhardt, C. (1994) Cross-reactivity studies between sera of patients with heparin associated thrombocytopenia and a new low molecular weight heparin, reviparin. *Thromb. Haemostasis* **72(4),** 644.

46. Altés, A., Rodrigo, M., Gari, M., et al. (1995) Heparin-induced thrombocytopenia and heart operation: management with tedelparin. *Ann. Thorac. Surg.* **59,** 508.

---

*Study shows an increase in thrombotic events at 1 yr follow-up in patients with anti-heparin/PF4 antibodies compared to those without antibodies, despite no evidence of thrombocytopenia.

47. Leroy, J., LeClerc, M. H., Delahousse, B., et al. (1985) Treatment of heparin-associated thrombocytopenia and thrombosis with low molecular weight heparin (CY 216). *Semin. Thromb. Hemost.* **11(3),** 326.

48. Robitaille, D., Leclerc, J. R., Laberge, R., et al. (1992) Cardiopulmonary bypass with a low-molecular-weight heparin fraction (enoxaparin) in a patient with a history of heparin-associated thrombocytopenia. *J. Thorac. Cardiovasc. Surg.* **103(3),** 597.

49. Roussi, J. H., Houbouyan, L. L., and Goguel, A. F. (1984) Use of low-molecular-weight heparin in heparin-induced thrombocytopenia with thrombotic complications. *Lancet* **(May 26),** 1183.

50. Eichinger, S., Kyrle, P. A., Brenner, B., et al. (1991) Thrombocytopenia associated with low-molecular-weight heparin. *Lancet* **337,** 1425.

51. Gouault-Heilmann, M., Payen, D., Contant, G., et al. (1985) Thrombocytopenia related to synthetic heparin analogue therapy. *Thromb. Haemostasis* **54(2),** 557.

52. Wallis, D. E., Quintos, R., Whermacher, W., and Messmore, H. (1999) Safety of warfarin anticoagulation in patients with heparin-induced thrombocytopenia. *Chest* **116,** 1333–1338.

53. Walenga, J. M., Fasanella, A. R., Iqbal, O., Hoppensteadt, D. A., Ahmad, S., Wallis, D. E., et al. (1999) Coagulation laboratory testing in patients treated with argatroban. *Semin. Thromb. Hemost.* **25 (Suppl. 1),** 61–66.

54. Sheth, S. B., DiCicco, R. A., Hursting, M. J., Montague, T., and Jorkasky, D. K. (2001) Interpreting the international normalized ratio (INR) in individuals receiving argatroban and warfarin. *Thromb. Haemostasis* **85,** 435–440.

55. Hursting, M. J., Zehnder, J. L., Joffrion, J. L., Becker, J. C., Knappenberger, G. D., and Schwarz, R. P. (1999) The interventional normalization ratio during concurrent warfarin and argatroban anticoagulation differential contributions of each agent and effects of the choice of the thromboplastin used. *Clin. Chem.* **45(13),** 409–412.

56. Lewis, B. E., Leya, F. S., Wallis, D., and Grassman, E. (1994) Failure of ancrod in the treatment of heparin-induced arterial thrombosis. *Can. J. Cardiol.* **10(5),** 559.

57. Chamberlin, J. R., Lewis, B., Leya, F., et al. (1995) Successful treatment of heparin-associated thrombocytopenia and thrombosis using hirulog. *Can. J. Cardiol.* **11(6),** 511.

57a. Reid, T., Alving, B. M. (1994) Hrulog therapy for heparin-associated thrombocytopenia and deep venous thrombosis. *Am. J. Hematol.* **45,** 352–353.

57b. Campbell, K. R., Mahaffey, K. W., Lewis, B. E., Weitz, J. I., Berkowitz, S. D., Ohman, E. M., et al. (2000) Bivalirudin in patients with heparin-induced thrombocytopenia underoing percutaneous coronary intervention. *J. Invas. Cardiol.* **12 (Suppl F),** 14F-9.

*58. Walenga, J. M., Lewis, B. E., Jeske, W. P., Leya, F., Wallis, D. E., Bakhos, M., et al. (1999) Combined thrombin and platelet inhibition treatment for HIT patients. *Hämostaseologie* **19,** 128–133.

---

*Describes the use of the combination of a GP IIb/IIIa inhibitor and a direct thrombin inhibitor for the treatment of acute thrombosis in patients with HIT.

*59. Lewis, B. E., Wallis, D. E., Berkowitz, S. D., Matthai, W. H., Fareed, J., Walenga, J. M., et al., for the ARG-911 Study Investigators (2001) Argatroban anticoagulant therapy in patients with heparin-induced thrombocytopenia. *Circulation* **103(14),** 1838–1843.

60. Lewis, B. E., Ferguson, J. J., Grassman, E. D., Fareed, J., Walenga, J. M., Joffrion, J. L., et al. (1996) Successful coronary interventions performed with argatroban anticoagulation in patients with heparin-induced thrombocytopenia and thrombosis syndrome. *J. Invas. Cardiol.* **8(9),** 410–417.

61. Lewis, B. E., Iqbal, O., Hoppensteadt, D., Ahsan, A., Ahmad, S., Messmore, H. L., et al. (1997) Clinical pharmacokinetic and pharmacodynamic studies on argatroban to optimize the anticoagulant dosage in interventional cardiovascular procedures [abstract]. *Thromb. Haemostasis* **(Suppl.),** 492.

62. Lewis, B. E., Rangel, Y., and Fareed, J. (1998) The first report of successful carotid stent implant using argatroban anticoagulation in a patient with heparin-induced thrombocytopenia and thrombosis syndrome: A case report. *Angiology* **49(1),** 61–67.

63. Lewis, B. E., Cohen, M., Moses, J., Matthai, W., for the ARG-216/310/311 investigators (2000) Argatroban anticoagulation during initial and repeat percutaneous coronary intervention in patients with heparin-induced thrombocytopenia [abstract]. *Am. J. Cardiol.* **86 (Suppl. 8A),** 141.

63a. Jang, I. K., Lewis, B. E., Matthai, W. H., and Kleiman, N. S. (2003) Combination of a direct thrombin inhibitor, argatroban, and glycoprotein IIb/IIIa inhibitor is effective and safe in patients undergoing percutaneous coronary intervention. *J. Am. Coll. Cardiol.* **41(6 Suppl A),** 68A.

64. Greinacher, A., Volpel, H., Janssens, U., Hach-Wunderle, V., Kemkes-Matthes, B., Eichler, P., et al., for the HIT Investigators Group (1999) Recombinant hirudin (lepirudin) provides safe and effective anticoagulation in patients with heparin-induced thrombocytopenia. A prospective study. *Circulation* **99, 73–80.

65. Greinacher, A., Janssens, U., Berg, G., Bock, M., Kwasny, H., Kemkes-Matthes, B., et al., for the HAT investigators (1999) Lepirudin (recombinant hirudin) for parenteral anticoagulation in patients with heparin-induced thrombocytopenia. *Circulation* **100(6),** 587–593.

66. Pötzsch, B. and Klovekorn, W. P. (2000) Use of heparin during cardiopulmonary bypass in patients with a history of heparin-induced thrombocytopenia. *N. Engl. J. Med.* **343,** 515.

67. Koster, A., Loebe, M., Mertzluftt, F., Kuppe, H., and Hetzer, R. (2000) Cardiopulmonary bypass in a patient with heparin-induced thrombocytopenia II and impaired renal function using heparin and the platelet GP IIb/IIIa inhibitor tirofiban as anticoagulant. *Ann. Thorac. Surg.* **70(6),** 2160–2161.

68. Kappa, J. R., Fisher, C. A., and Todd, B. (1990) Intraoperative management of patients with heparin-induced thrombocytopenia. *Ann. Thorac. Surg.* **49,** 714.

---

*Argatroban is shown to reduce all-cause death, all-cause amputation, and new thrombosis in patients with HIT.
**Clinical benefit of r-hirudin treatment in HIT patients is described.

69. Fabrizio, M. C. (2001) Use of the ecarin clotting time (ECT) with lepirudin therapy in heparin-induced thrombocytopenia and cardiopulmonary bypass. *J. Extracorp. Tech.* **33(2)**, 117–125.
70. Riess, F. C., Kormann, J., and Poetzsch, B. (2000) Recombinant hirudin as anticoagulant during cardiopulmonary bypass. *Anesthesiology* **93(6)**, 1551–1552.
71. Shah, A. C., Genoni, M., Niederhauser, U., Maloigne, M., and Turina, M. (2000) R-hirudin (lepirudin, refludan) as an alternative anticoagulant in heparin-induced thrombocytopenia during cardiopulmonary bypass connection (German). Schweizerische Medizinische Wocenschrift. *Journal Suisse de Medicine* **130(23)**, 896–899.
72. Rubens, F. D., Sabloff, M., Wells, P. S., and Bourke, M. (2000) Use of recombinant hirudin in pulmonary thromboendarterectomy. *Ann. Thorac. Surg.* **69(6)**, 1942–1943.
73. Koster, A., Loebe, M., Hansen, R., Bauer, M., Mertzlufft, F., Kuppe, H., et al. (2000) A quick assay for monitoring hirudin during cardiopulmonary bypass in patients with heparin-induced thrombocytopenia type II: adaptation of the ecarin clotting time to the ACT II device. *J. Thorac. Cardiovasc. Surg.* **119(6)**, 1278–1283.
74. Longrois, D., de Maistre, E., Bischoff, N., Dopff, C., Meistelman, C., Angioi, M., et al. (2000) Recombinant hirudin anticoagulation for aortic valve replacement in heparin-induced thrombocytopenia. *Can. J. Anaesthesiol.* **47(3)**, 255–260.
75. Latham, P., Revelis, A. F., Joshi, G. P., DiMaio, J. M., and Jessen, M. E. (2000) Use of recombinant hirudin in patients with heparin-induced thrombocytopenia with thrombosis requiring cardiopulmonary bypass. *Anesthesiology* **92(1)**, 263–266.
76. Koster, A., Pasic, M., Bauer, M., Kuppe, H., and Hetzer, R. (2000) Hirudin as anticoagulant for cardiopulmonary bypass: importance of preoperative renal function. *Ann. Thorac. Surg.* **69(1)**, 37–41.
77. Koster, A., Kuppe, H., Hetzer, R., Sodian, R., Crystal, G. J., and Mertzlufft, F. (1998) Emergent cardiopulmonary bypass in five patients with heparin-induced thrombocytopenia type II employing recombinant hirudin. *Anesthesiology* **89(3)**, 777–780.
77a. Lewis, B. E., Grassman, E. D., Wrona, L., Rangel, Y. (1997) Novastan anticoagulation during renal stent implant in a patient with heparin-induced thrombocytopenia. *Blood Coag. Fibrinol.* **8(1)**, 54–58.
77b. Lewis, B. E., Rangel, Y, Fareed, J. (1998) The first report of successful carotid stent implant using argatroban anticoagulation in a patient with heparin-induced thrombocytopenia and thrombosis syndrome. *Angiology* **49**, 61–67.
77c. Matsuo, T., Chikahira, Y., Yamada, T., Nakao, K., Ueshima, S., Matsuo, O., (1998) Effect of synthetic thrombin inhibitor (MD805) as an alternative drug on heparin-induced thrombocytopenia during hemodialysis. *Thromb. Res.* **52**, 165–171.
77d. Koide, M., Yamamoto, S., Matsuo, M., Suzuki, S., Arima, N., Matsuo, T., (1995) Anticoagulation for heparin-induced thrombocytopenia with spontaneous platelet

aggregation in a patient requiring haemodialysis. *Nephrol. Dial. Transplant* **10,** 2137–2140.

77e. Steuer, S., Boogen, C., Plum, J., Deppe, C., Reinauer, H., Grabensee, B. (1999) Anticoagulation with r-hirudin in a patient with acute renal failure and heparin-induced thrombocytopenia. *Nephrol. Dial. Transplant* **14,** 45–47.

77f. Schneider, T., Heuer, B., Deller, A., Boesken, W. H. (2000) Continuous hemofiltration with r-hirudin (lepirudin) as anticoagulant in a patient with heparin-induced thrombocytopenia (HIT II). *Wein. Klin. Wochenschr.* **112,** 552–555.

77g. Van Wyck, V., Badenhorst, P. N., Luus, H. G., Kotze, H. F. (1995) A comparison between the use of recombinant hirudin and heparin during hemodialysis. *Kidney Int.* **48,** 1338–1343.

77h. Manfredi, J. A., Wall, R. P., Sane, D. C., Braden, G. A. (2001) Lepirudin as a safe alternative for effective anticoagulation in patients with known heparin-induced thrombocytopenia undergoing percutaneous coronary intervention: case reports. *Cath. Cardiovasc. Intervent.* **52(4),** 468–472.

77i. Pinto, D. S., Sperling, R. T., Tu, T. M., Cohen, D. J., Carrozza, J. P. (2003) Combination platelet glycoprotein IIb/IIIa receptor and lepirudin administration during percutaneous coronary intervention in patients with heparin-induced thrombocytopenia. *Cath. Cardiovasc. Intervent.* **58(1),** 65–68.

78. Chong, B. H., Ismail, F., Cade, J., et al. (1989) Heparin-induced thrombocytopenia: studies with a new low molecular weight heparinoid, Org 10172. *Blood* **73(6),** 1592.

79. Haas, S., Walenga, J. M., Jeske, W. P., and Fareed, J. (1999) Heparin-induced thrombocytopenia: Clinical considerations of alternative anticoagulation with various glycosaminoglycans and thrombin inhibitors. *Clin. Appl. Thrombosis/ Hemostasis* **5 (Suppl. 1),** 52–59.

80. Magnani, H. N. (1993) Heparin-induced thrombocytopenia (HIT): an overview of 230 patients treated with orgaran (Org 10172). *Thromb. Haemostasis* **70(4),** 554.

81. Ortel, T. L., Gocherman, J. P., Califf, R. M., et al. (1992) Parenteral anticoagulation with the heparinoid Lomoparan (ORG 10172) in patients with heparin-induced thrombocytopenia and thrombosis. *Thromb. Haemostasis* **67(3),** 292.

82. Cohen, J. I., Cooper, M. R., and Greenberg, C. S. (1985) Streptokinase therapy of pulmonary emboli with heparin-associated thrombocytopenia. *Arch. Intern. Med.* **135,** 1725–1726.

83. Fiessinger, J. N., Aiach, M., Roncato, M., et al. (1984) Critical ischemia during heparin-induced thrombocytopenia. Treatment by intra-arterial streptokinase. *Thromb. Res.* **33,** 235.

84. Rao, R. C., Lewis, B. E., and Johnson, S. A. (1995) Thrombolytic experience for treatment of thrombosis in patients with post-operative heparin-induced thrombocytopenia. *Blood* **86(10)(Suppl. 1),** 551a.

85. Haas, S., Walenga, J. M., Jeske, W. P., and Fareed, J. (1999) Heparin-induced thrombocytopenia: the role of platelet activation and therapeutic implications. *Semin. Thromb. Hemost.* **25 (Suppl. 1),** 67–76.

7

Laboratory Methods for Heparin-Induced Thrombocytopenia

Margaret Prechel, Walter P. Jeske, and Jeanine M. Walenga

1. Introduction

Heparin-induced thrombocytopenia (HIT) is associated with high morbidity and mortality. Because the pathophysiology of this complex disorder has remained unclear, so has the development of supportive diagnostic laboratory assays. The currently available laboratory methods for HIT include platelet-function assays such as the platelet aggregation assay, the serotonin release assay (SRA) and flow-cytometric assays, and antigen assays (enzyme-linked immunosorbent assays [ELISAs]) that quantitate the titer of anti-heparin-platelet factor 4 antibody. In a clinically defined HIT population, the aggregation and SRA are highly specific, but the aggregation is usually less sensitive than the SRA. The flow-cytometric assay has not been tested clinically, although it shows promising data. The ELISA has a higher sensitivity than the functional assays, but it gives a high frequency of false-positive results (e.g., patients with no clinical signs or symptoms of HIT, yet the ELISA titer is positive). False-negative results, in which patients are clinically HIT-positive yet have negative ELISA titers, are also observed. Positive aggregation and SRA results are generally associated with a higher antibody titer; however, a minimum critical titer is not identifiable. There is no direct correlation between the positive responses of any of these assays, and clinically positive patients can be missed by all assays. With these limitations, the combination of aggregation, SRA, and ELISA testing with multiple samples offers the best chance of identifying a positive HIT patient. Caution is advised for all assays, as none is optimal. The clinical impression remains the most important factor for the diagnosis of HIT.

From: *Methods in Molecular Medicine, vol. 93: Anticoagulants, Antiplatelets, and Thrombolytics*
Edited by: S. A. Mousa © Humana Press Inc., Totowa, NJ

HIT is an immune reaction in which the formation of heparin-dependent antibodies can result in platelet activation *(1–4)*. The antibodies are targeted against the heparin-platelet factor 4 (PF4) complex and are typically IgG, although IgM and IgA antibodies have been identified *(3–9)*. The IgG antibodies bind to PF4 following a heparin-induced conformational change and cause platelet activation via platelet FcγRIIa receptor binding *(2,3,5,7,10–13)*. These antibodies are not heparin-specific, as they react when non-heparin glycosaminoglycans (GAGs) or other highly sulfated materials are used in place of heparin in test systems *(14,15)*.

HIT is a complex clinical syndrome with an overall incidence estimated at 2% of all patients exposed to heparin *(1,16–18)*. It is characterized by one or more of the following clinical features: development of thrombocytopenia to a platelet count of <100,000/µL or a 50% decrease from baseline, in the absence of any other reasonable cause of thrombocytopenia, and normalization of the platelet count following discontinuation of heparin. Nearly one-third of the patients progress to overt thrombosis, often resulting in amputation. The mortality from HIT is approx 30%.

Although the diagnosis of HIT may be considered based on clinical features alone, the decision to discontinue heparin in a patient with recent thrombosis— often in the face of few choices for continuing anticoagulation, may be difficult, especially when other potential causes of thrombocytopenia are present. Because of the potential clinical severity of HIT, it is desirable to support clinical suspicions with laboratory confirmation. Several assays based on the known pathophysiology of HIT have been developed *(3,19,20)*. Functional assays include platelet aggregometry, platelet aggregometry with simultaneous measurement of adenosine triphosphate (ATP) release (lumi-aggregometry), SRA, and flow-cytometric analysis. Following the discovery that antibodies that cause HIT are targeted against the heparin-PF4 complex, ELISAs were developed to quantitate this antibody titer.

2. Methods for HIT
2.1. Platelet Aggregation Assay
2.1.1. Assay Technique

Normal healthy donors are prescreened to identify those whose platelets are reactive in this assay *(19,21,22)*. A two-syringe technique is used to draw whole blood from the donor into sodium citrate (0.109 *M*) in a ratio of 1 part anticoagulant to 9 parts whole blood. The initial 3 mL of whole blood in the first syringe is discarded. The citrated blood is centrifuged at 80*g* for 15 min at room temperature to obtain platelet-rich plasma (PRP).

After removing the PRP, the remaining whole blood is re-centrifuged at 1200*g* for 15 min to prepare platelet-poor plasma (PPP). The platelet count of the PRP should be 250,000–300,000/mL. If it is too high, the PPP is used as diluent. If it is too low, the aggregation test will be less sensitive. Platelets should be maintained at room temperature, and covered to avoid exposure to air and thus pH change. PRP should be used within 4 h of blood collection.

Serum from patients who are clinically suspected of HIT is used as the test sample. Serum is pretreated at 56°C for 45 min to inactivate complement and nonspecific enzymes such as thrombin. The heat-inactivated serum is centrifuged at 600g for 10 min to remove any solid material. Serum can be frozen or kept at 4°C for several days. Freezing may decrease the platelet activation activity of the antibody in the serum.

Aggregation is detected by an increase in light transmission through the platelet suspension measured by a commercial aggregometer (e.g., BioData; Horsham, PA). After blanking the aggregometer with PPP, 140 µL of pre-warmed (37°C) PRP and 220 µL of serum is added to a cuvet containing a stir bar. This mixture is monitored for 3–5 min. If spontaneous aggregation occurs, the serum cannot be tested with heparin. If there is no spontaneous aggregation, 40 µL of heparin (or another test drug such as low molecular weight heparin) is added to the cuvet. Final concentrations of 0.1, 1.0, and 100 U/mL heparin are used. The aggregation response is monitored for 20 min. Sera are considered positive for HIT if the low heparin concentrations produce ≥10% aggregation response, but the 100 U/mL heparin does not cause aggregation. Appropriate positive and negative controls (stored patient sera previously tested) are run in parallel with test samples. For all negative responses, viability of platelets is verified using arachidonic acid activation.

Platelet aggregation with simultaneous measurement of ATP release—lumi-aggregometry—has also been used to assay for HIT *(23)*. This test is performed exactly as the aggregation test described previously, with the addition of the luciferin-luciferase reagent (Sigma, St. Louis, MO) to a final concentration of 4.0 mg/mL to detect released ATP.

2.1.2. Assay Precautions

Specificity of the platelet aggregation assay for HIT is >90%. Sensitivity is 40–60%, but in experienced hands, when optimizing each of the technical points described in **Subheading 2.1.1.**, it can be as high as 80% *(24)*. One of the most important factors is the responsiveness of donor platelets *(19)*. Assay sensitivity has been shown to range from 29–82%, depending on the platelets used. Because of this, it is recommended that donors be screened to demonstrate responsiveness, or that several donor platelets be used to assay one serum. Expert handling of platelets to maintain their function is critical.

The second most important condition is the heparin concentration in the assay *(19)*. Sensitivity and specificity are improved when multiple heparin concentrations are used. Low heparin concentration triggers the antibody-induced platelet activation response. High heparin levels inhibit the response. When combined with a potential heparin contaminant in the serum, the heparin added as a reagent in the assay may inhibit the activation response, as the total heparin level is too high. Heparinase is effective for removing heparin contamination in serum *(25)*.

Conditions must be controlled so that a positive result demonstrates a true heparin-dependent antibody. Because controls are not commercially available, previously identified HIT-negative and HIT-positive patient specimens must be used. One disadvantage is that such samples are typically in limited volume, and offer no batch-to-batch consistency.

False-positive aggregation responses are rare, but have been shown for patients with thrombotic thrombocytopenic purpura (TTP) and cocaine abuse. Platelets can also interact nonspecifically with heparin in the absence of HIT serum because of alloantibodies from other disease states. These are not HIT responses.

Although it has been reported by Stewart that the sensitivity and specificity of the lumi-aggregometry method is comparable to that of the SRA *(23)*, other studies have not confirmed that there is any advantage of the lumi-aggregation assay over the platelet aggregation assay for HIT.

2.2. Serotonin Release Assay

2.2.1. Assay Technique

The SRA is similar to the platelet aggregation assay for HIT, but uses the release of radioactive serotonin as the activation end point *(26)*. In brief, PRP is prepared from citrated whole blood as previously described. PRP is labeled with 0.1 μCi ^{14}C-serotonin/mL for 45 min at 37°C, then washed and resuspended in albumin-free Tyrode's solution to a count of 300,000 platelets/μL. Twenty μL of heat-inactivated test serum is incubated for 1 h with 70 μL of the platelet suspension and 10 μL of saline or heparin solution (final concentrations 0.1 and 100 U/mL). After ethylenediaminetetraacetic acid (EDTA) is added to stop the activation reaction, the mixture is centrifuged to pellet the platelets. ^{14}C-serotonin released into the supernatant is measured in a scintillation counter. Maximal release is measured following platelet lysis with 10% Triton X-100. Sera are designated as positive for heparin antibody if they cause the release of ≥20% serotonin with 0.1 U/mL heparin and <20% serotonin with 100 U/mL heparin. Controls as used in the platelet aggregation assay, are included in each assay.

2.2.2. Assay Precautions

The prerequisite for a high-quality, reproducible SRA test is training and experience of the laboratory technician. The SRA is a technically demanding, labor-intensive, and time-consuming procedure, and requires a license to use radioactivity. Many labs choose to have this test performed by a reference lab. If properly performed, the SRA is considered to have better sensitivity for HIT than the aggregation assay. The specificity and sensitivity of the assay have been reported to be as high as 90% and >80%, respectively *(20,24)*. False-positive results are obtained with samples from patients with idiopathic thrombocytopenic purpura (ITP) and TTP, as well as from thrombin and other contaminants that cause release from the platelet granules.

2.3. Flow Cytometry

2.3.1. Assay Technique

In an effort to develop an assay for the laboratory diagnosis of HIT that is more user-friendly than the platelet-activation assays yet provides clinically relevant results, the flow cytometer has recently been employed. There are several different approaches available for assays to diagnose HIT by flow cytometry, including both whole blood and washed platelet systems. Samples run on the flow cytometer can be analyzed for forward-angle light scatter, side-angle light scatter, and fluorescence. Parameters that can be measured include platelet microparticle formation, platelet aggregation, platelet-leukocyte interaction, and expression of cell-surface markers by fluorescent-tagged antibodies to markers of interest. For example, surface expression of P-selectin is minimal on resting platelets, but is increased on activated platelets.

An example of an assay that utilizes non-anticoagulated whole blood follows *(27,28)*. Although non-anticoagulated blood provides for the most optimal assay system, it is not practical in some settings. Hirudin can be used as a blood collection anticoagulant in this assay if needed. Freshly drawn whole blood (290 μL) is incubated with test serum (160 μL) and heparin (50 μL) at 37°C with stirring for 15 min. The cells are then fixed in 1% *p*-formaldehyde for 30 min at 4°C. The excess *p*-formaldehyde is removed, and an aliquot of cells is resuspended in 400 μL calcium-free Tyrode's solution (pH 7.4). This suspension is incubated with fluorescent-labeled antibodies (e.g., CD61: GPIIIa to identify platelets; and CD62: P-selectin to identify activated platelets) for 30 min at room temperature in the dark, then analyzed. Controls, as used in the platelet aggregation assay, are included in each assay. The test is considered positive for heparin antibody if the P-selectin expression on platelets or the platelet microparticle formation for platelets incubated with serum and low-dose heparin is significantly greater than control.

Other assays use citrated PRP *(29,30)*, and one assay *(29)* is performed as follows: To 70 μL adjusted PRP (300,000/μL), 20 μL test plasma and 10 μL heparin are added. After incubating at room temperature for 1 h, a 5 μL aliquot is removed, mixed with 10 μL CD41, 1 μL anti-annexin V antibody, and 50 μL

N-2-hydroxyethylpiperazine N'2-ethane sulfonic acid (HEPES) buffer. Following a 15-min incubation at room temperature, a 1 : 10 dilution in HEPES buffer is made, and the resulting mixture is analyzed by flow cytometry. CD41 (GPIIb/IIIa) identifies platelets, and the annexin V detects activated platelets.

2.3.2. Assay Precautions

At present, flow-cytometry assays are only being used in the research setting. They are still in development, and have not been verified for clinical relevance.

We have observed that the whole-blood assay provides better dose-dependent and reproducible responses with the lowest background noise than assays that use PRP or washed platelets. Compared to the pure platelet systems, whole blood has the added advantages of being more physiological, uses patient's own platelets, has a decreased turn-around time of the assay, and allows for the study of platelet-leukocyte interactions.

Use of flow cytometry requires technical expertise of the instrument and knowledge of cellular gating thresholds for platelets, as well as typical platelet activation responses. There are several important steps to be performed prior to flow-cytometric analysis of any test material. For example, one must establish the thresholds for each fluorescent marker, size calibrations must be done, gating control samples must be run, and amorphous regions need to be drawn for the cell populations being analyzed. In addition, all antibodies must be titrated against cells expressing their specific antigen prior to experimentation to determine their saturating concentration.

2.4. Antiheparin-PF4 Antibody ELISA

2.4.1. Assay Technique

There are two commercially available, sandwich-type HIT antibody ELISA assays: Asserachrom HPIA (Diagnostica Stago; Asnieres, France) and the GTI-HAT assay (GTI; Brookfield, WI).

For the GTI kit, two 30 min incubations at 37°C are required. Alkaline phosphatase-conjugated goat anti-human immunoglobulin is the detection antibody. All antibody isotypes are detected. After incubation with p-nitrophenyl phosphate (PNP) substrate, the optical density (OD) at 405 nm is determined for each test well. Test samples with OD $\geq$ 0.400 are regarded as positive for HIT antibody. If a test sample is positive, it should be repeat-tested in the presence of 100 U/mL heparin. Inhibition of the OD by 50% or more in the presence of excess heparin confirms a true heparin-PF4 antibody. Inhibition by less than 50% is an equivocal result. The kits provides a positive (OD $\geq$ 1.800) and negative (OD $\leq$ 0.300) control.

For the Stago HPIA kit *(3)*, there are two incubations of 60 min at room temperature. Peroxidase-conjugated goat anti-human immunoglobulin is the detection antibody. All antibody isotypes are detected. After incubation with ortho-phenylenediamine (OPD) substrate, OD is read at 490 nm. Results are interpreted in comparison to a reference standard included in each kit. ODs greater than a defined percentage of the reference standard OD are considered positive for heparin antibody. Positive and negative control plasmas are included in each kit.

2.4.2. Assay Precautions

The primary difference between the two kits is that Stago coats the microtiter wells with heparin-PF4 complex as the antigen, whereas GTI coats the wells with a polyvinyl sulfonate-PF4 complex as the antigen. This and other differences in reaction conditions ("heparin"-PF4 density on the microtiter plate, "heparin"-PF4 ratio, epitope of the detection antibody, sample dilution) and definition of a positive result contribute to the differences in sensitivity and specificity between these two ELISAs.

Relative to the SRA, the sensitivity and specificity of the Asserachrom HPIA assay were 73% and 77%, respectively *(31)*. The sensitivity and specificity of the GTI-HAT assay were 60% and 93%, respectively. Antibodies were detected by HPIA in 18% of the sera negative by both SRA and GTI-HAT.

These ELISAs provide a simpler alternative to the functional platelet assays for the diagnosis of HIT; however, they have limitations that must be understood for data interpretation. The ELISAs demonstrate the presence of the antibody, but are unable to demonstrate an ability of the antibody to cause platelet activation (a functional response associated with HIT). Sufficient data exists that shows a high incidence of antibody in patients exposed to heparin in the absence of any clinical symptoms associated with HIT *(19,21,32,33)*. Thus, antibody titer alone does not necessarily correspond with clinical symptoms of HIT. Other studies demonstrate a population of patients considered to clinically HIT-positive, for whom the ELISA test was negative. Additionally, the available ELISAs cannot be used to test the reactivity of the antibodies to low molecular weight heparins (LMWHs), heparinoids or any drug other than the heparin used by the manufacturer. This latter protocol modification can easily be performed in the functional platelet-based assays.

3. Conclusion

In comparative studies, the platelet-aggregation assay has less sensitivity than the SRA, and the ELISA has the highest sensitivity to identify patients who are positive for HIT *(34)*. Although the aggregation test was generally the least sensitive, it can identify HIT-positive patients in cases in which the SRA and the ELISA are negative. We believe that the pathophysiology of HIT is complex, and that each of the described assays provides different information related to the involved mechanisms. No one assay can stand alone as the optimum diagnostic assay. Moreover, the sensitivity of all assays is lower than desired, as patients with clinical signs and symptoms of HIT are often found negative by all tests.

Recommendations have been made, but not validated, to use the ELISA assay as a screening assay and a functional platelet assay to confirm a HIT diagnosis. However, caution is advised, as false-positive results—and, more importantly, false-negative results—are frequent, making the interpretation of the ELISA difficult. Antibody alone is not the cause of the clinical symptoms of HIT. These results suggest that other factors are involved in the pathogenesis of HIT and associated thrombosis.

Clearly, the clinical definition of HIT is not standardized. HIT is a complex syndrome that is manifested in numerous ways. In addition, the assays for HIT have never been tested in large-scale valid systems that truly determine their sensitivity and specificity in whole patient populations. The numbers reported reflect studies only from patients suspected of HIT. Thus, the true sensitivity and specificity of the assays for HIT is difficult to determine. The assays for HIT diagnosis should be used only in patients who have been previously examined clinically and are strongly suspected of having HIT.

All patterns of positive and negative results by the aggregation assay, SRA, and the ELISA were observed for HIT patients with and without thrombosis *(34)*. There was no direct correlation of ELISA titer to aggregation assay or SRA or clinical outcome; clinically ill patients had a wide range of titers. There was no relationship between any of the three assays. A significant number of patients were not identified as HIT-positive by any of the three assays.

Nevertheless, studies have shown that a positive assay response was more often obtained for HIT patients with thrombosis than for HIT patients without thrombosis *(34)*. Also, the ELISA antibody titer was higher for HIT patients with thrombosis. These were general findings that did not hold true on an individual patient basis, as even low titers could be found in thrombotic patients *(34)*. No assay was able to predict the thrombotic risk in patients with HIT.

All assays available for the laboratory diagnosis of HIT are of limited value. Today, the best that can be offered is to perform the combination of the aggregation, SRA, and ELISA tests on samples collected over multiple days for the best chance to identify a patient with HIT. Newer approaches to improve the laboratory diagnosis of HIT, including the use of flow cytometry, may offer a solution to the difficulties associated with the current tests. Further elucidation of the pathophysiology of HIT will also help to develop improved laboratory assays for HIT. Until that time, results obtained with the current assays should be interpreted with caution, and clinical impressions are best used to direct the treatment of patients with HIT.

References

1. Chong, B. H. (1995) Heparin-induced thrombocytopenia. *Br. J. Haematol.* **89,** 431–439.
2. Kelton, J. G., Sheridan, D., Santos, A., Smith, J., Steeves, K., Smith, C., et al. (1988) Heparin-induced thrombocytopenia: laboratory studies. *Blood* **72,** 925–930.
3. Amiral, J., Bridey, F., Dreyfus, M., Vissac, A. M., Fressinaud, E., Wolf, M., et al. (1992) Platelet factor 4 complexed to heparin is the target for antibodies generated in heparin-induced thrombocytopenia. *Thromb. Haemostasis* **68,** 95–96.
4. Greinacher, A., Pötzsch, B., Amiral, J., Dummel, V., Eichner, A., and Mueller-Eckhardt, C. (1994) Heparin-associated thrombocytopenia: Isolation of the antibody and characterization of a multimolecular PF4-heparin complex as the major antigen. *Thromb. Haemostasis* **71,** 247–251.
5. Amiral, J., Marfaing-Koka, M. P. D., and Meyer, D. (1998) The biological basis of immune heparin-induced thrombocytopenia. *Platelets* **9,** 77–91.
6. Suh, J. S., Malik, M. I., Aster, R. H., and Visentin, G. P. (1997) Characterization of the humoral response in heparin-induced thrombocytopenia. *Am. J. Hematol.* **54,** 196–201.
7. Visentin, G. P., Ford, S. E., Scott, J. P., and Aster, R. H. (1994) Antibodies from patients with heparin-induced thrombocytopenia/thrombosis are specific for platelet factor 4 complexed with the heparin or bound to endothelial cells. *J. Clin. Invest.* **93,** 81–88.
8. Amiral, J., Bridey, F., Wolf, M., Boyer-Neumann, C., Fressinaud, E., Vissac, A. M., et al. (1995) Antibodies to macromolecular platelet factor 4-heparin complexes in heparin-induced thrombocytopenia: a study of 44 cases. *Thromb. Haemostasis* **73,** 21–28.
9. Kelton, J. G., Smith, J. W., Warkentin, T. E., Hayward, C. P., Denomme, G. A., and Horsewood, P. (1994) Immunoglobulin G from patients with heparin-induced thrombocytopenia binds to a complex of heparin and platelet factor 4. *Blood* **83,** 3232–3239.
10. Mikhailov, D., Young, J. C., Linhardt, R. J., and Mayo, K. H. (1999) Heparin dodecasaccharide binding to platelet factor-4 and growth related protein-α. Induction of a partially folded state and implications for heparin-induced thrombocytopenia. *J. Biol. Chem.* **274,** 25,317–25,329.
11. Newman, P. M. and Chong, B. H. (1999) Further characterization of antibody and antigen in heparin-induced thrombocytopenia. *Br. J. Haematol.* **70,** 91–98.
12. Chong, B. H., Ismail, F., Chesterman, C. N., and Berndt, M. D. (1989) Heparin-induced thrombocytopenia: mechanism of interaction of the heparin-dependent antibody with platelets. *Br. J. Haematol.* **73,** 235–240.

13. Newman, P. M. and Chong, B. (2000) Heparin-induced thrombocytopenia: new evidence for the dynamic binding of purified anti-PF4-heparin antibodies to platelets and the resultant platelet activation. *Blood* **96**, 182–187.
14. Greinacher, A., Michels, I., and Mueller-Eckhardt, C. (1992) Heparin-associated thrombocytopenia: the antibody is not heparin specific. *Thromb. Haemostasis* **67**, 545–549.
15. Walenga, J. M., Koza, M. J., Lewis, B. E., and Pifarré, R. (1996) Relative heparin induced thrombocytopenic potential of low molecular weight heparins and new antithrombotic agents. *Clin. Appl. Thromb./Hemostasis* **2**, 521–527.
16. Wallis, D. E., Workman, D. L., Lewis, B. E., Pifarré, R., and Moran, J. F. (1999) Failure of early heparin cessation as a treatment for heparin-induced thrombocytopenia. *Am. J. Med.* **106**, 629–635.
17. Warkentin, T. E. and Kelton, J. G. (1996) A 14-year study of heparin-induced thrombocytopenia. *Am. J. Med.* **101**, 502–507.
18. Warkentin, T. E., Chong, B. H., and Greinacher, A. (1998) Heparin-induced thrombocytopenia: towards consensus. *Thromb. Haemostasis* **79**, 1–7.
19. Walenga, J. M., Jeske, W. P., Fasanella, A. R., Wood, J. J., and Bakhos, M. (1999) Laboratory tests for the diagnosis of heparin-induced thrombocytopenia. *Semin. Thromb. Hemost.* **25 (Suppl. 1)**, 43–49.
20. Warkentin, T. E. (2000) Laboratory testing for heparin-induced thrombocytopenia. *J. Thromb. Thrombolysis* **10**, S35–S45.
21. Walenga, J. M., Jeske, W. P., Fasanella, A. R., Wood, J. J., Ahmad, S., and Bakhos, M. (1999) Laboratory diagnosis of heparin-induced thrombocytopenia. *Clin. Appl. Thromb./Hemostasis* **5 (Suppl. 1)**, S21–S27.
22. Look, K. A., Sahud, M., Flaherty, S., and Zehender, J. L. (1997) Heparin-induced platelet aggregation vs platelet factor 4 enzyme-linked immunosorbent assay in the diagnosis of heparin-induced thrombocytopenia-thrombosis. *Coag. Transfus. Med.* **108**, 78–81.
23. Stewart, M. W., Etches, W. S., Boshkov, L. K., and Gordon, P. A. (1995) Heparin-induced thrombocytopenia: an improved method of detection based on lumi-aggregometry. *Br. J. Haematol.* **91**, 173–177.
24. Chong, B. H., Burgess, J., and Ismail, F. (1993) The clinical usefulness of the platelet aggregation test for the diagnosis of heparin-induced thrombocytopenia. *Thromb. Haemostasis* **69**, 344–350.
25. Pötzsch, B., Keller, M., Madlener, K., and Muller-Berghaus, G. (1996) The use of heparinase improves the specificity of cross-reactivity testing in heparin-induced thrombocytopenia. *Thromb. Haemostasis* **76(6)**, 1121.
26. Sheridan, D., Carter, C., and Kelton, J. G. (1986) A diagnostic test for heparin-induced thrombocytopenia. *Blood* **67**, 27–30.
27. Jeske, W., Szatkowski, E., Hoppensteadt, D., and Walenga, J. M. (1996) Development of a flow cytometric assay for the laboratory diagnosis of heparin induced thrombocytopenia. *Blood* **88(10)**, 317a.

28. Jeske, W. P., Walenga, J. M., Szatkowski, E., Ero, M., Herbert, J. M., Haas, S., et al. (1997) Effect of glycoprotein IIb/IIIa antagonists on the HIT serum induced activation of platelets. *Thromb. Res.* **88,** 271–281.
29. Tomer, A., Masalunga, C., and Abshire, T. C. (1999) Determination of heparin-induced thrombocytopenia: a rapid flow cytometric assay for direct demonstration of antibody medicated platelet activation. *Am. J. Hematol.* **61,** 53–61.
30. Lee, D. H., Warkentin, T. E., Denomme, G. A., Hayward, C. P. M., and Kelton, J. G. (1996) A diagnostic test for heparin-induced thrombocytopenia: detection of platelet microparticles using flow cytometry. *Br. J. Haematol.* **95,** 724–731.
31. Izban, K. F., Lietz, H., Hoppensteadt, D. A., Jeske, W. P., Fareed, J., Bakhos, M., et al. (1999) Comparison of two PF4/heparin ELISA assays for the laboratory diagnosis of heparin-induced thrombocytopenia. *Semin. Thromb. Hemost.* **2 (Suppl. 1),** 51–56.
32. Lindhoff-Last, E., Eichler, P., Stein, M., Plagemann, J., Gerdsen, F., Wagner, R., et al. (2000) A prospective study on the incidence and clinical relevance of heparin-induced antibodies in patients after vascular surgery. *Thromb. Res.* **97,** 387–393.
33. Bauer, T. L., Arepally, G., Konkle, B. A., Mestichelli, B., Shapiro, S. S., Cines, D. B., et al. (1997) Prevalence of heparin-associated antibodies without thrombosis in patients undergoing cardiopulmonary bypass surgery. *Circulation* **95,** 1242–1246.
34. Walenga, J. M., Jeske, W. P., Wood, J. J., Ahmad, S., Lewis, B. E., and Bakhos, M. (1999) Laboratory tests for heparin-induced thrombocytopenia: a multicenter study. *Semin. Hematol.* **36 (Suppl. 1),** 22–28.

8

Factor Xa Inhibitors

Jeanine M. Walenga, Walter P. Jeske, Debra Hoppensteadt, and Jawed Fareed

1. Introduction

Serine proteases play an important role in the process of thrombogenesis. In the coagulation network, various serine proteases are activated that facilitate the formation of factor Xa *(1)*. The serine protease factor Xa has a central role in coagulation and platelet activation. Factor Xa is an essential component of the prothrombinase complex, and leads to the formation of thrombin. Thus, the inhibition of factor Xa represents an important strategy in the development of new antithrombotic drugs.

A growing interest in the development of specific inhibitors of serine proteases is evident *(2)*. In addition, to the development of factor Xa inhibitors, there is also interest in the development of factor VIIa, factor VIIa-tissue factor (TF), factor XIIIa, factor XIIa, and factor IXa inhibitors. Although the development of these inhibitors represents a logical approach to control thrombogenesis, each of these enzymes or enzyme/activator complexes represents a specific site with limited activation potential. Eventually, all of these proteases, with the exception of factor XIIIa, augment the generation of factor Xa. The direct inhibition of factor Xa would offer a more collective control of thrombogenesis than individual site inhibition would.

The initial development of factor Xa inhibitors met with less interest than the development of thrombin inhibitors. These early inhibitors had low affinity to factor Xa, low selectivity, and low enzymatic activity *(3,4)*. Because of the increase in catalytic activity within the coagulation cascade, once the prothrombinase complex is formed (300,000-fold more activity over factor Xa alone), a potent factor Xa inhibitor is required with high affinity for the enzyme. The first factor Xa inhibitors did not fulfill this requirement.

From: *Methods in Molecular Medicine, vol. 93: Anticoagulants, Antiplatelets, and Thrombolytics*
Edited by: S. A. Mousa © Humana Press Inc., Totowa, NJ

Factor Xa inhibitors have several potential advantages over thrombin inhibitors. Factor Xa is in the common pathway of both the intrinsic and extrinsic systems, playing a central role in the coagulation pathway. Since it is formed at an earlier stage than thrombin, the catalytic effect of factor Xa is less than that of thrombin until it is highly amplified by the prothrombinase complex. Thus, less inhibitory activity would be required to reduce the procoagulant action of factor Xa. Factor Xa has no known activity other than as a procoagulant, as opposed to thrombin, which has multiple plasmatic and cellular activation functions, not the least of which is activation of protein C.

Factor Xa has slower activation kinetics in comparison to thrombin because of its position in the coagulation cascade. In addition, factor Xa inhibitors do not completely suppress the production of thrombin. Small amounts of thrombin generated, despite factor Xa inhibition, can initiate primary hemostasis by forming platelet hemostatic plugs. However, this small amount of thrombin is insufficient to catalyze the conversion of large amounts of fibrinogen to fibrin. For these reasons, it is assumed that the narrow safety/efficacy margin of thrombin inhibitors shown in clinical trials that lead to drug overdose with a resultant bleeding would not be as readily observed with Xa inhibitors *(5,6)*. Because of their different mechanisms of action, factor Xa inhibitors are expected to be safer than thrombin inhibitors, yet be effective antithrombotic agents.

2. Classification

Factor Xa inhibitors are structurally diverse, ranging from peptides and proteins to heparin saccharidic sequences *(7,8*; **Table 1)**. They can be naturally derived, recombinant, or synthetic. Molecular size, specificity, and kinetics of factor Xa inhibition differ between inhibitors. They can be direct binding to factor Xa or indirect via a cofactor such as antithrombin (ATIII) and binding can be reversible or irreversible. Protein inhibitors tend to be immunogenic; they can carry viral or animal contaminants and can become limited in supply. The structural diversity among the factor Xa inhibitors influences their mechanisms of action.

3. Mechanisms of Action
3.1. Coagulation

The different factor Xa inhibitors will affect the coagulation cascade at different points, possibly resulting in differing antithrombotic efficacies. Based on the amplification mechanisms within the coagulation cascade and the important role of the prothrombinase complex, highly effective and selective factor Xa inhibitors will inhibit the generation of thrombin. This is probably the most important mechanism of factor Xa inhibitors as antithrombotic agents. By their action, thrombin-mediated feedback reactions, such as the activation of the

Table 1
Factor Xa Inhibitors

Agent	Originator	Chemical nature	Source	Developmental status
Direct inhibitors				
Yagin	Bio-Technology General	Medicinal leech protein (85 a.a.)	Animal derived	Terminated
Antistasin	Merck	Mexican leech protein (119 a.a.)	Recombinant	Terminated
TAP	Bristol-Myers Squibb	Tick protein (60 a.a.)	Recombinant	Preclinical
rNAPc-2	Corvas	Hookworm protein	Recombinant	Phase II
TFPI	Pharmacia/Chiron	Human protein	Recombinant	Phase II/III
DX-9065a	Daiichi	Propanoic acid derivative	Synthetic	Phase II
SEL 2711	Selectide	Pentapeptide produced by combinatorial chemistry	Synthetic	Preclinical
YM-60828	Yamanouchi	Peptidomimetic	Synthetic	Preclinical
ZK-807834	Berlex/Pfizer	Peptidomimetic	Synthetic	Phase II
KFA 1411	Kissei	Peptidomimetic	Synthetic	Preclinical
RPR 120844	Rhone-Poulenc Rorer	Peptidomimetic	Synthetic	Preclinical
Bay-59-7939	Bayer	Peptidomimetic	Synthetic	Phase II
DPC-423	Bristol-Myers Squibb	Peptidomimetic	Synthetic	Phase I
Indirect inhibitors				
Heparin pentasaccharide	Sanofi/Organon	Oligosaccharide; requires binding to AT	Synthetic	Launched

cofactors V and VIII that amplify thrombin formation and the effect of thrombin on platelets and other cellular elements, will also be altered. Evidence for DX9065a, as described here, suggests that Xa inhibitors may also inhibit thrombin generation by blocking tissue factor (TF) induced coagulation.

A possible difference between the heparin-related and the synthetic low molecular weight factor Xa agents is the activation of vascular-bound ATIII by the heparin-like drugs. This may be a disadvantage for the synthetic agents that are unable to produce such a localized effect.

3.2. Free- vs Bound-Factor Xa

An important aspect of the antithrombotic mechanism of factor Xa inhibitors is their capacity to inhibit bound factor Xa. Because of the small size of some of these inhibitors (500–800 Daltons), they are able to inhibit prothrombinase-bound as well as free-factor Xa. Tick anticoagulant peptide (TAP) is particularly effective at inhibiting prothrombinase-bound factor Xa *(9)*. Tissue-factor pathway inhibitor (TFPI) and ATIII-dependent inhibitors are not effective in inhibiting prothrombinase-bound Xa *(10)*.

Small molecular weight drugs such as DX-9065a and TAP can penetrate the clot and inhibit Xa. On the other hand, the protein inhibitors are limited in their degree of activity, possibly because their size limits access to factor Xa bound within clots. Another possible mechanism is that when thrombin is bound to fibrin, the heparin-binding site on thrombin may be inaccessible to heparin. Larger molecules such as TFPI and antistasin do not inhibit clot-bound factor Xa. The activity of clot-bound factor Xa is also resistant to inhibition by ATIII- and ATIII-dependent inhibitors such as the heparin pentasaccharide (because of its size or other mechanisms) *(9,11–13)*.

Remnants of intravascular thrombi, known to induce activation of the coagulation system, may also play a role in rethrombosis, such as after coronary thrombolysis. Pre-existing thrombin, which is bound to fibrin and re-exposed during thrombolysis, has been believed to be the primary mediator of thrombus-associated procoagulant activity, and thus, thrombin inhibitors such as hirudin may be useful agents to prevent the recurrence of thrombosis after thrombolysis *(11)*. However, recent results indicate that other clotting factors such as factor Xa are also bound to whole blood clots, contributing to the procoagulant activity of intravascular thrombi *(12,14)*. Thus, Xa inhibitors may prove effective against rethrombosis.

3.3. Restenosis

Migration and proliferation of vascular smooth-muscle cells (VSMC) as a reaction to injury of the endothelium and the resulting formation of a neointima contribute to the development of restenosis and atherosclerosis. Platelets, thrombin, and other components of the thrombotic process are important factors in stimulation of VSMC and neointimal formation *(15–18)*. There is evidence that both direct and ATIII-mediated anti-Xa effects produce vascular effects. The inhibition of the proliferation of VSMC may be controlled by factor Xa inhibition. Aside from its action in the plasmatic coagulation system, the serine protease thrombin is known to exert several cellular effects via the reaction with its specific receptor *(16,18)*. Through this mechanism, it activates platelets and acts as a strong mitogen for endothelial cells, VSMC, fibroblasts, and macrophages. In limited studies on mitogenesis in cultured rat VSMC it was shown that factor Xa is also a potent mitogen that stimulates DNA synthesis and cell growth in VSMC *(19,20)*.

Factor Xa probably exerts its effect indirectly through the platelet-derived growth factor (PDGF)-receptor tyrosine kinase pathway. Factor Xa stimulates VSMC to release pre-existing PDGF which then, through the receptor tyrosine kinase pathway, leads to the activation of mitogen-activated protein kinases (MAPK), which are well-characterized intracellular mediators of cell proliferation *(19)*. This action of factor Xa on VSMC seems to be related to its serine protease activity, since in the presence of specific factor Xa inhibitors such as antistasin and TAP the mitogenic effect of factor Xa is blocked *(19,20)*. VSMC proliferation, which is mediated by factor Xa might also play an important role in restenosis after angioplasty. Therefore, specific inhibition of factor Xa can be expected to limit intimal hyperplasia after damage of the vascular endothelium.

Under experimental conditions, the specific factor Xa inhibitors antistasin and TAP have been shown to limit restenosis after balloon angioplasty *(21,22)*. A 2-h infusion of antistasin resulted in significantly less restenosis and less luminal narrowing by plaque measured 28 d after balloon angioplasty of atherosclerotic femoral arteries in rabbits compared with controls *(21)*. In a porcine model of severe coronary-artery injury, a short-term administration of TAP for 60 h resulted in a long term decrease in neointimal thickness measured 28 d after injury *(22)*. These results implicate specific factor Xa inhibitors as effective substances to reduce neointimal hyperplasia either by preventing the mitogenic effects of factor Xa and/or by inhibiting the generation of thrombin, which by itself is also a potent mitogen. These agents may be capable of producing anti-ischemic, antithrombotic, profibrinolytic, antiproliferative, anticoagulant, and anti-platelet effects.

4. Direct Inhibitors
4.1. Antistasin

Antistasin, purified several years ago from the Mexican leech *(Haementeria officinalis)*, has an apparent molecular weight of 17,000 Daltons *(23)*. Because of antibody formation, it has fallen out of developmental interest. It inhibits factor Xa by forming a stable enzyme-inhibitor complex *(24)*. Antistasin was more effective at prolonging the prothrombin time (PT) than hirudin, but only slightly less effective than hirudin at prolonging the activated partial thromboplastin time (aPTT) *(7)*.

4.2. Yagin

Yagin (Bio-Technology General), an 85 amino acid peptide isolated from the medicinal leech *(Hirudo medicinalis)*, has 50% homology with antistasin. It is a slow, tight-binding inhibitor of factor Xa, in which the inhibition is a time-dependent reaction effected by the order of addition of components *(25)*.

4.3. TAP

TAP was originally isolated from the tick *Ornithodorus moubata*. It is now produced through recombinant technology (Bristol-Myers Squibb Pharma Co.). This 60 amino acid peptide (6850 Daltons) is a slow, tight-binding inhibitor of factor Xa. Initially, it forms a relatively weak complex with factor Xa followed by a more stable enzyme-inhibitor complex in a second step *(26,27)*. TAP has a higher affinity to the enzyme when it is assembled in the prothrombinase complex with an appropriately lower inhibition constant (Ki value 0.006 nM vs 0.18 nM for free-factor Xa) *(28,29)*.

TAP, a very selective and highly effective factor Xa inhibitor, was shown to affect thrombosis and restenosis via the inhibition of thrombin generation. TAP inhibited the in vivo formation of venous thrombosis *(30–32)*, prevented platelet and fibrin deposition as well as thrombus formation in arterial thrombosis and in arteriovenous shunts *(32–34)* as well as in ex vivo, human non-anticoagulated blood *(35)*. It also accelerated perfusion during thrombolysis and prevented acute reocclusion in canines *(36–38)*.

TAP was much less potent than antistasin in prolonging the aPTT, despite nearly equal antithrombotic efficacies in a rabbit model of venous thrombosis *(29,30)*. This reflects kinetic differences in the rate of factor Xa inactivation between various inhibitors—e.g., TAP shows a time-dependent inhibition requiring an incubation period of 50–60 min to achieve maximal inhibition *(30)*. On the other hand, in the celite activated clotting time (ACT) assay, TAP showed the most potent anticoagulant activity in comparison to heparin and other factor Xa inhibitors. These differences show that the antithrombotic efficacy of a particular anticoagulant cannot always be predicted by clotting assay values.

Aside from the antithrombotic effectiveness of TAP, favorable actions against restenosis were demonstrated. TAP reduced angiographic restenosis and caused less luminal cross-sectional narrowing by plaque after short-term administration to rabbits *(21)*, produced a long-term decrease in neointimal thickness in damaged pig coronary arteries *(15)*, and inhibited mitogenesis in cultured rat aortic smooth-muscle cells *(20)*.

4.4. rNAPc-2

rNAPc-2 (Corvas), a recombinant anticoagulant protein, was originally isolated from hookworm nematodes. It has a molecular weight of 8700 Daltons and inhibits factor Xa and the factor VII/TF complex following prior binding to factor Xa *(39)*, and is undergoing Phase II investigations in acute coronary syndrome.

4.5. TFPI

TFPI is a human protein (43 kDa) identified more than 40 yr ago *(40,41)*. It is the endogenous inhibitor of the extrinsic coagulation pathway which, in addition to the inhibition of the factor VIIa/tissue factor (TF) complex in a final step, also binds to and inhibits factor Xa *(12,13)*. Because of its mechanism of action, TFPI is an important regulator of coagulation. The only physiologically significant inhibitor of factor VII is TFPI.

TFPI has been shown to inhibit venous and arterial thrombosis, including arterial reocclusion after thrombolysis, microvascular thrombosis, and disseminated intravascular and septic shock associated thrombosis *(42–44)*. Profound inhibition of cell proliferation and angiogenesis has also been demonstrated by several investigators *(44)*. Heparin and low molecular weight heparins release endogenous TFPI upon administration. None of the factor Xa inhibitors tested to date have been associated with the release of TFPI *(10,45)*.

A recombinant form has been studied in Phase II/III clinical trials with Pharmacia/Chiron. However, there have been reports of excessive bleeding in septic patients treated with TFPI. Because of its antithrombotic activity in various models of thrombosis, it has been suggested that TFPI would be an effective drug in unstable angina, MI, ischemic stroke, atherosclerosis, venous thrombosis, microvascular anastomosis, disseminated intravascular thrombosis, and septic shock *(44)*.

4.6. DX-9065a

DX-9065a is a synthetic, non-peptide, propanoic acid derivative, 571 Daltons, factor Xa inhibitor (Daiichi). It directly inhibits factor Xa in a competitive manner with an inhibition constant in the nanomolar range *(46,47)*. DX-9065a is highly selective for factor Xa *(47–50)*.

DX-9065a showed antithrombotic activity in models of venous and arterial thrombosis *(32,42,46,51,52)*, arteriovenous shunt thrombosis *(32,46,53,54)*, acute disseminated intravascular coagulation *(46,54–56)*, and disseminated intravascular coagulation in solid tumor-bearing rats *(57)* as well as hemodialysis in cynomologus monkeys *(58)*. After an intravenous (iv) dose of 1 mg/kg significant anticoagulant and anti-factor Xa activities could be measured in plasma up to 120 min in both rabbits and primates. Antithrombotic actions were also demonstrated after oral administration *(48,53–55)*.

DX-9065a caused a significant, dose-dependent prolongation of the aPTT, the prothrombin (PT) time test, and the ACT *(46,48,51,53–55,59)*. The PT was the most sensitive assay. Thrombin generation was inhibited by DX-9065a; however, the intrinsic pathway was more affected than the extrinsic pathway *(46,59)*. The anticoagulant action of DX-9065a is species-dependent showing much less activity in rat, dog, and mouse plasma than in human and common squirrel monkey plasma *(51,60)*.

Pharmacokinetic studies on DX-9065a revealed a biological half-life of approx 6 min for the alpha-phase and 99 min for the beta-phase when given intravenously *(53)*. Oral administration produced peak plasma concentrations at 30 min, and anticoagulant levels gradually declined over 6–8 h *(48,53)*. The bioavailability after oral administration was estimated to be approx 5–12% *(53)*.

DX-9065a does not affect platelet aggregation stimulated by epinephrine, collagen, and ADP *(48)*. However, tissue factor activation of platelets as measured by P-selectin expression can be inhibited by DX-9065a at a low concentration of 0.1 µg/mL *(59)*. This data suggests that factor Xa inhibitors may be able to block tissue factor-mediated generation of additional factor Xa, which subsequently results in the generation of thrombin. Thus, factor Xa inhibitors may produce their therapeutic effect not only by the inactivation of coagulation, but also by the inhibition of platelet activation induced by TF. Other studies by our group have demonstrated that DX-9065a does not produce a positive platelet aggregation effect in an in vitro heparin-induced thrombocytopenia (HIT) system (unpublished data).

DX-9065a has no significant effect in a rabbit ear bleeding model at doses higher than those shown to be effective for antithrombotic protection. At dosages up to 5 mg/kg, DX-9065a did not produce any bleeding, in contrast to heparin, which produced a concentration-dependent effect. This data is supported by similar findings in other animals *(46,48,54)*. In a recent study DX-9065a showed less bleeding in comparison to warfarin in a rat model of gastric ulcer *(61)*.

In a recent study of the effect of factor Xa inactivation on restenosis in rats, DX-9065a at single subcutaneous (sc) doses of 2.5 to 10 mg/kg given before vessel injury significantly reduced vascular smooth-muscle cell proliferation in terms of total cell number and incorporation of DNA precursor molecules *(62)*. Similarly, in cell culture, DX-9065a was able to inhibit endothelial-cell activation *(63)*. It is suggested that interactions of factor Xa with specific cell-surface receptors, such as effector-cell protease receptor-1 (EPR-1), protease-activated receptor (PAR-2), and mitogenic effects mediated via the PDGF-receptor tyrosine kinase pathway, are altered in the presence of factor Xa inhibitors *(62,63)*.

DX-9065a is in Phase II clinical trials. After iv administration to healthy males of doses ranging from 0.625 to 30 mg, a good correlation between linear pharmacokinetics and pharmacodynamics was found, with no adverse affects *(64)*. Bleeding time did not increase at the highest plasma concentration of 1640 ng/mL.

4.7. SEL Series

The SEL series of novel factor Xa inhibitors (SEL-1915, SEL-2219, SEL-2489, SEL-2711: Selectide) are pentapeptides based on L-amino acids produced by combinatorial chemistry *(65)*. They are highly selective for factor Xa and have potencies in the pM range. The Ki for SEL 2711, one of the most potent analogs, is 0.003 μM for factor Xa and 40 μM for thrombin *(66)*.

4.8. YM-60828

YM-60828 is a synthetic, orally active agent that is in preclinical studies at Yamanouchi. In animal models, it is effective against carotid arterial thrombosis and as an adjunct to thrombolysis after oral administration *(67)*.

4.9. RPR-120844

A non-peptide, synthetic factor Xa inhibitor, RPR-120844 (Rhone-Poulenc Rorer), is one of a series of novel inhibitors that incorporate 3-(S)-amino-2-pyrrolidinone as a central template *(68)*. This compound has a Ki of 7 nm with selectivity >150-fold over thrombin, activated protein C, plasmin and tissue plasminogen activator (tPA). It prolongs the PT and aPTT in a concentration-dependent manner, and is more sensitive to the aPTT. It is a fast-binding, reversible, and competitive inhibitor of factor Xa. The efficacy of antithrombotic activity has been demonstrated in a rabbit venous thrombosis model and a rat arterial thrombosis model.

4.10. BX-807834

BX-807834 is under development by Berlex *(69)*. This synthetic agent has a molecular weight of 527 Daltons and a Ki of 110 pM for factor Xa (compared to 180 pM for TAP and 40 nM for DX-9065a). Antithrombotic efficacy has been demonstrated in several animal models of thrombosis, including the carotid electrical vascular injury and copper wire or cotton thread in the superior vena

Table 2
Characteristics of DX-9065a and Pentasaccharide

Pentasaccharide	DX-9065a
Synthetic	Synthetic
Oligosaccharide	Propanoic acid derivative
1728 Daltons	571 Daltons
ATIII-pentasaccharide complex binds FXa	Direct binding to FXa
Limited inhibition of clot-bound/ prothrombinase-bound FXa	Inhibits clot-bound/ prothrombinase-bound FXa
Prolongs the Heptest	Does not prolong the Heptest
Does not prolong the aPTT or PT	Prolongs the aPTT and PT
No platelet interactions in normal and HIT[*] systems	No platelet interactions in normal and HIT[*] systems
IV and SC half-life about 18 h	IV half-life about 90 min
100% bioavailable subcutaneously	Orally bioavailable
Limited bleeding side effect	Limited bleeding side effect
Predictable dose response	Predictable dose response

[*]HIT = heparin-induced thrombocytopenia.

cava of rabbits. ED_{50} values for preventing arterial occlusion were 0.2 μM/kg, compared to 1 μM/kg for TAP and 5 μM/kg for DX-9065a. Bleeding was less than that observed for TAP-treated animals. ED_{50} values for preventing venous thrombosis were <0.008 μM/kg for BX-807834. PT and aPTT were unchanged only at the ED_{50} doses in the venous model.

5. Indirect Inhibitors

5.1. Heparin Pentasaccharides

The only available indirect factor Xa inhibitor is the heparin pentasaccharide (**Table 2**). This agent produces its antithrombotic effect via high-affinity binding to ATIII. It is the smallest heparin-based molecule (mol wt 1728 Daltons) that retains antithrombotic activity. It is composed of five saccharide units—two of the regular region of heparin and three of the irregular region *(70)*. Pentasaccharide was developed in 1983 as proof of the hypothesis that a five-member heparin chain was the most minimal saccharide sequence for antithrombotic activity, and that sole factor Xa inhibition was indeed antithrombotic *(71–73)*. It was shown in experimental models that inhibition of factor Xa controls excessive thrombin generation, produces an antithrombotic effect, and has less bleeding risk than heparin *(74–76)*.

SR-90107 is a synthetic heparin pentasaccharide produced in a cooperative effort by Sanofi and Organon. The chemical synthesis process permits the generation of structurally modified analogs. From this work, it was determined that the binding to ATIII was most critical for expression of antithrombotic activity *(77–80)*. The synthetic pentasaccharides have stronger antifactor Xa potencies and longer half-lives than the natural compound *(77,80–82)*. Because of its small size, pentasaccharide possesses antifactor Xa activity with no inhibitory actions against thrombin or other serine proteases. The pentasaccharide-ATIII complex has a potency of about 700 anti-factor Xa IU/mg in human plasma *(79)*. An equivalent amount of ATIII is required for complete expression of the antifactor Xa activity of pentasaccharide *(83)*. Recently, it has been shown that pentasaccharide inhibits the coagulant activity of the factor VIIa-TF complex *(84)*. The antithrombotic activity was found to be related to the inhibition of thrombin generation shown in in vitro and ex vivo settings, but the maximal inhibition was less than that for heparin *(75,85–87)*. The same result was obtained after administration of pentasaccharide to humans *(88)*. Thrombin generation inhibition following extrinsic pathway activation was stronger than the inhibition after intrinsic pathway activation.

The aPTT was minimally affected (about 100 s at a very high dose) by pentasaccharide, and the PT and ACT were not affected at all *(51,70)*. No platelet interactions have been observed for pentasaccharide in agonist-induced systems for aggregation or in heparin-induced thrombocytopenia (HIT) test systems *(89)*.

Pentasaccharide has dose-dependent antithrombotic activity in several animal models of thrombosis, and the degree of antithrombotic activity is dependent on the thrombogenic stimulus for venous thrombosis *(42,74,76,90)*. Pentasaccharide was also effective against arterial thrombosis in a rat arteriovenous shunt model *(76,91,92)*, a modified arteriovenous shunt model in baboons *(93)*, and in a laser-induced rat model *(70,92)*. This agent has also been shown to facilitate fibrinolysis induced by tPA in rabbits *(94)*.

Pharmacokinetic studies reveal a prolonged half-life in both iv (approx 4 h) and sc (approx 18 h) dosing regimens *(76,82,95)*. Subcutaneous bioavailability was near 100% *(96)*. Human pharmacokinetics revealed a similar half-life at about 13.5 h and a linear correlation with dose *(97)*. The majority of pentasaccharide was eliminated through the kidneys. In elderly subjects the half-life was prolonged to 14.5 h, and plasma clearance was decreased *(97)*. Bleeding studies in rats suggested very minor bleeding at dosages 100-fold higher than required for complete protection against induced thrombosis *(70,76)*.

SR-90107 (ORG-31540) has undergone successful clinical trials for the prophylaxis of venous thrombosis in orthopedic surgical patients using a once-daily single sc dose of 2.5 mg (Fondaparinux, Arixtra®). A brief study on the successful use of SR-90107 with percutaneous transluminal coronary angioplasty has recently been reported *(98)*. It is more attractive than low molecular weight heparins because it is a well-defined synthetic drug with a long half-life and 100% sc bioavailability. It does not appear to be related to the heparin-induced thrombocytopenic response, and may therefore be used as a substitute antithrombotic agent in patients with HIT *(99)*. SR-90107 appears to have a minimal bleeding risk.

Several analogs of pentasaccharide have recently been produced. SANORG-34006 is a more potent and longer-acting pentasaccharide than SR-90107. It has a higher affinity to ATIII ($Kd = 1.4 \pm 0.3$ vs 48 ± 11 nM) with an activity of 1240 anti-Xa U/mg *(100)*. Similar to SR-90107, this new analog demonstrated antithrombotic activity in venous and arterial thrombosis models, and enhanced thrombolysis during tPA therapy. It did not enhance bleeding in a rabbit ear bleeding model. The half-life in humans was as long as 120 h, with linear pharmacokinetics. Subcutaneous bioavailability was near 100%. Phase I studies in healthy young males and elderly males and females at doses of 2–10 mg (sc) and 2–14 mg (iv) showed the drug to be well-tolerated, without significant adverse events *(101,102)*.

Molecular modeling studies at Sanofi have led to the synthesis of SR123781A, a hexadecasaccharide constituted by two distinct domains: a pentasaccharide that binds ATIII and a thrombin-binding domain *(103)*. These two domains are separated by a central uncharged oligosaccharide. SR123781A showed high affinity for ATIII ($Kd = 58 \pm 22$ nM), high potency (297 ± 13 anti-Xa U/mg), and thrombin inhibition activity equal to heparin ($IC_{50} = 4.0 \pm 0.5$ ng/mL). Rat, rabbit, and baboon models of thrombosis showed better antithrombotic activity than heparin ($ED_{50} = 18 \pm 0.1$ µg/kg vs 77 ± 3 µg/kg for heparin) *(104)*.

6. Comparative Studies

A comparison of synthetic pentasaccharide SR 90107 and the synthetic peptidomimetic anti-Xa agent, DX 9065a is useful because both agents are at a similar stage of clinical development, yet are different in structure and mechanism *(47,48,76)*.

Both SR-90107 and DX-9065a are synthetic, low molecular weight agents. SR-90107 is a heparinomimetic drug, whereas DX-9065a is a peptidomimetic agent. SR-90107 requires endogenous ATIII for its effects, whereas DX-9065a is a direct anti-Xa agent (**Table 2**).

The initial studies carried out on the comparison of SR-90107 and DX-9065a revealed significant differences in the inhibition of clot-bound factor Xa, so that DX-9065a, but not SR-90107, was able to inhibit clot-bound factor Xa.

Interestingly, SR-90107 did not produce sizable prolongation of the PT and aPTT, although DX-9065a produced a concentration-dependent effect on both parameters. Although DX-9065a did not produce a strong effect on the Heptest, SR-90107 did. TAP and DX-9065a produced relatively stronger anticoagulant effects, whereas heparin at comparable concentrations produced a weaker effect. SR-90107 failed to produce any effect at concentrations up to 10 µg/mL. The different actions on the coagulation cascade may account for some of these variabilities. Although DX-9065a and SR-90107 produced no inhibition of agonist-induced platelet aggregation, both agents inhibited platelet activation by TF. All agents had strong in vivo antithrombotic effects in animal models. These results suggest that although anti-Xa agents have differing anticoagulant mechanisms, they can still be effective antithrombotic agents.

The pharmacokinetics of the factor Xa inhibitors also differs markedly. Previous reports on the long-lasting effects of SR-90107 have suggested that this agent shows an extended half-life because of its interaction with ATIII *(100)*. Many of the synthetic anti-Xa drugs exhibit a relatively short half-life. The biologic half-life of SR-90107 was markedly longer than that of DX-9065a. Both drugs were well-absorbed via the sc route, and both exhibited a predictable dose-response relationship in both iv and sc studies. However, pentasaccharide did not exhibit oral bioavailability, whereas DX-9065a exhibited 10–20% oral bioavailability.

At the present time, only limited data on the bleeding effects of these agents are available. In contrast to the antithrombin agents, these two factor Xa inhibitors produce relatively lesser bleeding effects.

These studies, although preliminary, demonstrate that each factor Xa inhibitor should be studied for its own merits as plasma and cellular interactions can differ as a result of individualized structure, size, physical constraints, and mechanisms of action for each drug.

7. Discussion

As the common point between the extrinsic and intrinsic pathways, factor Xa plays a pivotal role in the coagulation process. Although thrombin is an important enzyme, its generation is dependent on factor Xa. Thus, control of activated factor X would control excessive thrombin generation. With less thrombin, the rate of fibrin formation is slowed, and a regulated control of the activation of the coagulation cascade would be achieved. With factor Xa inhibitors, bleeding risk should be minimal, because some thrombin generation/clot formation is still possible under treatment, since thrombin generation is not completely blocked.

It is now well-recognized that drugs with sole anti-Xa activity are capable of producing antithrombotic effects. The early studies with pentasaccharide validated this hypothesis *(74,75)*. The factor Xa inhibitors presently undergoing preclinical and clinical development are a diverse class of new antithrombotic agents with direct and indirect mechanisms of inhibition. They possess differences in their mechanisms of action, molecular size, access to clot-bound factor Xa, access to prothrombinase-bound factor Xa, specificity, and kinetics of inhibition. Their small molecular weight provides better bioavailability and endovascular access. These agents inhibit thrombin generation, bind to preformed thrombi, bind to injured vessel walls, interact with specific cell-surface receptors, and seem to play a role in cell proliferation.

Factor Xa inhibitors can potentially be used for clinical indications in which heparin or low molecular weight heparins (LMWHs) are used such as for prophylaxis of the thrombotic processes. They may be particularly effective in less severe indications in which there is not a high degree of preformed thrombin. As antithrombotic agents, factor Xa inhibitors are expected to be weaker than thrombin inhibitors because they cannot inhibit generated thrombin. In comparison to LMWHs, factor Xa inhibitors can have a sc bioavailability of almost 100%, which may provide for more acceptable dosing regimens. Their pharmacodynamics differ significantly, and the half-life of some agents can be very long. These agents do not release endogenous TFPI as heparin does; the clinical significance of this must still be determined.

These agents may be useful not only as prophylactic agents against venous thrombosis, but also in cancer, DIC, sepsis, and inflammatory disorders. Factor Xa inhibitors may also be better adjunct drugs than heparin and thrombin inhibitors for the new antiplatelet agents. This would open developmental applications for factor Xa inhibitors in arterial thrombosis such as coronary thrombosis, unstable angina, and thrombotic stroke. As adjunct agents, these drugs may also be ideal for thrombolytic therapy in both cardiovascular and cerebrovascular indications. If used at higher doses as therapeutic agents, their selectivity and predictable pharmacokinetics should make them more controllable than heparin and antithrombin agents.

Studies are needed to determine the relative importance of inhibition of clot-associated factor Xa in the progression of thrombosis. One study has suggested that the inhibition of factor Xa, but not thrombin, results in sustained attenuation of thrombus associated procoagulant activity *(14)*. For effective suppression of the procoagulant activity and the resulting continuation of the thrombotic processes, it may be useful to combine the inhibition of factor Xa with the inhibition of thrombin. Factor Xa inhibitors are able to inhibit thrombin generation, but they do not have the capacity to inhibit pre-existing thrombin. Thrombin inhibitors can inhibit pre-existing thrombin as well as clot-bound thrombin and released thrombin upon clot lysis. The resulting antithrombotic effect of both factor Xa and thrombin inhibitors could provide a therapeutic benefit *(7,8,105)*. However, additive or synergistic effects must be addressed when combining drugs.

Both TAP and DX-9065a produce measurable in vitro anticoagulant effects. In contrast, pentasaccharide does not produce an anticoagulant effect by the typical clot-based assays. Thus, with factor Xa inhibitors there is not necessarily the same correlation between current lab assays and antithrombotic efficacy that occurs with heparin. Clinical monitoring for these drugs may require the development of new assay systems.

In contrast to thrombin inhibitors, factor Xa inhibitors are largely devoid of bleeding effects resulting in a dissociation between the bleeding and antithrombotic responses. None of the factor Xa inhibitors produce significant inhibition against agonist-induced platelet activation. Therefore, it can be projected that the safety/efficacy profile of factor Xa inhibitors should be better than that of heparin and anti-thrombin agents. Furthermore, factor Xa inhibitors are devoid of heparin-induced thrombocytopenia (HIT) and immunogenic responses, making them potentially useful alternative antithrombotic agents in patients in whom heparin is contraindicated. Thrombin inhibitors indiscriminately inhibit thrombin, and thus impair the cellular regulatory functions of this enzyme. Factor Xa inhibitors do not modulate the regulatory actions of thrombin, which should further contribute to the relative safety of these agents.

The limited data available on factor Xa inhibitors is favorable, and warrants additional investigations to demonstrate the efficacy of these agents in thrombotic and cardiovascular indications and to validate their true clinical potential. It should be emphasized that each of the factor Xa inhibitors represents a distinct drug that requires individual indication-specific dosage optimization. The future holds promise for factor Xa inhibitors as effective antithrombotic agents.

8. Developmental Perspective

In light of significant developments with LMWHs and anti-thrombin agents, the developmental approaches taken for the factor Xa inhibitors are somewhat ambiguous, and a clear strategy is not in sight. It has been suggested that the factor Xa inhibitors may be useful in the control of post-surgical thrombosis. However, none of the Xa inhibitors show any interaction with TFPI. Therefore, in post-surgical conditions where TF may be the primary trigger for thrombosis, the efficacy of these agents may be questionable. Similarly, there is a strong thrust in promoting these drugs for the management for acute coronary syndromes (ACS). Since there is no preclinical data on this subject at this time, such a use of factor Xa inhibitors also appears to be premature. However, synthetic Xa inhibitors may be useful as adjunct drugs, especially in cardiovascular indications. Most notably, these agents may show useful interactions with anti-platelet drugs such as GPIIb/IIIa inhibitors and ADP antagonists. Adjunct use of these drugs with thrombolytic agents may also be helpful in optimizing the use of lytic approaches in both cerebrovascular and cardiovascular indications. With the limited oral bioavailability and unpredictable pharmacodynamics after oral administration, iv or sc approaches currently appear to be most feasible for clinical development of factor Xa inhibitors.

References

1. Samama, M. M., Walenga, J. M., Kaiser, B., and Fareed, J. (1997) Specific factor Xa inhibitors, in *Cardiovascular Thrombosis: Thrombocardiology* (Verstraete, M., Fuster, V., and Topol, E., eds.), Lippincott-Raven, Brussels, Belgium, pp. 173–188.
2. Weitz, J. I. and Hirsh, J. (1998) New antithrombotic agents. *Chest* **114,** 715S–727S.
3. Stürzebecher, J., Stürzebecher, U., Vieweg, H., Wagner, G., Hauptmann, J., and Markwardt, F. (1989) Synthetic inhibitors of bovine factor Xa and thrombin. Comparison of their anticoagulant efficiency. *Thromb. Res.* **54,** 245–252.
4. Hauptmann, J., Kaiser, B., Nowak, G., Stürzebecher, J., and Markwardt, F. (1990) Comparison of the anticoagulant and antithrombotic effects of synthetic thrombin and factor Xa inhibitors. *Thromb. Haemostasis* **63,** 220–223.
5. The Global Use of Strategies to Open Occluded Coronary Arteries (GUSTO) IIb Investigators (1996) A comparison of recombinant hirudin with heparin for the treatment of acute coronary syndromes. *N. Engl. J. Med.* **335(11),** 775–782.
6. Antman, E. M., for the TIMI 9B Investigators (1996) Hirudin in acute myocardial infarction. Thrombolysis and thrombin inhibition in myocardial infarction (TIMI) 9B trial. *Circulation* **94,** 911–921.
7. Kaiser, B. and Hauptmann, J. (1994) Factor Xa inhibitors as novel antithrombotic agents: facts and perspectives. *Cardiovas. Drug Rev.* **12(3),** 225–236.
8. Kaiser, B. (1997) Factor Xa versus factor IIa inhibitors. *Clin. Appl. Thrombosis/ Hemostasis* **3(1),** 16–24.
9. Meddahi, S., Bara, L., Uzan, A., and Samama, M. M. (1996) Pharmacologic modulation of human clots associated thrombin and prothrombinase activities by a direct anti Xa drug, r-hirudin and low molecular weight heparin. *Haemostasis* **26 (Suppl. 3),** 578.
10. Hoppensteadt, D. (1996) Doctoral thesis: Tissue factor pathway inhibitor as a modulator of post-surgical thrombogenesis. Experimental and clinical studies. University of London, London, UK, October 1996.
11. Weitz, J. I., Hudoba, M., Massel, D., Maraganore, J., and Hirsh, J. (1990) Clot-bound thrombin is protected from inhibition by heparin-antithrombin III but is susceptible to inactivation by antithrombin III-independent inhibitors. *J. Clin. Investig.* **86,** 385–391.
12. Eisenberg, P. R., Siegel, J. E., Abendschein, D. R., and Miletich, J. P. (1993) Importance of factor Xa in determining the procoagulant activity of whole-blood clots. *J. Clin. Investig.* **91,** 1877–1883.
13. Prager, N. A., Abendschein, D. R., McKenzie, C. R., and Eisenberg, P. R. (1995) Role of thrombin compared with factor Xa in the procoagulant activity of whole blood clots. *Circulation* **92,** 962–967.

14. McKenzie, C. R., Abendschein, D. R., and Eisenberg, P. R. (1996) Sustained inhibition of whole-blood clot procoagulant activity by inhibition of thrombus-associated factor Xa. *Arterioscler. Thromb. Vasc. Biol.* **16,** 1285–1291.
15. Schwartz, R. S., Holmes, D. R., Jr., and Topol, E. J. (1992) The restenosis paradigm revisited: An alternative proposal for cellular mechanisms. *J. Am. Coll. Cardiol.* **20,** 1284–1293.
16. Kanthou, C. and Benzakour, O. (1995) Cellular effects of thrombin and their signaling pathways. *Cell Pharmacol.* **2,** 293–302.
17. Benzakour, O. and Kanthou, C. (1996) Cellular and molecular events in atherogenesis: Basis for pharmacological and gene therapy approaches to restenosis. *Cell Pharmacol.* **3,** 7–22.
18. McNamara, C. A., Sarembock, I. J., Bachhuber, B. G., et al. (1996) Thrombin and vascular smooth muscle cell proliferation: implications for atherosclerosis and restenosis. *Semin. Thromb. Hemost.* **22,** 139–144.
19. Ko, F. N., Yang, Y. C., Huang, S. C., and Ou, J. T. (1996) Coagulation factor Xa stimulates platelet-derived growth factor release and mitogenesis in cultured vascular smooth muscle cells of rat. *J. Clin. Investig.* **98,** 1493–1501.
20. Gasic, G. P., Arenas, C. P., Gasic, T. B., and Gasic, G. J. (1992) Coagulation factors X, Xa, and protein S as potent mitogens of cultured aortic smooth muscle cells. *Proc. Natl. Acad. Sci. USA* **89,** 2317–2320.
21. Ragosta, M., Gimple, L. W., Gertz, D., et al. (1994) Specific factor Xa inhibition reduces restenosis after balloon angioplasty of atherosclerotic femoral arteries in rabbits. *Circulation* **89,** 1262–1271.
22. Schwartz, R. S., Holder, D. J., Holmes, D. R., Jr., Veinot, J. P., Camrud, A. R., Jorgenson, M. A., et al. (1996) Neointimal thickening after severe coronary artery injury is limited by short-term administration of a factor Xa inhibitor. Results in a porcine model. *Circulation* **93,** 1542–1548.
23. Tuszynski, G. P., Gasic, T. B., and Gasic, G. J. (1987) Isolation and characterization of antistasin. *J. Biol. Chem.* **262,** 9718–9723.
24. Dunwiddie, C. T., Thornberry, N. A., Bull, H. G., et al. (1989) Antistasin, a leech-derived inhibitor of factor Xa. Kinetic analysis of enzyme inhibition and identification of the reactive site. *J. Biol. Chem.* **264(28),** 16,694–16,699.
25. Rigbi, M., Jackson, C. M., Atamna, H., et al. (1995) FXa inhibitor from the saliva of the leech *Hirudo medicinalis. Thromb. Haemostasis* **73,** 1306.
26. Jordan, S. P., Mao, S. S., Lewis, S. D., and Shafer, J. A. (1992) Reaction pathway for inhibition of blood coagulation factor Xa by tick anticoagulant peptide. *Biochemistry* **31,** 5374–5380.
27. Jordan, S. P., Waxman, L., Smith, D. E., and Vlasuk, G. P. (1990) Tick anticoagulant peptide: Kinetic analysis of the recombinant inhibitor with blood coagulation factor Xa. *Biochemistry* **29,** 11,095–11,100.
28. Krishnaswamy, S., Vlasuk, G. P., and Bergum, P. W. (1994) Assembly of the prothrombinase complex enhances the inhibition of bovine factor Xa by tick anticoagulant peptide. *Biochemistry* **33,** 7897–7907.

29. Vlasuk, G. P. (1993) Structural and functional characterization of tick anticoagulant peptide (TAP): A potent and selective inhibitor of blood coagulation factor Xa. *Thromb. Haemostasis* **70,** 212–216.

30. Vlasuk, G. P., Ramjit, D., Fujita, T., et al. (1991) Comparison of the in vivo anticoagulant properties of standard heparin and the highly selective factor Xa inhibitors antistasin and tick anticoagulant peptide (TAP) in a rabbit model of venous thrombosis. *Thromb. Haemostasis* **65,** 257–262.

31. Fioravanti, C., Burkholder, D., Francis, B., Siegl, P. K. S., and Gibson, R. E. (1993) Antithrombotic activity of recombinant tick anticoagulant peptide and heparin in a rabbit model of venous thrombosis. *Thromb. Res.* **71,** 317–324.

32. Wong, P. C., Crain, E. J., Jr., Nguan, O., Watson, C. A., and Racanelli, A. (1996) Antithrombotic actions of selective inhibitors of blood coagulation factor Xa in rat models of thrombosis. *Thromb. Res.* **83(2),** 117–126.

33. Lynch, J. J., Sitko, G. R., Lehman, E. D., and Vlasuk, G. P. (1995) Primary prevention of coronary arterial thrombosis with the factor Xa inhibitor rTAP in a canine electrolytic injury model. *Thromb. Haemostasis* **74,** 640–645.

34. Schaffer, L. W., Davidson, J. T., Vlasuk, G. P., and Siegl, P. K. S. (1991) Antithrombotic efficacy of recombinant tick anticoagulant peptide. A potent inhibitor of coagulation factor Xa in a primate model of arterial thrombosis. *Circulation* **84,** 1741–1748.

35. Ørvim, U., Barstad, R. M., Vlasuk, G. P., and Sakariassen, K. S. (1995) Effect of selective factor Xa inhibition on arterial thrombus formation triggered by tissue factor/factor VIIa or collagen in an ex vivo model of shear-dependent human thrombogenesis. *Arterioscler. Thromb. Vasc. Biol.* **15,** 2188–2194.

36. Mellott, M. J., Stranieri, M. T., Sitko, G. R., Stabilito, I. I., Lynch, J. J., and Vlasuk, G. P. (1993) Enhancement of recombinant tissue plasminogen activator-induced reperfusion by recombinant tick anticoagulant peptide, a selective factor Xa inhibitor, in a canine model of femoral arterial thrombolysis. *Fibrinolysis* **7,** 195–202.

37. Sitko, G. R., Ramjit, D. R., Stabilito, I. I., Lehmann, D., Lynch, J. J., and Vlasuk, G. P. (1992) Conjunctive enhancement of enzymatic thrombolysis and prevention of thrombotic reocclusion with the selective factor Xa inhibitor tick anticoagulant peptide. Comparison to hirudin and heparin in a canine model of acute coronary artery thrombosis. *Circulation* **85,** 805–815.

38. Lifkovits, J., Malycky, J. L., Rao, J. S., Hart, C. E., Plow, E. F., Topol, E. J., et al. (1996) Selective inhibition of factor Xa is more efficient than factor VIIa-tissue factor complex blockade at facilitating coronary thrombolysis in the canine model. *J. Am. Coll. Cardiol.* **28,** 1858–1865.

39. Vlasuk, G. P., Bergum, P. W., Brunck, T. K., et al. (1995) Anticoagulant repertoire of hematophagous nematodes. *Thromb. Haemostasis* **73,** 1305.

40. Broze, G. J., Jr. (1995) Tissue factor pathway inhibitor. *Thromb. Haemostasis* **74,** 90–93.

41. Jort, P. F. H. (1957) Intermediate reactions in the coagulation of blood with tissue thromboplastin. *Scan. J. Lab. Investig.* **9 (Suppl. 27),** 81–183.

42. Kaiser, B., Jeske, W., Hoppensteadt, D., Walenga, J. M., and Fareed, J. (1996) Anticoagulant and antithrombotic effects of the synthetic heparin pentasaccharide and the direct factor Xa inhibitor DX-9065a after i.v. administration in rabbits. *Blood* **88 (Suppl. 1),** 67b.

43. Wang, Z., Hebert, D., Kaplan, A. V., Creasy, A., and Galluppi, G. R. (1996) Persistent inhibition to 12 hours of mural platelet thrombosis after a single local infusion of tissue factor pathway inhibitor at the site of angioplasty. *Circulation* **94(8),** I–268.

44. Kaiser, B., Hoppensteadt, D., and Fareed, J. (2000) Tissue factor pathway inhibitor for cardiovascular disorders. *Emerging Drugs* **5(1),** 1–15.

45. Fareed, J., Callas, D., Hoppensteadt, D., and Walenga, J. (1995) Modulation of endothelium by heparin and related polyelectrolytes, in *The Endothelial Cell in Health and Disease* (Vane, J. R., Born, G. V. R., and Welzel, D., eds.), FK Schattauer Verlagsgesellschaft mbH, Stuttgart, Germany, pp. 165–182.

46. Herbert, J. M., Bernat, A., Dol, F., Hérault, J. P., Crepon, B., and Lormeau, J. C. (1996) DX 9065A, a novel, synthetic, selective and orally active inhibitor of factor Xa: in vitro and in vivo studies. *J. Pharmacol. Exp. Ther.* **276,** 1030–1038.

47. Nagahara, T., Katakura, S., Yokoyama, Y., et al. (1995) Design, synthesis and biological activities of orally active coagulation factor Xa inhibitors. *Eur. J. Med. Chem.* **30 (Suppl.),** 140s–143s.

48. Hara, T., Yokoyama, A., Ishihara, H., Yokoyama, Y., Nagahara, T., and Iwamoto, M. (1994) DX-9065a, a new synthetic, potent anticoagulant and selective inhibitor for factor Xa. *Thromb. Haemostasis* **1,** 314–319.

49. Katakura, S., Nagahara, T., Hara, T., and Iwamoto, M. (1993) A novel factor Xa inhibitor: structure-activity relationships and selectivity between factor Xa and thrombin. *Biochem. Biophys. Res. Commun.* **197,** 965–972.

50. Katakura, S., Nagahara, T., Hara, T., Kunitada, S., and Iwamoto, M. (1995) Molecular model of an interaction between factor Xa and DX-9065a, a novel factor Xa inhibitor: contribution of the acetimidoylpyrrolidine moiety of the inhibitor to potency and selectivity for serine proteases. *Eur. J. Med. Chem.* **30,** 387–394.

51. Fareed, D., Wyma, D., Ahmad, S., Iqbal, O., and Kunitada, S. (1997) Anticoagulant and antithrombotic effects of a synthetic factor Xa inhibitor (DX-9065a) [Abstract]. *Thromb. Haemostasis* **Supp. 292.**

52. Emaciate, T., Tsuji, T., Matsuoka, A., Giddings, J. C., and Yamamoto, J. (1997) The antithrombotic effect of synthetic low molecular weight human factor Xa inhibitor, DX-9065a, on He-Ne laser-induced thrombosis in rat mesenteric vessels. *Thromb. Res.* **85,** 45–51.

53. Yokoyama, T., Kelly, A. B., Marzec, U. M., Hanson, S. R., Kunitada, S., and Harker, L. A. (1995) Antithrombotic effects of orally active synthetic antagonists of activated factor X in nonhuman primates. *Circulation* **92,** 485–491.

54. Hara, T., Yokoyama, A., Tanabe, K., Ishihara, H., and Iwamoto, M. (1995) DX-9065a, an orally active, specific inhibitor of factor Xa, inhibits thrombosis without affecting bleeding time in rats. *Thromb. Haemostasis* **74,** 635–639.

55. Yamazaki, M., Asakura, H., Aoshima, K., et al. (1994) Effects of DX-9065a, an orally active, newly synthesized and specific inhibitor of factor Xa, against experimental disseminated intravascular coagulation in rats. *Thromb. Haemostasis* **72,** 393–396.

56. Yamazaki, M., Asakura, H., Saito, M., Aoshima, K., Morishita, E., and Matsuda, T. (1995) Effects of DX-9065a, an orally active, newly synthesized and specific inhibitor of factor Xa against experimental disseminated intravascular coagulation in rats. *Thromb. Haemostasis* **73,** 1312.

57. Tanabe, K., Terada, Y., Shibutani, T., Kunitada, S., and Kondo, T. (1999) A specific inhibitor of factor Xa, DX-9065a, exerts effective protection against experimental tumor induced disseminated intravascular coagulation in rats. *Thromb. Res.* **96,** 135–143.

58. Hara, T., Morishima, Y., and Kunitada, S. (1995) Selective factor Xa inhibitor, DX-9065a; suppressed hypercoagulable state during haemodialysis in cynomologus monkeys. *Thromb. Haemostasis* **73,** 1311.

59. Kaiser, B., Jeske, W., Walenga, J. M., and Fareed, J. (1999) Inactivation of factor Xa by the synthetic inhibitor DX-9065a causes strong anticoagulant and antiplatelet actions in human blood. *Blood Coagulation* **10(8),** 495–501.

60. Hara, T., Yokoyama, A., Morishima, Y., and Kunitada, S. (1995) Species differences in anticoagulant and anti-Xa activity of DX-9065a, a highly selective factor Xa inhibitor. *Thromb. Res.* **80,** 99–104.

61. Tanabe, K., Morishima, Y., Shibutani, T., Terada, Y., Hara, T., Shiohara, Y., et al. (1999) DX-9065a, an orally active factor Xa inhibitor, does not facilitate haemorrhage induced by tail transection or gastric ulcer at the effective doses in rat thrombosis model. *Thromb. Haemostasis* **81,** 828–834.

62. Kaiser, B., Paintz, M., Scholz, O., Kunitada, S., and Fareed, J. (2000) A synthetic inhibitor of factor Xa, DX-9065a, reduces proliferation of vascular smooth muscle cells in vivo in rats. *Thromb. Res.* **98(2),** 175–185.

63. Herbert, J.-M., Bono, F., Hérault, J.-P., Michaux, C., Nestor, A.-L., Guillemot, J.-C., et al. (1999) Activation of endothelial cells by factor Xa reveals a new mode of activation of the PAR-2 receptor [Abstract]. *Thromb. Haemostasis* **(Suppl.),** 693.

64. Murayama, N., Tanaka, M., Kunitada, S., Yamada, H., Inoue, T., Terada, Y., et al. (1999) Tolerability, pharmacokinetics, and pharmacodynamics of DX-9065a, a new synthetic potent anticoagulant and specific factor Xa inhibitor, in healthy male volunteers. *Clin. Pharmacol. Ther.* **66,** 258–264.

65. Ostrem, J. A., Stringer, S., Al-Obeidi, F., et al. (1995) Characterization of an orally available and highly specific synthetic factor Xa inhibitor. *Thromb. Haemostasis* **73,** 1306.

66. Al-Obeidi, F. and Ostrem, J. A. (1999) Factor Xa inhibitors. *Exp. Opin. Ther. Patents* **9(7),** 931–953.

67. Kawasaki, T., Sato, K., Hirayama, F., et al. (1998) Comparative studies of an orally-active factor Xa inhibitor, YM-60828, with various antithrombotic agents in a rat model of arterial thrombosis. *Thromb. Haemostasis* **79(4),** 859–864.

68. Ewing, W. R., Pauls, H. W., and Spada, A. P. (1999) Progress in the design of inhibitors of coagulation factor Xa. *Drugs of Future* **24(7),** 771–787.

69. Baum, P., Light, D., Verhallen, P., Sullivan, M., Eisenberg, P., and Abendschein, D. (1998) Antithrombotic effects of a novel antagonist of factor Xa. *Circulation* **98(17)(Suppl.),** I79.

70. Walenga, J. M., Jeske, W. P., Bara, L., Samama, M. M., and Fareed, J. (1997) State-of-the-art article. Biochemical and pharmacologic rationale for the development of a heparin pentasaccharide. *Thromb. Res.* **86(1),** 1–36.

71. Choay, J., Petitou, M., Lormeau, J. C., Sinay, P., Casu, B., and Gatti, G. (1983) Structure-activity relationship in heparin: A synthetic pentasaccharide with high affinity for antithrombin III and eliciting high anti-factor Xa activity. *Biochem. Biophys. Acta* **116(2),** 492–499.

72. Sinay, P., Jaquinet, J. E., Petitou, M., et al. (1984) Total synthesis of a heparin pentasaccharide fragment having high affinity for antithrombin III. *Carbohydr. Res.* **132,** C5–C9.

73. Petitou, M., Duchaussoy, P., Lederman, I., et al. (1986) Synthesis of heparin fragments. A chemical synthesis of the pentasaccharide 0-(2-deoxy-2-sulfamido-6-O-sulfo-alpha-D-glucopyranosyl)-1→4)-0-(beta-D-glucopyranosyluronic acid)-(1→4)-0-(2-deoxy-2-sulfamido-3, 6-di-0-sulfo-alpha-D-glucopyranosyl)-(1→4)-0-(2-O-sulfo-alpha-L-idopyranosyluronic acid)-(1→4)-2-deoxy-2-sulfamido-6-O-sulfo-D-glucopyranose decasodium salt, a heparin fragment having high affinity for antithrombin III. *Carbohydr. Res.* **147,** 221–236.

74. Walenga, J. M., Petitou, M., Lormeau, J. C., Samama, M., Fareed, J., and Choay, J. (1987) Antithrombotic activity of a synthetic heparin pentasaccharide in a rabbit stasis thrombosis model using different thrombogenic challenges. *Thromb. Res.* **46,** 187–198.

75. Walenga, J. M., Bara, L., Petitou, M., Samama, M., Fareed, J., and Choay, J. (1988) The inhibition of the generation of thrombin and the antithrombotic effect of a pentasaccharide with sole anti-factor Xa activity. *Thromb. Res.* **51,** 23–33.

76. Hobbelen, P. M. J., van Dinther, T. G., Vogel, G. M. T., van Boeckel, C. A. A., Moelker, H. C. T., and Meuleman, D. G. (1990) Pharmacological profile of the chemically synthesized antithrombin III binding fragment of heparin (pentasaccharide) in rats. *Thromb. Haemostasis* **63(2),** 265–270.

77. Petitou, M., and van Boeckel, C. A. A. (1992) Chemical synthesis of heparin fragments and analogues. *Prog. Chem. Org. Nat. Prod.* **60,** 143–210.

78. Van Boeckel, C. A. A., Beetz, T., Vos, J. N., de Jong, A. J. M., van Aelst, S. F., van den Bosch, R. H., et al. (1985) Synthesis of a pentasaccharide corresponding to the antithrombin III binding fragment of heparin. *J. Carbohydr. Chem.* **4,** 293–321.

79. Petitou, M., Lormeau, J. C., and Choay, J. (1993) A new synthetic pentasaccharide with increased anti-factor Xa activity: Possible role for anionic clusters in the interaction of heparin and antithrombin III. *Semin. Thromb. Res.* **19 (Suppl. 2),** 143–146.

80. Visser, A., Buiting, M. T., van Dinther, T. G., van Boeckel, C. A. A., Grootenhuis, P. G., and Meuleman, D. G. (1991) The AT-III binding affinities of a series of synthetic pentasaccharide analogues. *Thromb. Haemostasis* **65(6),** 1296.

81. Meuleman, D. G., Hobbelen, P. M. J., van Dinther, T. G., Vogel, G. M. T., van Boeckel, C. A. A., and Moelker, H. C. T. (1991) Anti-factor Xa activity and antithrombotic activity in rats of structural analogues of the minimal antithrombin III binding sequence: Discovery of compounds with a longer duration of action than of the natural pentasaccharide. *Semin. Thromb. Hemost.* **17 (Suppl. 1),** 112–117.

82. van Amsterdam, R. G. M., Vogel, G. M. T., Visser. A., Kop, W. J., Buiting, M. T., and Meuleman, D. G. (1995) Synthetic analogues of the antithrombin III-binding pentasaccharide sequence of heparin. Prediction of in vivo residence times. *Arterioscler. Thromb. Vasc. Biol.* **15(4),** 495–503.

83. Walenga, J. M., Bara, L., Hoppensteadt, D., Choay, J., Fareed, J., and Samama, M. (1991) AT III as a rate limiting factor for the measurement of pentasaccharide in laboratory assays. *Thromb. Haemostasis* **65(6),** 1314.

84. Lormeau, J. C., Hérault, J. P., and Herbert, J. M. (1996) Antithrombin mediated inhibition of factor VIIa-tissue factor complex by the synthetic pentasaccharide representing the heparin binding site to AT. *Thromb. Haemostasis* **76(1),** 5–8.

85. Dol, F., Gaich, C., Petitou, M., et al. (1993) The antithrombotic activity of synthetic pentasaccharides and fraxiparine is closely correlated with their respective ability to alter thromboplastin-triggered thrombin generation ex vivo. *Thromb. Haemostasis* **69(6),** 655.

86. Béguin, S., Choay, J., and Hemker, H. C. (1989) The action of a synthetic pentasaccharide on thrombin generation in whole plasma. *Thromb. Haemostasis* **61(3),** 397–401.

87. Lormeau, J. C. and Hérault, J. P. (1993) Comparative inhibition of extrinsic and intrinsic thrombin generation by standard heparin, a low molecular weight heparin, and a synthetic AT-III binding pentasaccharide. *Thromb. Haemostasis* **69(2),** 152–156.

88. Lormeau, J. C. and Hérault, J. P. (1995) The effect of the synthetic pentasaccharide SR 90107/ORG 31540 on thrombin generation ex vivo is uniquely due to AT-mediated neutralization of factor Xa. *Thromb. Haemostasis* **74(6),** 1474–1477.

89. Walenga, J. M., Koza, M. J., Lewis, B. E., and Pifarré, R. (1996) Relative heparin-induced thrombocytopenic potential of low molecular weight heparins and new antithrombotic agents. *Clin. Appl. Thrombosis/Hemostasis* **2 (Suppl. 1),** S21–S27.

90. Amar, J., Caranobe, P., Sie, P., and Boneu, B. (1990) Antithrombotic potencies of heparins in relation to their anti-factor Xa and antithrombin activities: An experimental study in two models of thrombosis in the rabbit. *Br. J. Haematol.* **76,** 94–100.

91. Vogel, G. M. T., van Amsterdam, R. G. M., Kop. W. J., and Meuleman, D. G. (1993) Pentasaccharide and Orgaran arrest, whereas heparin delays thrombus formation in a rat arteriovenous shunt. *Thromb. Haemostasis* **69(1),** 29–34.

92. Weichert, W. and Breddin, H. K. (1988) Effect of low molecular weight heparins on laser-induced thrombus formation in rat mesenteric vessels. *Haemostasis* **18 (Suppl. 3),** 55–63.

93. Hérault, J. P., Pflieger, A. M., Savi, P., et al. (1996) Comparative effects of two factor Xa inhibitors on prothrombinase assembled in different environments. *Haemostasis* **26**, S3.

94. Bernat, A., Hoffmann, P., Sainte-Marie, M., and Herbert, J. M. (1996) The synthetic pentasaccharide SR 90107A/Org 31540 enhances tissue-type plasminogen activator-induced thrombolysis in rabbits. *Fibrinolysis* **10(3)**, 151–157.

95. Crépon, B., Donat, F., Bârzu, T., and Hérault, J. P. (1993) Pharmacokinetic (PK) parameters of AT binding pentasaccharides in three animal species: predictive value for humans. *Thromb. Haemostasis* **69(6)**, 654.

96. Walenga, J. M. and Fareed, J. (1985) Preliminary biochemical and pharmacologic studies on a chemically synthesized pentasaccharide. *Semin. Thromb. Hemost.* **11(2)**, 89–99.

97. Boneu, B., Necciari, J., Cariou, R., et al. (1995) Pharmacokinetics and tolerance of the natural pentasaccharide (SR90107/ORG31540) with high affinity to antithrombin III in man. *Thromb. Haemostasis* **74**, 1468–1473.

98. Schiele, F. J., Vuillemenot, A. R., Meneveau, N. F., et al. (1996) Initial experience of a sulphated pentasaccharide, a pure factor Xa inhibitor, in coronary angioplasty. *Circulation* **94(8)**, I–742.

99. Elalamy, I., Lecrubier, C., Potevin, F., et al. (1995) Absence of in vitro cross-reaction of pentasaccharide with the plasma heparin dependent factor of twenty-five patients with heparin associated thrombocytopenia. *Thromb. Haemostasis* **74**, 1384–1385.

100. Herbert, J. M., Heravlet, J. P., Bernat, A., Van Amsterdam, R. G., Lormeau, J. C., Petitou, M., et al. (1998) Biochemical and pharmacologic properties of SanOrg 34006, a potent and long-acting synthetic pentasaccharide. *Blood* **91(11)**, 4197–4205.

101. Faaij, R. A., Burggraaf, J., Schoemaker, R. C., van Amsterdam, R. G. M., and Cohen, A. F. (1999) A phase 1 single rising dose study to investigate the safety, tolerance and pharmacokinetics of SANORG 34006 in healthy young male volunteers [Abstract]. *Thromb. Haemostasis* **(Suppl.)**, 853.

102. Faaij, R. A., Burggraaf, J., Schoemaker, R. C., van Amsterdam, R. G. M., and Cohen, A. F. (1999) A phase 1 single rising dose study to investigate the safety, tolerance and pharmacokinetics of subcutaneous SANORG 34006 in healthy male and female elderly volunteers. *Thromb. Haemostasis* **(Suppl.)**, 490.

103. Hérault, J. P., Bernat, A., Driguez, P. A., Duchaussoy, P., Petitou, M., and Herbert, J. M. (1999) New synthetic heparin mimetics—part 2: Biochemical and pharmacological properties. *Thromb. Haemostasis* **(Suppl)**, 722.

104. Herbert, J. M., Hérault, J. P., Bernat, A., Petitou, M. (1999) SR123781A, a synthetic heparin mimetic. *Thromb. Haemostasis* **(Suppl.)**, 414.

105. Fareed, J., Callas, D. D., Hoppensteadt, D., Jeske, W., and Walenga, J. M. (1995) Recent developments in antithrombotic agents. *Exp. Opin. Invest. Drugs* **4(5)**, 389–412.

9

Tissue Factor/VIIa in Thrombosis and Cancer

Shaker A. Mousa

1. Introduction

Tissue factor (TF) is a transmembrane glycoprotein that functions as a receptor and cofactor for activated factor VII (factor VIIa) to initiate blood coagulation. Although TF has been characterized best for its role in blood coagulation, recent studies have suggested a role for the molecule in physiologic processes that are distinct from hemostasis. Recently, this molecule has been shown to induce cellular signaling and promote angiogenesis and tumor metastasis (*1–6*).

TF is a 47-kDa transmembrane glycoprotein that consists of a 219 amino acid extracellular domain, a 23 amino acid single transmembrane domain, and a 21 amino acid cytoplasmic domain (**Fig. 1**). The protein function as a cofactor for the serine protease factor VIIa, and formation of the TF-VIIa complex initiates the blood coagulation pathway (*7*). Procoagulant activity is localized in the extracellular domain of TF (*8*). The cytoplasmic domain, which is not required for procoagulant function, contains three serine residues that can be phosphorylated (*9,10*). Because the structure of the extracellular domain of TF is similar to several hematopoietic and cytokine receptors, TF has been believed to participate in other physiologic processes (**Fig. 1**) apart from the initiation of blood coagulation (*11–13*).

Factor VII is the zymogen form (inactive precursor), and factor VIIa is the active enzyme form (serine protease). In plasma, about 99% of the factor VII circulates in the zymogen form and about 1% circulates as factor VIIa, the active enzyme. Factor VIIa lacks the Gla domain, and the active site is inhibited with a peptidyl-chloromethylketone inhibitor (Gla-domainless factor VIIai).

TF and factor VIIa are multidomain proteins. TF, the triggering agent of the blood clotting system, is a member of the class 2 cytokine receptor superfamily. The extracellular portion of TF is composed of two fibronectin type III

From: *Methods in Molecular Medicine, vol. 93: Anticoagulants, Antiplatelets, and Thrombolytics*
Edited by: S. A. Mousa © Humana Press Inc., Totowa, NJ

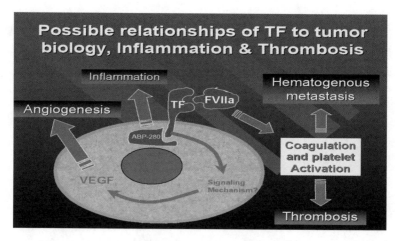

Fig. 1. Illustration of role of TF/VIIa in thrombosis, angiogenesis, and inflammation.

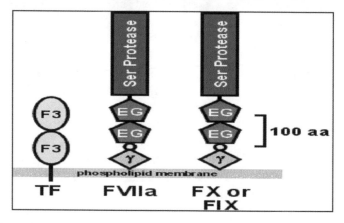

Fig. 2. Illustration of TF, factor VIIa, X, or IX Membrane Assembly.

domains (F3). This is followed by a membrane-spanning domain and a short cytoplasmic tail on the C-terminus. FVIIa is the ligand for TF, and the resulting TF:VIIa complex is the first enzyme in the clotting cascade. FVIIa contains an N-terminal domain that is rich in the modified amino acid, gamma-carboxyglutamic acid (the Gla domain; indicated in **Fig. 2** by the Greek letter gamma). The Gla domain confers the ability to bind, in a reversible and calcium-dependent manner, to membranes containing negatively charged phospholipids. Next is the aromatic or hydrophobic stack, followed by two epidermal growth factor-like domains (EGF domains; indicated by the letters "EG" in **Fig. 2**). Last is the serine protease domain, which is structurally related to

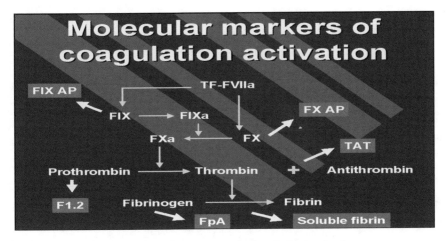

Fig. 3. Molecular markers of coagulation activation.

trypsin and chymotrypsin. The major protein substrates for the TF: VIIa complex, factors IX and X **(Fig. 2)** have the same domain structure as factor VII. Molecular markers of coagulation activation are as shown in **Fig. 3.**

2. Role of TF-VIIa Complex in Cellular Signaling

TF has been shown to have a role in cellular signaling. Treatment of cells that express TF with factor VIIa has been shown to induce an array of cellular events. Camerer et al. showed that factor VIIa induced calcium fluxes in tumor cells and endothelial cells that expressed TF *(14)*. Subsequently, other investigators showed that factor VIIa treatment of cells that express TF induces: i) tyrosine phosphorylation in monocytes *(15)*; ii) *p44/p42* mitogen-activated protein kinase (MAPK) phosphorylation in variety of cell lines *(16)*; iii) activation of Src family members c-Src, Lyn, and Yes followed by stimulation of phosphatidylinositol 3-kinase and activation of c-Akt/protein kinase B, Rac, Cdc 42, p44/p42 MAPK, and *p38* MAPK in fibroblasts *(17)*; iv) expression of poly (A) polymerase in a fibroblast cell line *(18)*; v) induction of vascular endothelial growth factor (VEGF) secretion in fibroblasts *(19)*; vi) increased expression of the urokinase receptor in a pancreatic tumor-cell line *(20)*, vii) activation of phospholipase C and chemotaxis in fibroblasts *(21)*; viii) upregulation of genes such as egr-1, Cyr61 and connective-tissue growth factor *(22,23)*. However, the physiologic consequences of these signaling events, which require catalytically active factor VIIa, are not fully known.

Activation of the blood coagulation system stimulates the growth and dissemination of cancer cells through multiple mechanisms, and anticoagulant drugs inhibit the progression of certain cancers. Laboratory data on the effects of anticoagulants in various tumors suggest that this treatment approach has considerable potential in some cancers, but not others. For example, renal-cell carcinoma (RCC) is one of a small number of human tumor types in which the tumor cell contains an intact coagulation pathway, leading to thrombin generation and conversion of fibrinogen to fibrin immediately adjacent to viable tumor cells *(41)*. Similar observations have been made in melanoma and ovarian and small-cell lung cancers, but not in breast, colorectal, and nonsmall-cell lung cancers *(42)*. This is of considerable relevance to the finding that growth of melanoma and small-cell lung cancer is inhibited by anticoagulants, but that no such effect has been observed in those other tumor types *(43)*. We hypothesize that, based on the relatively unique features of the interaction of the coagulation system with RCC, RCC will respond to anticoagulation therapy similarly to small-cell lung cancer and melanoma. Therefore, we propose that an anticoagulant that inhibit at TF/VIIa level would have an improved efficacy and safety in inhibiting tumor-associated thrombosis, angiogenesis, and metastasis. We would also predict that a combination of that type of anticoagulant, that inhibits TF/VIIa, such as anti-TF, anti-VIIa, anti-TF/VIIa, tissue-factor pathway inhibitor (TFPI), or TFPI-releasing low-molecular-weight heparin (LMWH), with various angiogenesis inhibitors (e.g., Thalidomide, anti-VEGF, anti-$\alpha_v\beta_3$ integrin antagonist, and MMP inhibitors) and chemotherapeutic agents would have greater impact on thrombosis, tumor growth, tumor angiogenesis, tumor metastasis, and eventually, survival and quality of life.

3. Coagulation and Cancer

The association between coagulation system activation (**Fig. 3**) and systemic thrombosis in human cancers has been recognized for more than a century since Trousseau's original description of migratory thrombophlebitis complicating gastrointestinal malignancy *(27)*. In recent years, an improved appreciation of the interdependency of the coagulation system and malignant behavior has led to an understanding of how an activated coagulation system in turn may enhance cancer-cell growth *(28)*. Although this does not establish causality or even a biologic association, it is of interest that a recent Danish study showed that patients with cancer who developed venous thrombosis during the course of their disease had significantly shorter cancer-related survival than similar patients who remained thrombosis-free *(29)*. Conversely, and resting on greater strength of evidence, several studies, including randomized clinical trials, have documented improved cancer-related survival in patients treated with anticoagulants compared to those who did not receive anticoagulants *(26,30–32)*.

4. Tumor Factors That Predict Sensitivity to Anticoagulants

The various tumor types differ in the nature of their interactions with the coagulation system, and in this regard there are two types of tumors: those that activate the coagulation system directly and those that mediate coagulation activation indirectly via a paracrine mechanism. Tumors in the first group include RCC, melanoma, ovarian, and small-cell lung cancers. These tumors overexpress procoagulant molecules such as TF, cancer procoagulant—or, in the case of RCC—hepsin on their cell surfaces. The entire coagulation pathway is assembled on the surface of these tumor cells, leading to fibrin formation in close proximity to the tumors. This at least partly explains the occasional finding in RCC of clot emanating from the tumor and extending into the renal vein and inferior vena cava (IVC). Tumors in the second group, however, tend to activate systemic coagulation by releasing cytokines (e.g., TNF-alpha, IL-1-beta) that in turn stimulate the production procoagulant molecules on the surface of circulating monocytes. Examples of these tumor types include breast, colorectal, and nonsmall-cell lung cancers. Based on this difference in the biology of coagulation activation, tumors in the first group might be predicted to be more likely to respond to anticoagulation that interferes with TF/VIIa than tumors in the second group. In support of this hypothesis, anticoagulants have had significant activity in melanoma and small-cell lung cancer, but not in breast, colorectal, and nonsmall-cell lung cancers in prospective trials *(30–33)*.

5. The Role of the Coagulation System in Angiogenesis

The processes of blood coagulation and the generation of new blood vessels both play crucial roles in wound healing. For example, platelets are the first line of defense during vascular injury, and contain at least a dozen promoters of angiogenesis, which they may be induced to secrete into the surrounding vasculature upon activation by thrombin *(34)*. It follows that these pathways are also intricately linked within human tumors. Targeting both the coagulation and angiogenesis pathways may provide more potent antitumor effect than targeting either pathway alone. Elucidation of the TF signaling pathway using tumor cells as a model system should provide new insights into the cellular biology of TF that might be applied to signaling in endothelial cells, smooth-muscle cells, and fibroblasts. Also, since new classes of anticoagulant molecules have been developed over the past several years *(35–37)*, which selectively target TF and/or TF-VIIa complex, an understanding of this pathway might provide the rational basis for the development of new agents to prevent and/or reduce angiogenesis-related disorders, tumor-associated thrombosis, and the positive feedback loop between thrombosis and cancer *(4)*. TF-factor/VIIa and tumor-associated hypercoagulation. Under normal physiological conditions, TF is expressed only on extravascular sites and perivascularly in the adventitial layer of blood vessels. Although not normally expressed by cells within the circulation, TF can be induced in monocytes and endothelial cells. Also, several malignant cells express high levels of TF. Recent reports have shown that FVIIa binding to TF can influence a number of biological functions, such as angiogenesis and cancer metastasis. As previously described, TF appears to play an important role in cell adhesion and migration. The intracellular signaling is independent of downstream activation of the blood coagulation cascade. FVIIa/TF seems to transduce signaling by two distinct mechanisms: one independent of the cytoplasmic domain but dependent on the proteolytic activity of FVIIa, and one dependent on the cytoplasmic domain of TF.

Idiopathic thrombosis often precedes the diagnosis of occult cancer by several years. Whether hyper-coagulability predisposes for malignancy or the converse holds true is an unresolved paradigm that stems from the known vicious cycle of clot formation and tumor growth. Central to this paradigm is the interplay between TF, the initiator of coagulation, and angiogenesis, and the life support of tumors. Both clotting-dependent and -independent mechanisms of TF-induced angiogenesis have been elucidated that may signal through distinct pathways.

TF expression is a hallmark of cancer progression. The procoagulant functions of TF that lead to thrombin generation are critically important to support metastasis, in part through the generation of fibrin that assures prolonged arrest of tumor cells in target organs. In addition, the coagulation initiation complex— e.g., TF-VIIa-Xa, generates autocrine cell signaling though protease-activated receptors. A cooperation of the TF cytoplasmic domain with protease signaling may explain the diverse contributions of TF to metastasis and angiogenesis.

The anticoagulant heparin and LMWH has many actions that may affect the malignant process, especially metastasis. Thrombin is generated by tumors, and the resultant fibrin formation impedes natural killer cell activity. Heparin prevents the formation of thrombin and neutralizes its activity at various levels (4,95). Angiogenesis plays an important role in metastasis; heparin minimizes angiogenesis via the inhibition of VEGF, TF, and platelet-activating factor. It decreases tumor-cell adhesion to vascular endothelium as it inhibits selectin and chemokine actions, and it also decreases the replication and activity of some oncogenic viruses. Matrix metalloproteinases, serine proteases, and heparinases all play an important role in metastasis. Heparin decreases their activation and limits their effects. It competitively inhibits tumor-cell attachment to heparinsulfate proteoglycans. It blocks the oncogenic action of ornithine decarboxylase and enhances the antineoplastic effect of transforming growth factor-beta. Heparin inhibits activator protein-1, which is the nuclear target of many oncogenic signal-transduction pathways, and it potently inhibits casein kinase

II, which has carcinogenic activity. PDGF, which has oncogenic effects, is also inhibited by heparin, as are reverse transcriptase, telomerase, and topoisomerase pro-oncogenic actions.

6. Angiogenesis Inhibitors and TF-Mediated Hypercoagulation

The angiogenesis inhibitor SU5416 is a potent inhibitor of VEGF receptor-1 and -2. VEGF may be involved in hemostasis by altering the hemostatic properties of endothelial cells. The effects of SU5416 on the coagulation cascade and the vessel wall in patients with advanced cancer were examined by Kuernen et al. *(38)*. Markers for thrombin generation, activation of the protein C pathway, fibrinolysis, and endothelial-cell activation were measured in patients with RCC, soft-tissue sarcoma, or melanoma on d 0, 14, and 28 of treatment with SU5416. Three of 17 sampled patients developed a thromboembolic event in the fifth week of treatment. Significant increase in endogenous thrombin potential and of parameters reflecting endothelial-cell activation in all patients was demonstrated *(38)*. In patients who experience a thromboembolic event, endogenous thrombin potential, soluble TF, and soluble E-selectin increased to a significantly greater extent *(38)*.

Certain angiogenesis inhibitors, such as anti-VEGF and thalidomide were documented to promote thrombosis when given alone, and more so when combined with chemotherapeutic agent. Anti-TF/VIIa is an upstream mechanism for the inhibition of angiogenesis and cancer or cancer-related therapies that increase thromboembolic events. Thus, the strategy of inhibiting TF/VIIa as an upstream mechanism might provide an improved efficacy and safety over other anti-angiogenesis strategies.

7. Tissue Factor Pathway Inhibitor (TFPI)

TFPI contains three Kunitz-type protease-inhibitor domains. The first Kunitz domain reacts with the active site of factor VIIa, and the second Kunitz domain reacts with the active site of factor Xa **(Fig. 4)**. The solution structure of the second Kunitz domain of TFPI has been solved by NMR, as has the X-crystal structure of the second Kunitz domain of TFPI in complex with porcine trypsin (in the latter, the structure of TFPI was solved to a resolution of 2.6 Angstroms).

A key plasma inhibitor of the TF:VIIa complex is TFPI. TFPI is composed of three Kunitz-type domains (K1-K3), which are homologous to bovine pancreatic trypsin inhibitor (BPTI). The first Kunitz domain binds to the active site of FVIIa, and the second Kunitz domain binds to the active site of FXa. The function of the third Kunitz domain is unknown. The C-terminal domain (represented by "C" in the above **Fig. 4**) can bind to cell-surface proteoglycans and also to the low-density lipoprotein receptor-related protein (LRP). TFPI inhibits both FXa and FVIIa (when the latter is bound to TF). Ultimately, this results in the

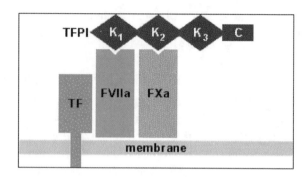

Fig. 4. Sketch of TFPI-binding domains to factor Xa, TF/VIIa.

formation of an inhibited tetra-molecular complex on the cell surface, composed of TF, FVIIa, FXa and TFPI. Additionally, based initial studies conducted in our laboratory heparin fractions with specific molecular weight and a high degree of sulfation were shown to induce optimal endothelial-cell TFP release *(39)*.

8. TF/Factor VIIa and Chemotaxis: Mechanisms Beyond Coagulation

Protease-activated receptor 2 (PAR2) is one of the G-protein-coupled receptors capable of being activated by trypsin and coagulation factor VIIa. Marutsuka et al. *(40)* reported that TF/factor VIIa (TF/FVIIa) complex was a strong chemotactic factor for cultured vascular smooth-muscle cells (SMCs). The migratory response was dependent on a catalytic activity of FVIIa, and did not involve factor Xa and thrombin generation. Trypsin and PAR2-activating peptide (AP; SLIGKV) stimulated SMC migration in a dose-dependent manner, and their abilities were comparable to those of TF/FVIIa complex and PDGF-BB, but PAR1-AP (TFLLR or SFLLR) or PAR4-AP (AYPGOV) did not elicit the migration *(40)*. The anti-sera against PAR2-AP significantly inhibited TF/FVIIa-induced SMC migration, but that of PAR1-AP did not. In immuno-staining, both intimal SMCs of the human coronary arteries and cultured SMCs showed a positive reaction for PAR2-AP *(40)*. These results suggest that PAR2 in SMCs plays a crucial role in the cell migration induced by TF/FVIIa complex. This may or may not be the case with other cells.

9. TF/Factor VIIa and Fibroblast Chemotaxis: Mechanisms Beyond Coagulation

The effects of FVIIa binding to TF on cell migration and signal transduction of human fibroblasts, which express high amounts of TF, were studied by Siegbahn et al. *(41)*. Fibroblasts incubated with FVIIa migrated toward a concentration gradient of PDGF-BB at approx 100× lower concentration than do fibroblasts not ligated with FVIIa. Anti-TF antibodies inhibited the increase in chemotaxis induced by FVIIa/TF. Moreover, a pronounced suppression of chemotaxis induced by PDGF-BB was observed with active site-inhibited FVIIa (FFR-FVIIa). The possibility that TF/VIIa-mediated hyper-chemotaxis to be induced by a putative generation of FXa and thrombin activity was excluded *(41)*.

10. Regulation of VEGF Production by TF

Abe et al. *(42)* demonstrated a significant correlation between TF and VEGF production in 13 human malignant melanoma cell lines. Two of these cell lines, RPMI-7951—a high TF and VEGF producer—and WM-115—a low TF and VEGF producer—were grown subcutaneously in severe combined immunodeficient mice. The high-producer cell line generated solid tumors characterized by intense vascularity, whereas the low producer generated relatively avascular tumors, as determined by immuno-histological staining of tumor vascular endothelial cells with anti-von Willebrand factor antibody *(42)*. Cells transfected with the full-length sequence produced increased levels of both TF and VEGF. Transfectants with the full-length sequence and the extracellular domain mutant produced approximately equal levels of VEGF mRNA. However, cells transfected with the cytoplasmic deletion mutant construct produced increased levels of TF, but little or no VEGF. Thus, the cytoplasmic tail of TF may play a key role in the regulation of VEGF expression in some tumor cells.

11. TF, Integrin, and VEGF

VEGF is a potent angiogenic factor in human gliomas. VEGF-induced proteins in endothelial cells, TF, osteopontin (OPN) and $\alpha_v\beta_3$ integrin have been implicated as important molecules by which VEGF promotes angiogenesis in vivo. Takano et al. *(43)* showed TF as well as VEGF to be a strong regulator of human glioma angiogenesis. First, TF expression in endothelial cells—which was observed in 74% of glioblastomas, 54% of anaplastic astrocytomas, yet no low-grade astrocytomas—correlated with the microvascular density of the tumors *(43)*. Double staining for VEGF and TF demonstrated co-localization of these two proteins in the glioblastoma tissues. Second, there was a correlation between TF and VEGF mRNA expression in the glioma tissues. Third, glioma cell-conditioned medium containing a large amount of VEGF upregulated the TF mRNA expression in human umbilical-vein endothelial cells *(43)*. OPN and alphavbeta3 integrin, were also predominantly observed in the microvasculature of glioblastomas associated with VEGF expression. Microvascular expression of these molecules suggests that an upstream regulation of TF/VIIa might be an effective anti-angiogenesis strategy for human gliomas and other tumors.

12. TF/VIIa and Tumor Metastasis

It has been suggested that TF plays an important role in tumor metastasis. Its expression in sarcoma cells was reported to upregulate the VEGF gene and thereby enhance tumor angiogenesis, which is essential to tumor metastasis. Although many malignant tumors have been reported to express this protein constitutively, recent clinical studies have focused mainly on the correlations among TF expression, tumor progression, and histological grade. Therefore, to address the role of TF and the underlying mechanism of hematogenous metastasis of colorectal carcinoma, the authors analyzed the correlations among TF expression, hepatic metastasis, and VEGF gene expression in surgical specimens. Furthermore, they analyzed the prognostic significance of TF expression with respect to overall patient survival. Univariate and multivariate analyses showed TF expression to be a significant and independent risk factor for hepatic metastasis, whereas a weak but insignificant correlation was observed between TF and VEGF gene expression (44). The outcomes in the TF-positive group were significantly worse in all cases and in the cases without synchronous hepatic metastasis. The study concluded that TF expression is a suitable indicator of both hepatic metastasis and prognosis for colorectal carcinoma patients. Again, these data provide further support for the key role of TF in tumor metastasis that is associated with a worsened clinical outcome.

We have established and utilized several angiogenesis and cancer-related models (45–50) as well as several biomarkers to determine the relationship between the progression of tumor growth, clinical outcome, and various pro-angiogenesis and pro-inflammatory biomarkers (51).

References

1. Bromberg, M. E., Konigsberg, W. H., Madison, J. F., et al. (1995) Tissue factor promotes metastasis by a pathway independent of blood coagulation. *Proc. Natl. Acad. Sci. USA* **92,** 8205–8209.
2. Bromberg, M. E., Sundaram, R., Homer, R. J., et al. (1999) Role of tissue factor in metastasis: function of the cytoplasmic and extracellular domains of the molecule. *Thromb. Haemostasis* **82,** 88–92.
3. Bromberg, M. E., Bailly, M. A., and Konigsberg, W. H. (2001) Role of protease-activated receptor 1 in tumor metastasis promoted by tissue factor. *Thromn. Haemostasis* **86,** 1210–1214.
4. Mousa, S. A. (2002) Anticoagulants in thrombosis and cancer: the missing link. *Semin. Thromb. Hemost.* **28(1),** 45–52.
5. Mousa, S. A. and Mohamed, S. (2001) Anti-angiogenesis efficacy & mechanism of the low molecular weight heparin, tinzaparin and tissue factor pathway inhibitor (TFPI): potential anti-cancer benefits. *Thromb. Haemostasis* P1981.

6. Amirkhosravi, A., Francis, J., and Mousa, S. A. (2001) Anti-metastatic effect of low molecular weight heparin and tissue factor pathway inhibitor. *Thromb. Haemostasis* P1409.

7. Nemerson, Y. (1988) Tissue factor and hemostasis. *Blood* **71**, 1–8.

8. Paborsky, L. R., Caras, I. W., and Fisher, K. L. (1991) Lipid association, but not the transmembrane domain, is required for tissue factor activity. Substitution of the transmembrane domain with a phosphatidylinositol anchor. *J. Biol. Chem.* **266**, 21,911–21,916.

9. Zioncheck, T. F., Roy, S., and Behar, G. A. (1992) The cytoplasmic domain of tissue factor is phosphorylated by a protein kinase C-dependent mechanism. *J. Biol. Chem.* **267**, 3561–3564.

10. Mody, R. S. and Carson, S. D. (1997) Tissue factor cytoplasmic domain peptide is multiply phosphorylated in vitro. *Biochemistry* **36**, 7869–7875.

11. Bazan, J. F. (1990) Structural design and molecular evolution of a cytokine receptor superfamily. *Proc. Natl. Acad. Sci. USA* **87**, 6934–6938.

12. Muller, Y. A., Ultsch, M. N., and deVos, A. M. (1996) The crystal structure of the extracellular domain of human tissue factor refined to 1.7 A resolution. *J. Mol. Biol.* **256**, 144–159.

13. Broze, G. J. (1998) The tissue factor pathway of coagulation, in *Thrombosis and Hemorrhage*, Baltimore, MD, Williams and Wilkins, pp. 77–104.

14. Camerer, E., Rottingen, J. A., Iversen, J. G., et al. (1996) Coagulation factor VII and coagulation factor X induce Ca^{2+} oscillations in Madin-Darby canine kidney cells only when proteolytically active. *J. Biol. Chem.* **271**, 29,034–29,042.

15. Masuda, M., Nakamura, S., Murakami, T., et al. (1996) Association of tissue factor with a gamma-chain homodimer of the IgE receptor-type I in cultured human monocytes. *Eur. J. Immunol.* **26**, 2529–2532.

16. Poulsen, L. K., Jacobsen, N., Sorensen, N. C. H., et al. (1998) Signal transduction via the mitogen-activated protein kinase pathway induced by binding of coagulation factor VIIa to tissue factor. *J. Biol. Chem.* **273**, 6228–6232.

17. Versteeg, H. H., Hoedemaeker, I., Diks, S. H., et al. (2000) FactorVIIa/tissue factor-induced signaling via activation of Src-like kinases, phosphatidylinositol 3-kinase, and Rac. *J. Biol. Chem.* **275**, 28,750–28,756.

18. Pendurthi, U. R., Alok, D., and Rao, L. V. M. (1997) Binding of factor VIIa to tissue factor induces alterations in gene expression in human fibroblast cells: up-regulation of poly(A) polymerase. *Proc. Natl. Acad. Sci. USA* **94**, 12,598–12,603.

19. Ollivier, V., Bentolia, S., Chabbat, J., et al. (1998) Tissue factor-dependent vascular endothelial growth factor production by human fibroblasts in response to activated factor VII. Blood **91**, 2698–2703.

20. Taniguchi, T., Kakkar, A. K., Tuddenham, E. G. D., et al. (1998) Enhanced expression of urokinase receptor induced through the tissue factor-factor VIIa pathway in human pancreatic cancer. *Cancer Res.* **58**, 4461–4467.

21. Siegbahn, A., Johnell, M., Rorsman, C., et al. (2000) Binding of factor VIIa to tissue factor on human fibroblasts leads to activation of phopholipase C and enhanced PDGF-BB-stimulated chemotaxis. *Blood* **96,** 3452–3458.

22. Camerer, E., Rottingen, J.-A., Gjernes, E., Larsen, K., Skartlien, A. H., Iversen, J.-G., et al. (1999) Coagulation factors VIIa and Xa induce cell signaling leading to up-regulation of the egr-1 gene. *J. Biol. Chem.* **274,** 32,225-32,233.

23. Pendurthi, U. R., Allen, K. E., Ezban, M., et al. (2000) Factor VIIa and thrombin induce the expression of Cyr61 and connective tissue growth factor, extra-cellular matrix signaling proteins that could act as possible downstream mediators in factor VIIa-tissue factor-induced signal transduction. *J. Biol. Chem.* **14,** 632–641.

24. Wojtukiewicz, M., Zacharski, L., Memoli, V., et al. (1990) Fibrinogen-fibrin trans-formation in situ in renal cell carcinoma. *Anticancer Res.* **10,** 579–582.

25. Zacharski, L., Wojtukiewicz, M., Costantini, V., et al. (1992) Pathways of coagulation/fibrinolysis activation in malignancy. *Sem. Thromb. Hemost.* **18,** 104–116.

26. Zacharski, L., Henderson, W., Rickles, F., et al. (1984) Effect of warfarin antico-agulation on survival in carcinoma of the lung, colon, head and neck and prostate. *Cancer* **53,** 2046–2052.

27. Trousseau, A. (1865) Phlegmasia alba dolens. Clinique medicale de l'hotel-dieu de Paris. *New Sydenham Society, London* **3,** 94.

28. Zacharski, L. and Meehan, K. (1993) Anticoagulants and cancer therapy. *The Cancer Journal* **6,** 16–20.

29. Sorensen, H., Mellemkjaer, L., Olsen, J., and Baron, J. (2000) Prognosis of cancers associated with venous thromboembolism. *N. Engl. J. Med.* **343,** 1846–1850.

30. Lebeau, B., Chastang, C., Brechot, J.-M., et al. (1994) Subcutaneous heparin treat-ment increases survival in small cell lung cancer. *Cancer* **74,** 38–45.

31. Chahinian, A., Propert, K., Ware, J., et al. (1989) A randomized trial of anticoag-ulation with warfarin and of alternating chemotherapy in extensive small-cell lung cancer by the Cancer and Leukemia Group B. *J. Clin. Oncol.* **7,** 993–1002.

32. Thornes, R. (1983) Coumarins, melanoma and cellular immunity, in *Protective Agents in Cancer* (McBrien, D. and Slator, T., eds.), London, Academic Press, pp. 43–56.

33. Levine, M., Hirsh, J., Gent, M., et al. (1994) Double-blind randomised trial of a very-low-dose warfarin for prevention of thromboembolism in stage IV breast cancer. *Lancet* **343,** 886–889.

34. Pinedo, H., Verheul, H., D'Amato, R., and Folkman, J. (1998) Involvement of platelets in tumour angiogenesis? *Lancet* **352,** 1775–1777.

35. Ruf, W. and Edgington, T. S. (1991) An anti-tissue factor monoclonal antibody which inhibits TF-VIIa complex is a potent anticoagulant in plasma. *Thromb. Haemostasis* **66,** 529–533.

36. Fiore, M. M., Neuenschwander, P. F., and Morrissey, J. H. (1992) An unusual anti-body that blocks tissue factor/factor VIIa function by inhibiting cleavage only of macromolecular substrates. *Blood* **80,** 3127–3134.

37. Wun, T. C., Kretzmer, K. K., Palmier, M. O., et al. (1992) Comparison of recombinant tissue factor pathway inhibitors expressed in human SK hepatoma, mouse C127, baby hamster kidney, and Chinese hamster ovary cells. *Thromb. Haemostasis* **68,** 54–59.

38. Kuenen, B. C., Levi, M., Meijers, J. C., Kakkar, A. K., van Hinsbergh, V. W., Kostense, P. J., et al. (2002) Analysis of coagulation cascade and endothelial cell activation during inhibition of vascular endothelial growth factor/vascular endothelial growth factor receptor pathway in cancer patients. *Arterioscler. Thromb. Vasc. Biol.* **22(9),** 1500–1505.

39. Mousa, S. A., Bozarth,, J., Larnkjaer, A., and Johanson, K. (2000) Vascular effects of heparin molecular weight fractions and LMWH on the release of TFPI from human endothelial cells. *Blood* **16(11),** 59, 3928.

40. Marutsuka, K., Hatakeyama, K., Sato, Y., Yamashita, A., Sumiyoshi, A., and Asada, Y. (2002) Protease-activated receptor 2 (PAR2) mediates vascular smooth muscle cell migration induced by tissue factor/factor VIIa complex. *Thromb. Res.* **107(5),** 271–276.

41. Siegbahn, A., Johnell, M., Rorsman, C., Ezban, M., Heldin, C. H., and Ronnstrand, L. (2000) Binding of factor VIIa to tissue factor on human fibroblasts leads to activation of phospholipase C and enhanced PDGF-BB-stimulated chemotaxis. *Blood* **96(10),** 3452–3458.

42. Abe, K., Shoji, M., Chen, J., Bierhaus, A., Danave, I., Micko, C., et al. (1999) Regulation of vascular endothelial growth factor production and angiogenesis by the cytoplasmic tail of tissue factor. *Proc. Natl. Acad. Sci. USA* **96(15),** 8663–8668.

43. Takano, S., Tsuboi, K., Tomono, Y., Mitsui, Y., and Nose, T. (2000) Tissue factor, osteopontin, alphavbeta3 integrin expression in microvasculature of gliomas associated with vascular endothelial growth factor expression. *Br. J. Cancer* **82(12),** 1967–1973.

44. Seto, S., Onodera, H., Kaido, T., Yoshikawa, A., Ishigami, S., Arii, S., et al. (2000) Tissue factor expression in human colorectal carcinoma: correlation with hepatic metastasis and impact on prognosis. *Cancer* **88(2),** 295–301.

45. Dupont, E., Falardeau, P., Mousa, S. A., Dimitriadou, V., Pepin, M. C., Wang, T., et al. (2002) Antiangiogenic and antimetastatic properties of Neovastat (AE-941), an orally active extract derived from cartilage tissue. *Clin. Exp. Metastasis* **19(2),** 145–153.

46. Kim, S., Mousa, S. A., and Varner, J. (2000) Requirement of integrin $\alpha_5\beta_1$ and its ligand fibronectin in angiogenesis. *Am. J. Pathol.* **156,** 1345–1362.

47. Colman, R. W., Pixley, R. A., Sainz, I. M., Song, J. S., Isordia-Salas, Mohamed, S., et al. (2003) Inhibition of angiogenesis by antibody blocking the action of proangiogenic high-molecular-weight kininogen. *J. Thromb. Haemostasis* **1(1),** 164–173.

48. Van Waes, C., Enamorado, D., Hecht, I., Sulica, L., Chen, Z., Batt, D., et al. (2000) Effects of the novel αv integrin antagonist SM256 and cis-platinum on growth of murine squamous cell carcinoma PAMLY8. *Int. J. Oncol.* **16(6),** 1189–1195.

49. Ali, S., O'Dounell, A., Balu, D., Pohl, M., Seyler, M., Mohamed, S., et al. (2000) Estrogen receptor-α in the inhibition of cancer growth and angiogenesis. *Cancer Res.* **60,** 7094–7098.
50. Luna, J., Tobe, T., Mousa, S. A., Reilly, T., and Campochiaro, P. (1996) Antagonist of Integrin α$_v$β$_3$ Inhibit Retinal Neovascularization in Murine Model. *Lab. Investig.* **75(4),** 563–573.
51. Chen, Z., Malhotra, P., Thomas, G., Ondrey, F., Duffey, D., Smith, C., et al. (1999) Expression of pro-inflammatory and pro-angiogenic cytokines in patients with head and neck cancer. *Clinical Cancer Res.* **(5),** 1369–1379.

10

Tissue Factor Pathway Inhibitor in Thrombosis and Beyond

Shaker A. Mousa, Jawed Fareed, Omer Iqbal, and Brigitte Kaiser

1. Introduction

Tissue factor (TF) plays a crucial role in the pathogenesis of thrombotic, vascular, and inflammatory disorders, and thus, the inhibition of this membrane protein provides a unique therapeutic approach for prophylaxis and/or treatment of various diseases. In recent years, tissue-factor pathway inhibitor (TFPI), the only endogenous inhibitor of the TF/FVIIa complex, has been characterized biochemically and pharmacologically. Studies in patients have demonstrated that both TF and TFPI may be indicators for the course and the outcome of cardiovascular and other diseases. Based on experimental and clinical data, TFPI may become an important drug for several clinical indications. TFPI is expected to inhibit the development of postinjury intimal hyperplasia and thrombotic occlusion in atherosclerotic vessels, and to be effective in acute coronary syndromes (ACS) such as unstable angina (UA) and myocardial infarction (MI). Of special interest is the inhibition of TF-mediated processes in sepsis and disseminated intravascular coagulation, which are associated with the activation of various inflammatory pathways as well as the coagulation system. A phase II trial of the efficacy of TFPI in patients with severe sepsis showed a mortality reduction in TFPI- compared to placebo-treated patients and an improvement of organ dysfunctions. TFPI can be administered exogenously in high doses to suppress TF-mediated effects, or high amounts of TFPI can be released from intravascular stores by other drugs such as heparin and low molecular weight heparins (LMWHs). In this way, high concentrations of the inhibitor are provided at sites of tissue damage and ongoing thrombosis. At present clinical studies with TFPI are rather limited, and the clinical potential of the drug cannot

From: *Methods in Molecular Medicine, vol. 93: Anticoagulants, Antiplatelets, and Thrombolytics*
Edited by: S. A. Mousa © Humana Press Inc., Totowa, NJ

be evaluated properly. However, TFPI and its variants are expected to undergo further development and to find indications in various clinical states.

The cascade or waterfall model of blood coagulation is undergoing some changes with regard to the role of cellular components for the clotting process. In the so-called cell-based model, hemostasis is believed to occur in three overlapping phases—e.g., the initiation that occurs on TF-bearing cells or particles; the amplification in which platelets and cofactors are activated, thus leading to thrombin generation; and the propagation, in which large amounts of thrombin are generated on the platelet surface (1). In both the cascade and the cell-based model of hemostasis, TF—which is a member of the cytokine-receptor super-family—is considered to be the primary physiologic initiator of blood coagulation. The clotting process proceeds when TF is brought into close proximity to activated platelets and coagulation factors. In addition to its essential role in physiologic hemostasis, TF—which is exposed to the blood following vascular injury—also triggers a wide variety of thrombotic diseases and other hypercoagulable states, including disseminated intravascular coagulation induced by sepsis, and arterial thrombosis overlying an atherosclerotic plaque, a process known to be the final event in acute myocardial infarction (AMI) and UA. New studies indicate that TF can function as a signaling receptor and, upon binding of factor VIIa (FVIIa) to TF, a signaling cascade can be initiated. Furthermore, it is suggested that this integral membrane protein exerts important non-hemostatic functions. Assembly of the TF-FVIIa complex on cellular surfaces may be important in mediating intimal hyperplasia as well as for tumor metastasis and angiogenesis. TF has also been shown to play an important role in early embryonic development (for review, see 2–5). Because of the pathophysiological role of TF in various disease states, the inhibition of the TF pathway represents an attractive therapeutic target for the development of new pharmacologic or biologic agents (5).

TF-mediated plasmatic and cellular reactions can be influenced by the TFPI, the only known physiologically significant inhibitor of the TF-initiated coagulation pathway. As described earlier, TFPI consists of 276 amino acid residues with 18 cysteine residues and three potential N-linked glycosylation sites, after removal of a 28-residue signal peptide. It contains an acidic N-terminal region followed by three tandemly repeated Kunitz-type serine protease inhibitory domains and a basic C-terminal region. Post-translational modifications in the TFPI molecule include partial phosphorylation of serine-2 as well as N-linked glycosylation (6–8). These modifications can influence pharmacokinetic/pharmacodynamic properties of TFPI. Recombinant TFPI lacking post-translational modifications may show functional differences to TFPI that is endogenously synthesized or released from endothelium (9). TFPI produces a FXa-dependent feedback inhibition of the TF/FVIIa catalytic complex through the formation

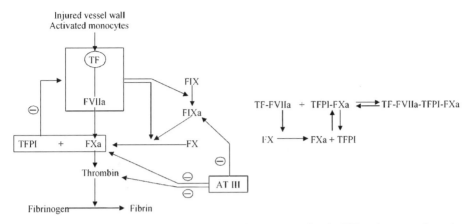

Fig. 1. Scheme of the initiation of the clotting process by the TF pathway and mechanism of action of TFPI.

of a final, quarternary inhibitory complex consisting of TFPI/FXa/TF/FVIIa. In the first step, TFPI binds and directly inhibits activated FX via the second Kunitz-domain. In the second step, the TFPI/FXa complex binds and inhibits FVIIa in the TF/FVIIa complex via the first Kunitz-domain *(10–15)*. See **Figs. 1** and **2** for the interactions between TFPI, Xa, and TF/VIIa. A kinetic analysis of the regulation of the extrinsic pathway by TFPI suggested that FXa is initially inhibited when it is bound to or near TF/FVIIa on the membrane surface. This leads to an unexpectedly rapid inactivation of TF/FVIIa and a resulting inhibition of factor X activation by the TF/FVIIa complex *(16)*.

Intensive studies have been done in the past to characterize TFPI regarding its biochemical actions and pharmacological properties (for review, *see 17,18*). During the past few years, studies with TFPI have focused on the direct or indirect use of the inhibitor for various clinical indications, especially in the cardiovascular field. The goal of this chapter is to review newer experimental and clinical results obtained with TFPI, and further aspects of its use in clinical states.

2. Role of TFPI in Cardiovascular Disorders

2.1. Atherosclerosis/Restenosis

The most important underlying mechanisms for the development of acute coronary syndromes are atherosclerotic plaques. Spontaneous plaque rupture or acute interventions such as balloon angioplasty, coronary atherectomy, or stent placement may increase the procoagulant activity of the vessel wall, and especially expose TF to circulating blood, resulting in the initiation of the clotting process with the formation of intravascular thrombi. As previously men-

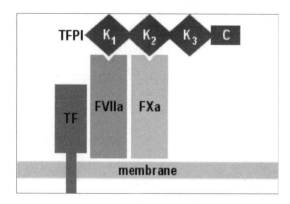

Fig. 2. Schematic illustration of the assembly of TFPI binding to factor Xa, TF/VIIa.

tioned, the effects of TF in vivo are very complex, and this membrane protein may play an important role in inflammatory processes such as those associated with atherosclerosis and restenosis. Because TF is upregulated after vascular injury and in atherosclerotic plaques, TFPI is expected to inhibit the development of postinjury intimal hyperplasia and thrombotic occlusion in atherosclerotic vessels.

2.1.1. Preclinical Studies

2.1.1.1. IN VITRO STUDIES

Various studies on the role of TFPI in hyperplasia of vascular smooth muscle cells (VSMCs) have been done using cell-culture systems. In human pulmonary arteries, the expression of TFPI in smooth-muscle cells (SMCs) is upregulated by treatment with serum or basic fibroblast growth factor (bFGF)/heparin, indicating that growth factors that can stimulate the vessel wall in vivo may locally regulate TFPI expression. The upregulation of TFPI may be pathophysiologically important for the regulation of TF-mediated coagulation within the vessel wall, and thus for the course of hyperplasia associated with pulmonary hypertension and atherosclerosis *(19)*. An increased expression of TFPI after an initial expression of TF was also found in serum-stimulated cultured fibroblasts, VSMCs, and cardiac myocytes *(20)*. The in vitro findings suggest that TFPI regulates the TF-initiated clotting and is also involved in inhibiting VSMC proliferation. Various studies have demonstrated the antiproliferative effectiveness of TFPI both in vitro and in vivo **(Table 1)**. TFPI was found to inhibit the FVIIa/TF-induced migration of cultured VSMCs *(21)*, and the proliferation of cultured human neonatal aortic SMCs *(22)*, as well as the growth of human umbilical-vein endothelial cells *(23)*. Newer studies demonstrated that the antiproliferative activity of TFPI is mediated by the very low-density lipoprotein (VLDL) receptor. In addition, for the inhibition of the proliferation of bFGF-stimulated endothelial cells, the C-terminal region of TFPI seems to be responsible because a truncated form of TFPI that only contains the first two Kunitz-type inhibitor domains is relatively ineffective *(24)*.

2.1.1.2. IN VIVO STUDIES

In animal experiments, the effect of TFPI on the proliferation of VSMCs as well as on atherosclerotic processes was investigated (**Table 1**). TFPI was shown to reduce angiographic restenosis and intima hyperplasia in a rabbit atherosclerotic femoral-artery injury model *(25)* and to inhibit neointima formation and stenosis in pigs after deep arterial injury of the carotid artery *(26)* as well as the procoagulant activity and the upregulation of TF at injured sites *(27)*, and to inhibit mural thrombus formation, neointima formation, and growth after repeated balloon angioplasty of the rabbit thoracic aorta *(28)*. In a model of small autografts in the rabbit femoral artery, topically applied TFPI significantly increased the patency rates of the grafts, and reduced the intimal area as well as the percentage of stenosis and the intima/media areas ratio *(29)*. In the last few years, experimental studies demonstrated the antithrombotic and antiproliferative effectiveness of an overexpression of TFPI achieved by local gene transfer *(30–35)*. Retrovirus-mediated TFPI gene transfer to the arterial wall effectively inhibited intravascular thrombus formation in stenotic and injured rabbit carotid arteries *(30)*. Adenovirus-mediated local expression of TFPI inhibited shear stress-induced recurrent thrombosis in balloon-injured carotid arteries of rabbits *(31)* and pigs *(32)*. The combination of brief irrigation with recombinant TFPI and adenovirus-mediated TFPI gene transfer fully suppressed TF activity and reduced fibroproliferative changes in rabbit carotid arteries, as shown by the reduction of intima/media ratios *(33)*. Recently published results obtained in a model of balloon-injured atherosclerotic arteries in rabbits demonstrated that an overexpression of TFPI markedly inhibited intimal hyperplasia *(34)*. In a murine model of flow cessation, adenoviral delivery of TFPI decreased vascular TF activity and inhibited neointima formation *(35)*. The TFPI overexpression by gene transfer and the resulting effects on thrombosis and restenosis were achieved without impairment of systemic hemostasis or excess bleeding. The local regulation of TF activity may be considered a target for a gene transfer-based antirestenosis therapy. The development of atherosclerosis in mice with a homozygous apolipoprotein E (ApoE) deficiency and an additional heterozygous TFPI deficiency was significantly greater than that seen in ApoE knockout mice with a normal TFPI genotype, indicating that TFPI provides protection from atherosclerosis and is an important regulator of thrombotic events in atherosclerosis *(36)*.

Table 1
In Vitro and In Vivo Studies on the Effect of TFPI on VSMC

	Effect	Reference
In vitro	Synthesis and secretion of TFPI by human pulmonary SMCs and upregulation of TFPI expression by serum or bFGF.	*19*
	Increased expression of TF and TFPI by serum-stimulated fibroblasts, VSMCs, and cardiac myocytes.	*20*
	Inhibition of TF/FVIIa-induced migration of cultured VSMCs.	*21*
	Inhibition of the proliferation of cultured human neonatal aortic SMCs (mediated by the C-terminal region of TFPI).	*22*
	Inhibition of the growth of cultured HUVECs by inducing apoptosis (no inhibition of DNA synthesis).	*23*
	Expression of TFPI protein and mRNA in atherosclerotic arteries, in internal carotid plaques from patients undergoing endarterectomy + in fatty-streak lesions in rabbits fed a high-cholesterol diet.	*37*
	Presence of biologically active TFPI and co-localization with TF in human atherosclerotic plaques of carotid and coronary arteries.	*38–40*
In vivo	Reduction of angiographic restenosis and decrease of neointimal hyperplasia in a rabbit atherosclerotic femoral-artery injury model.	*25*
	Inhibition of neointimal formation and stenosis in minipigs after deep arterial injury of the carotid artery.	*26*
	Inhibition of the procoagulant activity and the upregulation of TF at balloon-induced arterial injury in pigs.	*27*
	Inhibition of mural thrombus formation and neointimal growth after repeated balloon angioplasty of the rabbit thoracic aorta.	*28*
	Reduction of intimal thickness and increase of long-term patency of small arterial autografts in rabbits.	*29*
	Inhibition of intravascular thrombus formation and recurrent thrombosis in carotid arteries of rabbits and pigs by gene transfer-mediated overexpression of TFPI.	*30–32*
	Inhibition of intimal hyperplasia in balloon-injured atherosclerotic arteries in rabbits by gene-transfer of TFPI.	*33,34*
	Inhibition of neointima formation by adenoviral-mediated overexpression of TFPI in a murine model of vascular remodeling.	*35*
	Increase of atherosclerotic changes in arteries of ApoE-knockout mice with a heterozygous TFPI deficiency.	*36*

2.1.2. Studies in Human Vessels

Active TF is present in the atherosclerotic vessel wall, where it is believed to be responsible particularly for acute thrombosis after plaque rupture, the major complication of primary atherosclerosis. In addition to TF, TFPI is also expressed in atherosclerotic plaques *(37–40)*. In atherosclerotic lesions of human coronary arteries, a co-localization of TF and TFPI was found in endothelial cells, macrophages, macrophage-derived foam cells, and SMCs in intimal lesions. In type III and IV of atherosclerotic lesions, the number of TF- and TFPI-positive cells is increased, accompanied by extracellular localization of TF and TFPI in the lipid core of atherosclerotic plaques *(38)*. In human carotid atherosclerotic plaques, biologically active TFPI was found in endothelial cells, VSMCs, and macrophages *(39)*. Similar results were seen in other studies using human coronary arteries, popliteal arteries, and saphenous vein grafts. In the atherosclerotic vessels, TFPI frequently colocalized with TF in endothelial cells overlying the plaque and in microvessels, as well as in the medial and neointimal SMCs, and in macrophages and T cells in areas surrounding the necrotic core *(40)*. TFPI was found to be largely expressed in the normal vessel wall and enhanced in atherosclerotic vessels. TFPI was active against the TF-dependent procoagulant activity, suggesting a significant role for the inhibitor in the regulation of TF activity. It is assumed that upregulation of TFPI in atherosclerotic plaques may control their thrombogenicity or even prevent the complications associated with plaque rupture *(40)*. **Figure 3** illustrates the release of TFPI from endothelium by heparin and its circulation in free and bound forms.

In the TFPI gene, three polymorphisms have been recently identified that are associated with a significant variation in plasma TFPI levels *(41,42)*. However, studies in patients who underwent angioplasty, with or without stent implantation, revealed that—despite significant variations in TFPI levels—there was no evidence that the polymorphism of the TFPI gene influenced the risk of angiographic restenosis after angioplasty *(43)*.

2.2. UA and MI

Several clinical studies have been performed to evaluate the significance of measuring various parameters with regard to their diagnostic and prognostic value for cardiovascular disorders, especially for ischemic heart diseases such as UA and AMI. In patients with ischemic heart diseases, an excess of thrombin formation was demonstrated by increased plasma concentrations of prothrombin fragment F1.2 and thrombin-antithrombin III-complexes. This could be related to the elevated levels of circulating TF also found. In these patients,

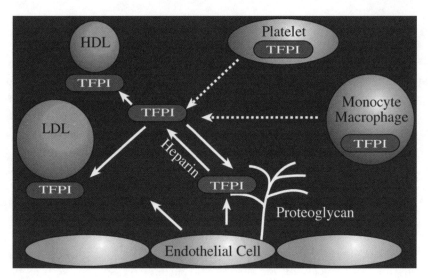

Fig. 3. Endothelial release of TFPI by heparin and its distribution in free and bound forms.

plasma levels of TFPI were also increased, but were not sufficient to interrupt the TF-induced coagulation activation *(44,45)*. Increased plasma concentrations of both total and free TFPI measured in AMI patients may result from their release by ischemic tissues *(46)*. Patients with AMI show an increased procoagulant activity of monocytes which is believed to be caused by an upregulation of TF and can be partially inhibited by surface-bound TFPI, suggesting that a direct inhibition of TF activity by a specific therapy may be particularly effective for the treatment of AMI *(47)*. The prognostic importance of TF and TFPI for recurrent coronary events was investigated in a long-term follow-up study over 4 yr in patients after AMI *(48)*. There were no statistical differences in TF or in total and free TFPI levels between patients and controls, demonstrating that the TF/TFPI system is not a useful prognostic marker. However, in middle-aged men with no history of coronary heart disease (CHD), a significant positive correlation was found between free TFPI plasma levels and atherogenic lipids such as total cholesterol and triglycerides, as well as factor VII and fibrinogen, which can be considered as a compensatory increase in plasma-free TFPI to the occurrence of risk factors for atherothrombotic diseases in apparently healthy men *(49)*. A large population study on the association between plasma levels of free and total TFPI, conventional cardiovascular risk factors, and endothelial-cell markers showed that plasma levels of free TFPI correlated poorly with that of total TFPI, indicating that free and lipid-bound TFPI are regulated differently. Free TFPI strongly correlates to endothelium-derived molecules such as thrombomodulin, von Willebrand's factor, and tissue-type plasminogen activator (t-PA), whereas total TFPI is more related to conventional risk factors such as low-density lipoprotein (LDL) cholesterin *(50)*.

2.3. Sepsis and Disseminated Intravascular Coagulation (DIC)

Severe sepsis is associated with the activation of various inflammatory pathways, and especially with the activation of the coagulation system. Because of endotoxin and the production of proinflammatory cytokines, TF is expressed on activated monocytes and vascular endothelial cells. TF-mediated coagulation activation can lead to microvascular thrombosis and further endothelial activation, which appear to play an important role in the development of multiple organ failure associated with severe sepsis. Based on the role of TF in sepsis and DIC, it is expected that TFPI can provide a new therapeutic rationale for the treatment of sepsis. Experimental findings suggest a significant role of TFPI in DIC and severe sepsis. Rabbits that have been immunodepleted of plasma TFPI activity are sensitized to substantial intravascular coagulation induced by an infusion of TF at doses that were essentially without effect in control animals *(51)*. Similar results were found after an injection of endotoxin, which induced extensive DIC in immunodepleted rabbits, but only minimal or moderate intravascular clotting in animals with normal TFPI levels *(52)*. The effectiveness of TFPI in DIC and septic shock has been investigated in various animal models (for review, *see 17,18,53)*. The results suggest that TFPI may offer benefits when used to treat severe sepsis. In various studies in humans, plasma concentrations of TF and TFPI have been determined to define the pathophysiological role of these molecules in DIC and septic shock. In patients with DIC, plasma concentrations of both TF and TFPI were seen to be significantly higher than in patients without DIC *(54,55)*. The increase of TF in plasma of DIC patients is followed by an increase in TFPI, which is most likely based on its release from vascular endothelium resulting from endothelial-cell injury *(54)*. In patients with DIC, plasma concentrations of truncated TFPI were significantly elevated as compared to pre- and nonDIC patients. Reduced levels of the intact form of TFPI found in preDIC patients may suggest a hypercoagulable state in those patients with a consumption of TFPI *(56,57)*.

In animal models of sepsis, TFPI was able to completely block the coagulant response and to prevent death as well as reduce the cytokine response. In a human model of endotoxemia, recombinant human TFPI effectively and dose-dependently attenuated the endotoxin-induced coagulation activation. However, in contrast to animal experiments, it did not influence leukocyte activation, chemokine release, endothelial-cell activation, or the acute phase responses. Thus, the complete prevention of coagulation activation by TFPI does not inhibit activation of inflammatory pathways during human endotoxemia

(58,59). In posttrauma patients with DIC, the TF-dependent coagulation acti-vation could not be sufficiently prevented by TFPI, which remained at normal levels. The DIC was associated with thrombotic and inflammatory responses, leading to multiple organ dysfunction and a poor outcome in these patients *(60)*.

In normal volunteers, TFPI was found to be well-tolerated, with no clinically significant bleeding *(53)*. Recently, recombinant human TFPI (Chiron, Emeryville, CA) was examined in small phase II clinical studies in patients with severe sepsis *(53,61)*. In the first trial, some of the patients showed an increase in the incidence of serious adverse events involving bleeding that might be caused by the relatively high doses of TFPI (0.33 and 0.66 mg/kg/h) adminis-tered. In the two following studies, lower doses of TFPI (0.025–0.1 mg/kg/h) were used, and then adverse events did not differ between placebo and TFPI groups *(53)*. A recently completed phase II study in 210 patients with sepsis showed a trend toward a relative reduction in d 28 all-cause mortality in TFPI-treated patients as compared with placebo. There was also an improvement in selected organ dysfunction scores and biochemical evidence of TFPI activity in these patients *(53,61)*. A large, international phase III study now underway will evaluate TFPI therapy for severe sepsis *(53)*.

2.4. Other Disorders

The role of TFPI as a possible diagnostic or prognostic marker or as a patho-genetic factor was also investigated in studies involving other diseases (for review, *see 18*). In patients with ischemic stroke, TFPI activity was significantly lower in atherothrombotic and lacunar infarction than in control subjects, which might be attributed to atherosclerotic changes in endothelial cells. In patients with venous thrombosis, an association between TFPI deficiency and throm-bosis has not been clearly demonstrated. Increased TFPI levels in patients with end-stage chronic renal failure are considered to be a compensatory mechanism for the activation of the clotting process. Increased levels of TFPI in patients with non-insulin- and insulin-dependent diabetes mellitus could indicate an imbalance between procoagulant and anticoagulant mechanisms in diabetic patients, or may reflect a vascular damage with an endothelial dysfunction. The increased TFPI levels seen in patients with malignancies cannot yet be explained.

3. Interactions Between TFPI, Unfractionated Heparin, and LMWHs

TFPI is synthesized in the vascular endothelium and is released from there after injection of either unfractionated heparin (UFH) or LMWHs, thus pro-viding high concentrations of TFPI at sites of tissue damage and ongoing throm-bosis (**Fig. 3**). The endogenous, cell-associated TFPI may be more important for maintaining the anticoagulant properties of the endothelium than the circulating TFPI *(62)*. Endothelial cell-released TFPI—which, in contrast to plasma TFPI, still contains the basic C-terminal tail—is considered to significantly contribute to the anticoagulant effect of heparin. UFH and LMWH, which were originally developed for prophylaxis of venous thromboembolic diseases, are now also used for the treatment of thrombotic disorders of both the venous and especially the arterial type *(63,64)*. Intravenous (iv) or subcutaneous (sc) administration of heparin reduced the elevated levels of TF observed in patients with UA and AMI and increased the concentrations of free TFPI *(65–67)*. In large, randomized clinical trials, the antithrombotic effectiveness of different LMWHs has been demonstrated *(68–74)*. LMWHs were observed to be superior to UFH in the treatment of both arterial and venous thrombosis, an effect that may be particularly based on the differential action of UFH and LMWHs on intravascular pools of TFPI *(75,76)*. At therapeutic doses, UFH but not LMWH is associated with a progressive depletion of both circulating and endothelial-bound TFPI, which may lead to a strong rebound activation of coagulation after cessation of treatment with UFH *(77–80)*. A depletion of intracellular TFPI was also observed in endothelial-cell culture systems in which the depletion was also significantly stronger with UFH than with LMWH *(62)*. This difference may be responsible for the higher antithrombotic efficacy of LMWH as compared to UFH The cellular mechanisms of the effect of heparin on endothelium-associated TFPI appears to involve not only a simple displacement of TFPI from the cell surface, but a more specific mechanism that includes increased secretion as well as redistribution of cellular TFPI induced by heparin *(62)*. In vitro studies on the effect of UFH on the synthesis and secretion of TFPI in endothelial cells demonstrated that heparin dose-dependently increased the expression of TFPI mRNA in endothelial cells, followed by a synthesis-dependent increase in TFPI release *(81)*. After heparin stimulation, the major portion of TFPI appears to be secreted from intracellular stores and not displaced from the membrane surface. An alternative explanation would be that when TFPI is displaced from the membrane surface, it is rapidly replaced from intracellular stores *(81)*.

In contrast to the differences between UFH and LMWH described here, recently published studies comparing the TFPI releasing effect of therapeutic doses of UFH and the LMWH dalteparin in hospitalized patients demonstrated that dalteparin caused significantly less TFPI induction, and, thus it is suggested that TFPI may not be a major contributor to the antithrombotic effect of heparin *(82)*. In patients with ACS such as UA and AMI, the measurements of markers of thrombin generation, endothelial function, and acute phase reaction revealed similar responses to UFH and the LMWH enoxaparin. The increase in plasma levels of total TFPI also did not show significant differences between UFH and the LMWH. In particular, after both heparins, a depletion of TFPI was observed that may indicate that the constitutive synthesis of TFPI is surpassed by its elimination in these patients *(83)*.

4. Comparison With Other Anticoagulants/Antithrombotics

Antithrombotic agents such as heparin and aspirin have been used for a long time for prophylaxis and therapy of thromboembolic disorders in both the venous and arterial system. New drugs developed during recent years represent a wide spectrum of natural, synthetic, and semi-synthetic as well as biotechnologically produced agents and include especially LMWHs, serine proteinase inhibitors such as direct and indirect thrombin and factor Xa inhibitors, endogenous anticoagulants such as antithrombin III, and platelet function inhibitors such as GPIIb/IIIa-receptor antagonists or ADP-receptor blockers.

With special emphasis on TFPI, it must be stated that—based on the central role of the TF/FVIIa complex in the initiation of blood coagulation—other therapeutic strategies for regulating the TF pathway are currently being evaluated. Recombinant inactivated FVIIa (FVIIai)—which at least has similar or even higher binding capacity to TF than FVIIa but blocks the catalytic activity of the TF/FVIIa complex—was investigated in various animal models *(84,85)*. When administered intravenously or topically, FVIIai prevented or diminished immediate thrombus formation after vessel-wall injury both in the venous and arterial system, and reduced the long-term intima thickening and narrowing of the vessel lumen. Furthermore, it attenuated coagulant and inflammatory responses in septic shock and reduced an experimental ischemia/reperfusion injury. In humans, FVIIai was studied in dose-escalation trials in healthy volunteers and as an adjunct to heparin in patients undergoing percutaneous transluminal balloon angioplasty (PTCA). The combination with FVIIai revealed a trend toward a reduction in the number of ischemia events as well as a lowering of heparin doses required to reach the same effect *(85)*.

Another potent inhibitor of the TF/FVIIa complex is the recombinant nematode anticoagulant protein c2 (NAPc2), which binds to factor Xa at a site distinct from the active site, and then the resultant binary complex inhibits the TF/FVIIa complex *(86,87)*. A multicenter dose-response study for the prevention of venous thromboembolism in patients undergoing knee replacement showed the antithrombotic efficacy of NAPc2 after sc administration, thus encouraging further clinical trials *(88)*. In healthy human volunteers, the anticoagulant action of NAPc2 could be reversed by the infusion of recombinant FVIIa, resulting in an increased generation of thrombin. FVIIa may be used as an antidote for inhibitors of the TF/FVIIa complex in cases of adverse effects such as bleeding events *(89)*.

An important clinical indication for TFPI is the treatment of severe sepsis that results from a generalized inflammatory and procoagulant response to an infection (*see* **Subheading 2.2.**). However, in addition to the TF pathway the other anticoagulant pathways—e.g., the antithrombin pathway and the protein C system—are also defective in sepsis and DIC *(90)*. Because the natural anticoagulants exhibit specific cellular interactions that appear to provide anti-inflammatory as well as anticoagulant activities, it is expected that restoration of the anticoagulant pathways may be associated with an improved clinical outcome in patients with sepsis and DIC *(91)*. The protein C system appears to play a central role in the pathogenesis of severe sepsis because of its antithrombotic/profibrinolytic actions, the modulation of vascular functions, and the anti-inflammatory properties *(92,93)*. In various animal models of sepsis and DIC, activated protein C (APC) has been shown to be an effective therapeutic agent *(94)*. In humans, the efficacy and safety of recombinant human APC for severe sepsis was studied in a multicenter phase 3 trial involving patients with systemic inflammation and organ failure resulting from acute infection. Administration of APC significantly reduced the rate of death from all causes at 28 d in patients with a clinical diagnosis of severe sepsis, but this may be associated with an increased risk of bleeding *(95)*. From the theoretical basis, replacement therapy with antithrombin III (ATIII), which is an important inhibitor of thrombin as well as of other proteases of the coagulation system, could be useful for the treatment of DIC and severe sepsis *(96,97)*. However, there have been no convincing clinical trial results demonstrating the efficacy of ATIII in these diseases. As shown in a randomized, placebo-controlled, double-blind multicenter phase II trial as well as in a meta-analysis on all trials with ATIII in patients with severe sepsis, there was a positive trend with ATIII for reduction of mortality and organ failure, but no statistically significant difference between ATIII- and placebo-treated groups *(98)*. In another study, ATIII replacement therapy significantly reduced mortality only in the subgroup of septic shock patients *(99)*. In the clinical trials, a relatively low number of patients was included. Therefore, a final evaluation of the therapeutic value of ATIII for DIC, and severe sepsis requires additional and larger clinical trials *(100)*.

TFPI demonstrated potent anti-angiogenesis efficacy vs many growth factors that might mediate the heparin anti-angiogenesis effects (**Fig. 4**).

5. Clinical Perspectives

It can be expected that, because of the various biological functions of TF and the role of this protein in the pathomechanism of many diseases, the inhibitor TFPI may have a broad spectrum of therapeutic use. However, until now TFPI has only found indications in severe sepsis in which defined trials have been

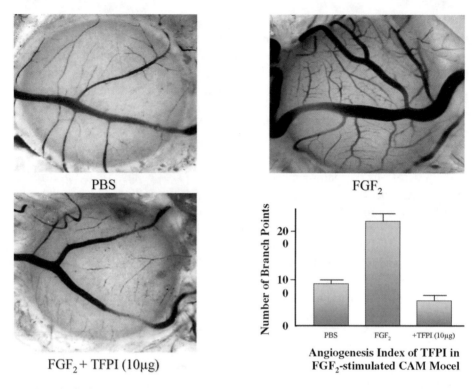

PBS

FGF$_2$

FGF$_2$ + TFPI (10µg)

**Angiogenesis Index of TFPI in
FGF$_2$-stimulated CAM Mocel**

Fig. 4. Potent inhibition of FGF2-induced angiogenesis by r-TFPI in the chick chorioallantoic membrane (CAM) model.

carried out that demonstrated the effectiveness of the drug by an improved outcome in terms of surrogate markers and mortality reduction in the patients. Numerous studies in patients suffering from cardiovascular and other disorders showed that both TF and TFPI may be indicators for the course and the outcome of certain diseases. Based on experimental and clinical findings, it may be assumed that TFPI could become an important drug for several clinical indications **(Table 2)**. The prevention of thrombotic complications of atherosclerosis after plaque rupture, and thus, the development of ACS, may represent a very promising indication for TFPI. In addition, in animal studies, TFPI was found to even protect vascular sites from atherosclerosis. Topical application of TFPI has been shown to improve capillary blood flow, which could be beneficial for patients with microangiopathic disorders. This is consistent with the observation that defibrotide enhances the release of TFPI. TFPI affects the inflammation cycle that contributes to microvascular thrombosis, and in this way it may be of value in the acute respiratory distress syndrome. TFPI could

Table 2
Clinical Relevance of TFPI and Potential Therapeutic Applications

Acute coronary syndromes (unstable angina, AMI)
Prevention of reocclusion and restenosis after successful PTCA or lysis
Disseminated intravascular coagulation and sepsis
Prophylaxis and therapy of deep venous thrombosis
Microvascular anastomosis
Ischemic stroke (especially atherothrombotic and lacunar infarction) and ischemia-
    reperfusion injury

Detailed references in *17,18* and herein.

also be useful for the prevention of thrombosis associated with stroke or transient ischemic attacks, as an antithrombotic drug in microvascular surgery and for the reduction of ischaemia/reperfusion injury *(18)*. TFPI may have important therapeutic value for various clinical indications, but it is important to recognize that the preclinical and especially the clinical investigations of TFPI are rather limited. Therefore, the clinical potential of the drug cannot yet be evaluated properly, and requires further study.

6. Conclusion

TF plays a crucial role in the pathogenesis of thrombotic, vascular, and inflammatory disorders **(Fig. 5)**. Targeting of this mediator provides a unique therapeutic approach to influence the underlying pathophysiologic processes and to prevent or treat the respective diseases. The development of recombinant TFPI and its molecular variants has provided a new dimension in the management of various disorders such as atherosclerosis, ACS including UA and MI, thrombotic stroke, and microangiopathic disorders, as well as for inflammation-associated pathogenetic processes. Although the development of recombinant TFPI is currently limited to sepsis, this agent and its variants are expected to find multiple indications. Molecular manipulation of the currently available TFPI forms will provide drugs with varying pharmacokinetic and pharmacodynamic properties and with relatively stronger affinity to endothelial or subendothelial target sites. As TFPI is present in several forms, the identification of these forms and their differential function may lead to the development of additional TFPI variants for specific indications. In addition, TFPI conjugates with drugs and chemicals may provide agents with a broader spectrum for the management of various diseases and a desirable duration of action. Because of the unique nature of TFPI, genomic manipulation of the vascular system will be an important consideration to enhance the endogenous synthesis and release of

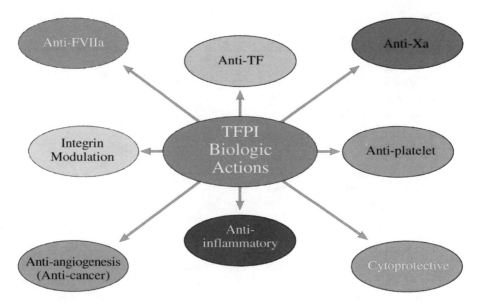

Fig. 5. Biologic actions of TFPI based on the inhibition of FXa and the TF/FVIIa complex.

TFPI. The TFPI gene can be readily introduced at various sites using different vectors, which may be an important approach to modulate thrombotic and vascular disorders.

References

1. Hoffmann, M. and Monroe, D. M., III (2001) A cell-based model of hemostasis. *Thromb. Haemostasis* **85(6),** 958–965.
2. Morissey, J. H. (2001) Tissue factor: an enzyme cofactor and a true receptor. *Thromb. Haemostasis* **86(1),** 66–74.
3. Ruf, W. and Mueller, B. M. (1999) Tissue factor signalling. *Thromb. Haemostasis* **82(2),** 175–182.
4. Rur, W., Fischer, E. G., Huang, H. Y., et al. (2000) Diverse functions of protease receptor tissue factor in inflammation and metastasis. *Immunol. Res.* **21(2–3),** 289–292.
5. Key, N. S. and Bach, R. R. (2001) Tissue factor as a therapeutic target. *Thromb. Haemostasis* **85(3),** 375–376.
6. Broze, G. J., Jr., Girard, T. J., and Novotny, W. F. (1990) Regulation of coagulation by a multivalent Kunitz-type inhibitor. *Biochemistry* **29(33),** 7539–7546.
7. Girard, T. J., Warren, L. A., Novotny, W. F., et al. (1989) Functional significance of the Kunitz-type inhibitory domains of lipoprotein-associated coagulation inhibitor. *Nature* **338(6215),** 518–520.

8. Girard, T. J., McCourt, D., and Novotny, W. G. (1990) Endogenous phosphorylation of the lipoprotein-associated coagulation inhibitor at serine-2. *Biochem. J.* **270(3),** 621–625.

9. Ho, G., Narita, M., Broze, G. J., Jr., and Schwartz, A. L. (2000) Recombinant full-length tissue factor pathway inhibitor fails to bind to the cell surface: implications for catabolism in vitro and in vivo. *Blood* **95(6),** 1973–1978.

10. Broze, G. J., Jr., Warren, L. A., Novotny, W. G., et al. (1988) The lipoprotein-associated coagulation inhibitor that inhibits the factor VII-tissue factor complex also inhibits factor Xa: insights into its possible mechanism of action. *Blood* **71(2),** 335–343.

11. Huang, Z. F., Wun, T. C., and Broze, G. J., Jr. (1993) Kinetics of factor Xa inhibition by tissue factor pathway inhibitor. *J. Biol. Chem.* **286(36),** 26,950–26,955.

12. Lindhout, T., Franssen, J., and Willems, G. (1995) Kinetics of the inhibition of tissue factor-factor VIIa by tissue factor pathway inhibitor. *Thromb. Haemostasis* **74(3),** 910–915.

13. Rapaport, S. I. (1989) Inhibition of factor VIIa/tissue factor-induced blood coagulation with particular emphasis upon a factor Xa-dependent inhibitory mechanism. *Blood* **73(2),** 359–365.

14. Rapaport, S. I. (1991) The extrinsic pathway inhibitor: a regulator of tissue factor-dependent blood coagulation. *Thromb. Haemostasis* **66(1),** 6–15.

15. Yoneda, T., Komooka, H., and Umeyama, H. (1997) A computer modeling study of the interaction between tissue factor pathway inhibitor and blood coagulation factor Xa. *J. Protein Chem.* **16(6),** 597–605.

16. Baugh, R. J., Broze, G. J., Jr., and Krishnaswamy, S. (1998) Regulation of extrinsic pathway factor Xa formation by tissue factor pathway inhibitor. *J. Biol. Chem.* **273(8),** 4378–4386.

17. Kaiser, B., Hoppensteadt, D. H., and Fareed, J. (1988) Recombinant TFPI and variants. Potential implications in the treatment of cardiovascular disorders. *Exp. Opin. Investig. Drugs* **7(7),** 1121–1137.

18. Kaiser, B., Hoppensteadt, D. H., and Fareed, J. (2000) Tissue factor pathway inhibitor for cardiovascular disorders. *Emerging Drugs* **5(1),** 73–87.

19. Pendurthi, U. R., Rao, L. V. M., Williams, J. T., and Idell, S. (1999) Regulation of tissue factor pathway inhibitor expression in smooth muscle cells. *Blood* **94(2),** 579–586.

20. Bajaj, M. S., Steer, S., Kuppuswamy, M. N., Kisiel, W., and Bajaj, P. (1999) Synthesis and expression of tissue factor pathway inhibitor by serum-stimulated fibroblasts, vascular smooth muscle cells and cardiac myocytes. *Thromb. Haemostasis* **82(6),** 1663–1672.

21. Sato, Y., Asada, Y., Marutsuk, A. K., et al. (1997) Tissue factor pathway inhibitor inhibits aortic smooth muscle cell migration induced by tissue factor/factor VIIa complex. *Thromb. Haemostasis 78(3),* 1138–1141.

22. Kamikumo, Y., Nakahara, Y., Takemoto, S., et al. (1997) Human recombinant tissue factor pathway inhibitor prevents the proliferation of cultured human neonatal aortic smooth muscle cells. *FEBS Lett.* **407(1),** 116–120.

23. Hamuro, T., Kamikubo, Y., Nakahara, Y., Miyamoto, S., and Funatsu, A. (1998) Human recombinant tissue factor pathway inhibitor induces apoptosis in cultured human endothelial cells. *FEBS Lett.* **421(3),** 197–202.

24. Hembrough, T. A., Ruiz, J. F., Papathanassiu, A. E., Green, S. J., and Strickland, D. K. (2001) Tissue factor pathway inhibitor inhibits endothelial cell proliferation via association with the very low density lipoprotein receptor. *J. Biol. Chem.* **276(15),** 12,241–12,248.

25. Jang, Y., Guzman, L. A., Lincoff, A. M., et al. (1995) Influence of blockade at specific levels of the coagulation cascade on restenosis in a rabbit atherosclerotic femoral artery injury model. *Circulation* **92(10),** 3041–3050.

26. Oltrona, L., Speidel, C. M., Recchia, D., et al. (1997) Inhibition of tissue factor-mediated coagulation markedly attenuates stenosis after balloon-induced arterial injury in minipigs. *Circulation* **96(2),** 646–652.

27. St. Pierre, J., Yang, L. Y., Tamarisa, K., et al. (1999) Tissue factor pathway inhibitor attenuates procoagulant activity and upregulation of tissue factor at the site of balloon-induced arterial injury in pigs. *Arterioscler. Thromb. Vasc. Biol.* **19(9),** 2263–2268.

28. Asada, Y., Hara, S., Tsuneyoshi, A., et al. (1998) Fibrin-rich and platelet-rich thrombus formation on neointima: recombinant tissue factor pathway inhibitor prevents fibrin formation and neointimal development following repeated balloon injury of rabbit aorta. *Thromb. Haemostasis* **80(3),** 506–511.

29. Sun, L. B., Utoh, J., Moriyama, S., Tagami, H., Okamoto, K., and Kitamura, N. (2001) Topically applied tissue factor pathway inhibitor reduced intimal thickness of small arterial autografts in rabbits. *J. Vasc. Surg.* **34(1),** 151–155.

30. Golino, P., Cirillo, P., Calabro, P., et al. (2001) Expression of exogenous tissue factor pathway inhibitor in vivo suppresses thrombus formation in injured rabbit carotid arteries. *J. Am. Coll. Cardiol.* **38(2),** 569–576.

31. Nishida, T., Ueno, H., Atsuchi, N., et al. (1999) Adenovirus-mediated local expression of human tissue factor pathway inhibitor eliminates shear stress-induced recurrent thrombosis in the injured carotid artery of the rabbit. *Circ. Res.* **84(12),** 1446–1452.

32. Zoldhelyi, P., McNatt, J., Shelat, H. S., Yamamoto, Y., Chen, Z. Q., and Willerson, J. T. (2000) Thromboresistance of balloon-injured porcine carotid arteries after local gene transfer of human tissue factor pathway inhibitor. *Circulation* **101(3),** 289–295.

33. Atsuchi, N., Nishida, T., Marutsuka, K., et al. (2001) Combination of a brief irrigation with tissue factor pathway inhibitor (TFPI) and adenovirus-mediated local TFPI gene transfer additively reduces neointima formation in balloon-injured rabbit carotid arteries. *Circulation* **103(4),** 570–575.

34. Zoldhelyi, P., Chen, Z. Q., Shelat, H. S. McNatt, J. M., and Willerson, J. T. (2001) Local gene transfer of tissue factor pathway inhibitor regulates intimal hyperplasia in atherosclerotic arteries. *Proc. Natl. Acad. Sci. USA* **98(7),** 4078–4083.

35. Singh, R., Pan, S., Mueske, C. S., et al. (2001) Role for tissue factor pathway in murine model of vascular remodeling. *Circ. Res.* **89(1),** 71–76.

36. Westrick, R. J., Bodary, P. F., Xu, Z., Shen, Y. C., Broze, G. J., and Eitzman, D. T. (2001) Deficiency of tissue factor pathway inhibitor promotes atherosclerosis and thrombosis in mice. *Circulation* **103(25)**, 3044–3046.

37. Drew, A. F., Davenport, P., Apostolopoulos, J., and Tipping, P. G. (1997) Tissue factor pathway inhibitor expression in atherosclerosis. *Lab. Investig.* **77(4)**, 291–298.

38. Caplice, N. M., Mueske, C. S., Kleppe, L. S., and Simari, R. D. (1998) Presence of tissue factor pathway inhibitor in human atherosclerotic plaques is associated with reduced tissue factor activity. *Circulation* **98(11)**, 1051–1057.

39. Kaikita, K., Takeya, M., Ogawa, H., et al. (1999) Co-localization of tissue factor and tissue factor pathway inhibitor in coronary atherosclerosis. *J. Pathol.* **188(2)**, 180–188.

40. Crawley, J., Lupu, F., Westmuckett, A. D., Severs, N. J., Kakkar, V. V., and Lupu, C. (2000) Expression, localization, and activity of tissue factor pathway inhibitor in normal and atherosclerotic human vessels. *Arterioscler. Thromb. Vasc. Biol.* **20(5)**, 1362–1373.

41. Moatti, D., Haidar, B., Fumeron, F., et al. (2000) A new T-287C polymorphism in the 5′ regulatory region of the tissue factor pathway inhibitor gene. Association study of the T-287C and C-399T polymorphisms with coronary artery disease and plasma TFPI levels. *Thromb. Haemostasis* **84(2)**, 244–249.

42. Moatti, D., Seknadji, P., Galand, C., et al. (1999) Polymorphisms of the tissue factor pathway inhibitor (TFPI) gene in patients with acute coronary syndromes and in healthy subjects: impact of the V264M substitution on plasma levels of TFPI. *Arterioscler. Thromb. Vasc. Biol.* **19(4)**, 862–869.

43. Moatti, D., Meirhaeghe, A., Ollivier, V., Bauters, C., Amouyel, P., and De Prost, D. (2001) Polymorphisms of the tissue factor pathway inhibitor gene and the risk of restenosis after coronary angioplasty. *Blood Coagul. Fibrinolysis* **12(4)**, 317–323.

44. Falciani, M., Gori, A. M., Fedi, S., et al. (1998) Elevated tissue factor and tissue factor pathway inhibitor circulating levels in ischaemic heart disease patients. *Thromb. Haemostasis* **79(3)**, 495–499.

45. Soejima, H., Ogawa, H., Yasue, H., et al. (1999) Heightened tissue factor associated with tissue factor pathway inhibitor and prognosis in patients with unstable angina. *Circulation* **99(22)**, 2908–2913.

46. Kamikura, Y., Wada, H., Yamada, A., et al. (1997) Increased tissue factor pathway inhibitor in patients with acute myocardial infarction. *Am. J. Hematol.* **55(4)**, 183–187.

47. Ott, I., Andrassy, M., Zieglgansberger, D., Geith, S., Schmömig, A., and Neumann, F. J. (2001) Regulation of monocyte procoagulant activity in acute myocardial infarction: role of tissue factor and tissue factor pathway inhibitor-1. *Blood* **97(12)**, 3721–3726.

48. Roldan, V., Marin, F., Fernandez, P., et al. (2001) Tissue factor/tissue factor pathway inhibitor system and long-term prognosis after acute myocardial infarction. *Int. J. Cardiol.* **78(2)**, 115–119.

49. Hansen, J., Grimsgaard, S., Huseby, N., Sandset, P. M., and Bonaa, K. H. (2001)
    Serum lipids and regulation of tissue factor-induced coagulation in middle-aged
    men. *Thromb. Res.* **102(1),** 3–13.
50. Morange, P. E., Renucci, J. F., Charles, M. A., et al. (2001) Plasma levels of free
    and total TFPI, relationship with cardiovascular risk factors and endothelial cell
    markers. *Thromb. Haemostasis* **85(6),** 999–1003.
51. Sandset, P. M., Warn-Cramer, B. J., Rao, L. V. M., Maki, S. L., and Rapaport,
    S. I. (1991) Depletion of extrinsic pathway inhibitor (EPI) sensitizes rabbits to
    disseminated intravascular coagulation induced with tissue factor: evidence
    supporting a physiologic role for EPI as a natural anticoagulant. *Proc. Natl. Acad.
    Sci. USA* **88(3),** 708–712.
52. Sandset, P. M., Warn-Cramer, B. J., Maki, S. L., and Rapaport, S. I. (1991)
    Immunodepletion of extrinsic pathway inhibitor sensitizes rabbits to endotoxin-
    induced intravascular coagulation and the generalized Shwartzman reaction. *Blood*
    78(6), 1496–1502.
53. Creasey, A. A. and Reinhart, K. (2001) Tissue factor pathway inhibitor activity in
    severe sepsis. *Crit. Care Med.* **29 (7 Suppl.),** S126–S129.
54. Shimura, M., Wada, H., Wakita, Y., et al. (1997) Plasma tissue factor and tissue
    factor pathway inhibitor levels in patients with disseminated intravascular coagu-
    lation. *Am. J. Hematol.* **55(4),** 169–174.
55. Takahashi, H., Sato, N., and Shibata, A. (1995) Plasma tissue factor pathway
    inhibitor in disseminated intravascular coagulation: comparison of its behavior with
    plasma tissue factor. *Thromb. Res.* **80(4),** 339–348.
56. Yamamuro, M., Wada, H., Kumeda, K., et al. (1998) Changes in plasma tissue
    factor pathway inhibitor levels during the clinical course of disseminated intravas-
    cular coagulation. *Blood Coagul. Fibrinolysis* **9(6),** 491–497.
57. Shimura, M., Wada, H., Nakasaki, T., et al. (1999) Increased truncated form of
    plasma tissue factor pathway inhibitor levels in patients with disseminated intravas-
    cular coagulation. *Am. J. Hematol.* **60(2),** 94–98.
58. De Jonge, E., Dekkers, P. E. P., Creasey, A. A., et al. (2000) Tissue factor pathway
    inhibitor dose-dependently inhibits coagulation activation without influencing the
    fibrinolytic and cytokine response during human endotoxemia. *Blood* **95(4),**
    1124–1129.
59. De Jonge, E., Dekkers, P. E. P., Creasey, A. A., et al. (2001) Tissue factor pathway
    inhibitor does not influence inflammatory pathways during human endotoxemia.
    J. Infect. Dis. **183(12),** 1815–1818.
60. Gando, S., Nanzaki, S., Norimoto, Y., Ishitani, T., and Kemmotsu, O. (2001) Tissue
    factor pathway inhibitor response does not correlate with tissue factor-induced dis-
    seminated intravascular coagulation and multiple organ dysfunction syndrome in
    trauma patients. *Crit. Care Med.* **29(2),** 262–266.
61. Abraham, E. (2000) Tissue factor inhibition and clinical trial results of
    tissue factor pathway inhibitor in sepsis. *Crit. Care Med.* **28 (9 Suppl.),**
    S31–S33.

62. Lupu, C., Poulsen, E., Roquefeuil, S., et al. (1999) Cellular effects of heparin on the production and release of tissue factor pathway inhibitor in human endothelial cells in culture. *Arterioscler. Thromb. Vasc. Biol.* **19(9)**, 2251–2262.

63. Cohen, M., Demers, C., Gurfinkel, E. P., et al. (1997) A comparison of low-molecular-weight heparin with unfractionated heparin for unstable coronary artery disease. *N. Engl. J. Med.* **337(7)**, 447–452.

64. Fareed, J., Hoppensteadt, D. H., and Bick, R. L. (2000) An update on heparins at the beginning of the new millenium. *Semin. Thromb. Hemost.* **26 (Suppl. 1)**, 5–21.

65. Soejima, H., Ogawa, H., Yasue, H., et al. (1999) Plasma tissue factor pathway inhibitor and tissue factor antigen levels after administration of heparin in patients with angina pectoris. *Thromb. Res.* **93(1)**, 17–25.

66. Gori, A. M., Pepe, G., Attanasio, M., et al. (1999) Tissue factor reduction and tissue factor pathway inhibitor release after heparin administration. *Thromb. Haemostasis* **81(4)**, 589–593.

67. Yamamoto, N., Ogawa, H., Oshima, S., et al. (2000) The effect of heparin on tissue factor and tissue factor pathway inhibitor in patients with acute myocardial infarction. *Int. J. Cardiol.* **75(2–3)**, 267–274.

68. Fox, K. A. (2001) Antithrombotic therapy in acute coronary syndromes: key notes from the ESSENCE and TIMI 11B. *Semin. Hematol.* **38 (2 Suppl. 5)**, 67–74.

69. Goodman, S. G., Cohen, M., Bigonzi, F., et al. (2000) Randomized trial of low molecular weight heparin (enoxaparin) versus unfractionated heparin for unstable coronary artery disease: one-year results of the ESSENCE study. Efficacy and safety of subcutaneous enoxaparin in non-Q wave coronary events. *J. Am. Coll. Cardiol.* **36(3)**, 693–698.

70. Husted, S., Becker, R., and Kher, A. (2001) A critical review of clinical trials for low-molecular-weight heparin therapy in unstable coronary artery disease. *Clin. Cardiol.* **24(7)**, 492–499.

71. Kereiakes, D. J., Grines, C., Fry, E., et al. (2001) Enoxaparin and abciximab adjunctive pharmacotherapy during percutaneous coronary intervention. *J. Invasive Cardiol.* **13(4)**, 272–278.

72. Mismetti, P., Laporte, S., Darmon, J. Y., Buchmuller, A., and Decousus, H. (2001) Meta-analysis of low molecular weight heparin in the prevention of venous thromboembolism in general surgery. *Br. J. Surg.* **88(7)**, 913–930.

73. Wallentin, L. (2000) Low molecular weight heparin in unstable coronary artery disease. *Expert Opin. Investig. Drugs* **9(3)**, 581–592.

74. Young, J. J., Kereiakes, D. J., and Grines, C. L. (2000) Low-molecular-weight heparin therapy in percutaneous coronary intervention: the NICE 1 and NICE 4 trials. National investigators collaborating on enoxaparin investigators. *J. Invasive Cardiol.* **12 (Suppl. E)**, E14–E18.

75. Hansen, J. B., Sandset, P. M., Huseby, K. R., et al. (1998) Differential effect of unfractionated heparin and low molecular weight heparin on intravascular tissue factor pathway inhibitor: evidence for a difference in antithrombotic action. *Br. J. Haematol.* **101(4)**, 638–646.

76. Hansen, J. B. and Sandset, P. M. (1998) Differential effects of low molecular weight heparin and unfractionated heparin on circulating levels of antithrombin and tissue factor pathway inhibitor (TFPI): a possible mechanism for difference in therapeutic efficacy. *Thromb. Res.* **91(4)**, 177–181.

77. Bendz, B., Hansen, J. B., Andersen, T. O., Ostergaard, P., and Sandset, P. M. (1999) Partial depletion of tissue factor pathway inhibitor during subcutaneous administration of unfractionated heparin, but not with two low molecular weight heparins. *Br. J. Haematol.* **107(4)**, 756–762.

78. Hansen, J. B., Naalsund, T., Sandset, P. M., and Svensson, B. (2000) Rebound activation of coagulation after treatment with unfractionated heparin and not with low molecular weight heparin is associated with partial depletion of tissue factor pathway inhibitor and antithrombin. *Thromb. Res.* **100(5)**, 413–417.

79. Sandset, P. M., Bendz, B., and Hansen, J. B. (2000) Physiological function of tissue factor pathway inhibitor and interaction with heparins. *Haemostasis* **30 (Suppl. 2)**, 48–56.

80. Theroux, P., Waters, D., Lam, J., Juneau, M., and McCans, J. (1992) Reactivation of unstable angina after the discontinuation of heparin. *N. Engl. J. Med.* **327(3)**, 141–145.

81. Hansen, J. B., Svensson, B., Olsen, R., Ezban, M., Østerud, B., and Paulssen, R. H. (2000) Heparin induces synthesis and secretion of tissue factor pathway inhibitor from endothelial cells in vitro. *Thromb. Haemostasis* **83(6)**, 937–943.

82. Brown, J. R. and Kuter, D. J. (2001) The effect of unfractionated vs. low molecular weight heparin on tissue factor pathway inhibitor levels in hospital inpatients. *Thromb. Haemostasis* **85(6)**, 979–985.

83. Vila, V., Martinez-Sales, V., Reganon, E., et al. (2001) Effects of unfractionated and low molecular weight heparins on plasma levels of hemostatic factors in patients with acute coronary syndromes. *Haematologica* **86(7)**, 729–734.

84. Sorensen, B. B. and Rao, L. V. (1988) Interaction of activated factor VII and active site-inhibited factor VII with tissue factor. *Blood Coagul. Fibrinolysis* **9 (Suppl. 1)**, S67–S71.

85. Hedner, U. and Erhardtsen, E. (2000) Future possibilities in the regulation of the extrinsic pathway: rFVIIa and TFPI. *Ann. Med.* **32 (Suppl. 1)**, 68–72.

86. Bergum, P. W., Cruikshank, S., Maki, S. L., Kelly, C. R., Ruf, W., and Vlasuk, G. P. (2001) Role of zymogen and activated factor X as scaffolds for the inhibition of the blood coagulation factor VIIa-tissue factor complex by recombinant nematode anticoagulant protein c2. *J. Biol. Chem.* **276(13)**, 10,063–10,071.

87. Duggan, B. M., Dyson, H. J., and Wright, P. E. (1999) Inherent flexibility in a potent inhibitor of blood coagulation, recombinant nematode anticoagulant protein c2. *Eur. J. Biochem.* **265(2)**, 539–548.

88. Lee, A., Agnelli, G., Buller, H., et al. (2001) Dose-response study of recombinant factor VIIa/tissue factor inhibitor recombinant nematode anticoagulant protein c2 in prevention of postoperative venous thromboembolism in patients undergoing total knee replacement. *Circulation* **104(1)**, 74–78.

89. Friederich, W., Levi, M., Bauer, K. A., et al. (2001) Ability of recombinant factor VIIa to generate thrombin during inhibition of tissue factor in human subjects. *Circulation* **103(21)**, 2555–2559.

90. Levi, M., De Jonge, E., and van der Poll, T. (2001) Rationale for restoration of physiological anticoagulant pathways in patients with sepsis and disseminated intravascular coagulation. *Crit. Care Med.* **29 (7 Suppl.)**, S90–S94.

91. Esmon, C. T. (2001) Role of coagulation inhibitors in inflammation. *Thromb. Haemostasis 86(1),* 51–56.

92. Faust, S. N., Heyderman, R. S., and Levin, M. (2001) Coagulation in severe sepsis: a central role for thrombomodulin and activated protein C. *Crit. Care Med.* **29 (7 Suppl.)**, discussion S67–S68.

93. Grinnell, B. W. and Joyce, D. (2001) Recombinant human activated protein C: a system modulator of vascular function for treatment of severe sepsis. *Crit. Care Med.* **29 (7 Suppl.)**, discussion S60–S61.

94. Esmon, T. (2001) Protein C anticoagulant pathway and its role in controlling microvascular thrombosis and inflammation. *Crit. Care Med.* **29 (7 Suppl.)**, discussion 51–52.

95. Bernard, G. R., Vincent, J. L., Laterre, P. F., et al. (2001) Efficacy and safety of recombinant human activated protein C for severe sepsis. *N. Engl. J. Med.* **344(10)**, 699–709.

96. De Jonge, E., Levi, M., Stoutenbeek, C. P., and Van Deventer, S. J. (1998) Current drug treatment strategies for disseminated intravascular coagulation. *Drugs* **55(6)**, 767–777.

97. Dickneite, G. (1998) Antithrombin III in animal models of sepsis and organ failure. *Semin. Thromb. Hemostasis* **24(1)**, 61–69.

98. Eisele, B., Lamy, M., Thijs, L. G., et al. (1998) Antithrombin III in patients with severe sepsis. A randomized, placebo-controlled, double-blind multicenter trial plus a meta-analysis on all randomized, placebo-controlled, double-blind trials with antithrombin III in severe sepsis. *Intensive Care Med.* **24(7)**, 663–672.

99. Baudo, F., Caimi, T. M., De Cataldo, F., et al. (1998) Antithrombin III (ATIII) replacement therapy in patients with sepsis and/or postsurgical complications: a controlled double-blind, randomized, multicenter study. *Intensive Care Med.* **24(4)**, 336–342.

100. Mammen, E. F. (1998) Antithrombin III and sepsis. *Intensive Care Med.* **24(7)**, 649–650.

11

Cell Adhesion Molecules

Potential Therapeutic and Diagnostic Implications

Shaker A. Mousa

1. Introduction

The role of cell adhesion molecules (CAM) and extracellular matrix (ECM) proteins in various pathological processes, including angiogenesis, thrombosis, apoptosis, cell migration, and proliferation, is well-documented. These processes can lead to both acute and chronic disease states such as ocular diseases, metastasis, unstable angina (UA), myocardial infarction (MI), stroke, osteoporosis, a wide range of inflammatory diseases, vascular remodeling, and neurodegenerative disorders. One key milestone in this field is evident from the potential role of the platelet GPIIb/IIIa integrin in the prevention and diagnosis of various thromboembolic disorders. Additionally, soluble adhesion molecules as potential diagnostic markers for acute and chronic leukocyte, platelet, and endothelial cellular insult are increasingly utilized. In this chapter, the development of various therapeutic and diagnostic candidates based on the key role of CAM—with special emphasis on integrins in various diseases as well as the structure-function aspects of cell adhesion and signaling of the different CAM and ECM—is highlighted.

Many physiological processes, including cell activation, migration, proliferation, and differentiation, require direct contact between cells or ECM proteins. Cell–cell and cell–matrix interactions are mediated through several different families of CAM, including the selectins, the integrins, the cadherins, and the immunoglobulins. Newly discovered CAM, along with the discovery of new roles for integrins, selectins, and immunoglobulins in certain disease states, provide ideal opportunities for the development of therapeutic and perhaps diagnostic modalities.

From: *Methods in Molecular Medicine, vol. 93: Anticoagulants, Antiplatelets, and Thrombolytics*
Edited by: S. A. Mousa © Humana Press Inc., Totowa, NJ

Intensified drug discovery efforts, directed at manipulating CAM activity through monoclonal antibodies (MAbs), peptides, peptidomimetics, and non-peptide small molecules for diagnostic and therapeutics, continue to broaden the scope of key clinical applications. This chapter focuses on the current advances in the discovery and development of novel anti-integrins for potential therapeutic and diagnostic applications, as well as methods required in studying these different CAM members.

CAM plays a critical role in normal as well as various pathophysiological disease states. For this reason, the selection of specific and relevant CAM to target certain disease conditions without interference in other normal cellular functions is a very important prerequisite for the ultimate success in developing truly active and safe therapeutic strategies *(1,2)*. Exciting advances in our understanding of several CAMs—most notably, the $\alpha_v\beta_3$, $\alpha_v\beta_5$, $\alpha_4\beta_1$, $\alpha_5\beta_1$, and $\alpha IIb/\beta_3$ integrin receptors—and their direct relationships to different disease states represent a tremendous therapeutic and diagnostic opportunities *(1–7)*. CAMs are believed to play a role in different disease states including: cardio-vascular, cancer, inflammatory, ocular, pulmonary, bone, central nervous system (CNS), kidney, and the gastrointestinal (GI) system. For example, the role of the integrin $\alpha IIb/\beta_3$ in the prevention, treatment, and diagnosis of various thromboembolic disorders provides excellent proof of this concept *(3–7)*. The potential prophylactic role of antiselectins, the role of β_1 along with other leukointegrins in various inflammatory conditions, the potential utility of various soluble adhesion molecules as surrogate markers for acute and chronic endothelial injury, and the potential role of $\alpha_v\beta_3$ in angiogenesis and osteoporosis, have all been implicated *(8,9)*.

CAMs for Therapeutic and Diagnostic Utility:
Selected CAM Receptors

2. Anti-Selectins

The families of cell adhesion receptors include: the selectins, consisting of three CAMs unified structurally by the inclusion of lectin (L), EGF-like (E), and complement (C) binding-like domains (LEC-CAMs). Functionally, the selectins are unified by their ability to mediate cell binding through interactions between their lectin domains and cell-surface carbohydrate ligands *(10)*. These include the E-, L-, and P- selections. The P- and E- selections are calcium-dependent on platelets or endothelial-cell surface lectins that mediate leukocyte adhesion by recognition of cell-specific carbohydrate ligands. L- selections are found on all leukocytes, and bind to its counter receptors on endothelial cells (Gly-CAM-1), a mucin-like endothelial glycoprotein *(11)*. E-selectin is an

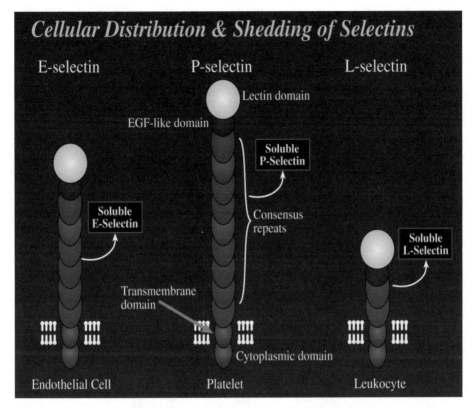

Fig. 1. Diagrammatic sketch for soluble selectins.

endothelial adhesion molecule whose expression is induced by various inflammatory stimuli, which recognizes cell-surface carbohydrate, Sialyl Lewis^x (SLe^x) *(12)*. P-selectin is found stored in alpha granules of platelets, as well as Weible-palade bodies of endothelial cells, and recognizes a carbohydrate that is closely related to SLe^x *(13)*.

The selectin family of CAMs plays a key role in the mediation of early neutrophil (PMN) rolling on and adherence to endothelial cells. P-selectin on platelet (P) and endothelial cells surfaces and L-selectin on the leukocyte surface act in concert to promote PMN-endothelial cells and PMN-P interactions. Monoclonal antibodies, which neutralize either P-selectin or L-selectin, have been found to preserve endothelial- and monocyte-cell function in a myocardial ischemia/reperfusion injury model *(14,15)*. Additionally, in a primate model of carotid-artery restenosis, GA-6 resulted in a 25% reduction in the neointimal-medial ratio after 14 d *(16)*. L-selectin is involved in mediating neutrophil rolling interactions at sites of inflammation *(17;* **Fig. 1***)*.

2.1. Human Soluble Selectin Assays (sP-, sL-, or sE-Selectins)

The most commonly used assay employs the quantitative sandwich immunoassay technique. A MAb specific for sP-, sL-, or sE-selectins precoated onto a microplate. Standard, samples, and control are pipetted into the wells, together with a polyclonal antibody that is specific for sP-, sL, or sE-selectins conjugated to horseradish peroxidase (HRP). After removal of unbound conjugated antibody, a substrate is added and color is developed that is proportional to sP-selectin concentration.

2.1.1. Assay Procedure

1. Dilute all samples. For most samples (serum or plasma), a dilution of 1 in 100 should be adequate. For cell-culture supernatant samples, a dilution of 1 in 25 is appropriate.
2. Remove excess microtiter-plate strips from the frame and store in the resealed foil pouch with the silica gel sachet.
3. Add 100 µL standard diluted sample or diluted parameter control to each well in duplicate.
4. Cover the plate with a plate sealer and incubate at room temperature for 1 h.
5. Add 100 µL anti-selectin/HRP conjugate to each well with sufficient force to ensure mixing. Conjugate is red-colored to facilitate correct addition.
6. Cover the plate with a new plate sealer provided and incubate at room temperature for 30 min.
7. Aspirate or decant contents from each well and wash by adding 400 µL of wash buffer per well. Repeat the process 5× for a total of six washes. After the last wash, aspirate or decant the contents and remove any remaining wash buffer by tapping the inverted plate firmly on clean paper toweling.
8. Add 100 µL substrate to each well. Cover the plate and incubate at room temperature for 30 min.
9. Add 100 µL of Stop Solution to each well. The Stop Solution should be added to the wells in the same order as the Substrate.
10. Determine the optical density (OD) of each well within 30 min using a microtiter-plate reader of Photometer set at 450 nm with a correction wavelength of 620 nm. If the wavelength correction facility is not available, read plates at 450 nm and then separately at 620 nm. Subtract the OD_{620} from the OD_{450}.

3. Integrins

Integrins are a widely expressed family of cell adhesion receptors that enable cells to attach to extracellular matrices, to each other, or to different cells. All integrins are composed of $\alpha\beta$ heterodimeric units that are expressed on a wide variety of cells, and most cells express several integrins. The interaction of integrins with the cytoskeleton and ECM appears to require the presence of both subunits. The binding of integrins to their ligands is a cation-dependent.

Integrins appear to recognize specific amino acid sequences in their ligands. The most extensively studied is the RGD sequence found within a number of matrix proteins including fibrinogen, vitronectin, fibronectin, thrombospondin, osteopontin, VWF, and others. However, other integrins bind to ligands via non-RGD-binding domains such as the $\alpha_4\beta_1$ integrin receptors that bind and recognize the LDV sequence within the CS-1 region of fibronectin. There are at least eight known β subunits and 14 α subunits *(1,2)*.

3.1. Coordinate Regulation of Cell Adhesion and Signaling Through Integrins

Integrin adhesion receptors contain an extracellular face that engages adhesive ligands and a cytoplasmic face that engages intracellular proteins. These interactions are critical for cell adhesion and for anchorage-dependent signaling reactions in normal and pathological states. For example, platelet activation induces a confirmational change in integrin $\alpha IIb/\beta_3$, thereby converting it into a high-affinity fibrinogen receptor. Fibrinogen binding then triggers a cascade of protein tyrosine kinases and phosphatases, and recruitment of numerous other signaling molecules into F-actin-rich cytoskeletal assemblies in proximity to the cytoplasmic tails of αIIb and β_3. These dynamic structures appear to influence platelet functions by coordinating signals emanating from integrins and G-protein-linked receptors. Studies of integrin mutations confirm that the cytoplasmic tails of $\alpha II/\beta_3$ are involved in integrin signaling, presumably through direct interactions with cytoskeletal and signaling molecules. Blockade of fibrinogen binding to the extracellular face of $\alpha IIb/\beta_3$ has been shown to be an effective way to prevent platelet-rich arterial thrombi after coronary angioplasty *(18)*. Once proteins that interact with the cytoplasmic tails of $\alpha IIb/\beta_3$ are fully identified, it may also be possible to develop selective inhibitors of integrin adhesion or signaling with a locus of action that is inside the cell.

3.2. Anti-Integrins as a Potential Drug Discovery Target

The commercial and therapeutic potential of CAMs is on the rise. Newly discovered CAM and the discovery of new roles for integrins, selectins, and immunoglobulins in certain disease states provide ideal opportunities to develop therapeutic and diagnostic drugs. Integrin represents the best opportunity to achieve small-molecule antagonist for both therapeutic and diagnostic utility in various key diseases with unresolved medical needs.

3.3. β_1 Integrins

The largest group of integrins is the β_1 integrin family, which are also known as the VLA subfamily because of the late appearance of VLA after activation.

There are at least seven receptors characterized from this subfamily, each with different ligand specificity. Among the most studied include the $\alpha_4\beta_1$, $\alpha_5\beta_1$, $\alpha_6\beta_1$, and $\alpha_2\beta_1$ receptors. The leukocyte integrin $\alpha_4\beta_1$ (also known as VLA-4, and CD49d/CD29) is a cell adhesion receptor, which is predominantly expressed on lymphocytes, monocytes, and eosinophil *(19)*. The leukocyte integrin $\alpha_4\beta_1$ (also known as VLA-4, and CD49d/CD29) is a potential target for therapeutics in chronic inflammatory diseases.

3.3.1. Potent and Selective Small-Molecule Antagonists of α_4 Integrins

The α_4 integrins are heterodimeric cell-surface molecules that are central to leukocyte-cell and leukocyte-matrix adhesive interactions. The integrin $\alpha_4\beta_7$, expressed on all leukocytes except neutrophils, interacts with the immunoglobulin (Ig) superfamily member VCAM-1, and with an alternately spliced form of fibronectin. The integrin $\alpha_4\beta_7$ is also restricted to leukocytes, and can bind not only to VCAM1 and fibronectin, but also to MAdCAM the mucosal addressin or homing receptor, which contains Ig-like domains related to VCAM-1. Certain MAbs to the α_4 chain and $\alpha_4\beta_7$ can block their in vitro adhesive function. In vivo studies with these MAbs in several species demonstrate that the interactions between these integrins and their ligands play a key pathophysiologic role in immune and inflammatory reactions. Thus, α_4 integrin-dependent adhesive interactions with VCAM-1, MAdCAM, and fibronectin appear to play a central role in the recruitment priming, activation, and apoptosis of certain leukocyte subsets, and offer novel targets for drug intervention. For this reason, a selective and potent anti-α_4 MAb and small-molecule antagonists were designed. These molecules demonstrated in vivo efficacy in several animal models *(20,21)*. The mucosal vascular addressin MAdCAM-1 is an immunoglobulin-like adhesion receptor that is preferentially expressed by venular endothelial cells that define sites of lymphocyte extravasation in mucosal lymphoid tissues and lamina propria. MAdCAM-1 binds lymphocyte integrin $\alpha_4\beta_7$ *(22)*. Peptide-based analogs based on various regions in the first and second domains of MAdCAM-1 for the binding to $\alpha_4\beta_7$ have been identified.

3.3.2. The Leukocyte Integrin $\alpha_4\beta_1$ as a Potential Target for Therapeutics

These leukocyte populations primarily mediate chronic inflammatory disease (e.g., rheumatoid arthritis, asthma, and psoriasis and allergy). In contrast, VLA-4 is not present on circulating unstimulated neutrophils, which constitute a first line of defense against acute infections. Eosinophils selectively accumulate at sites of chronic allergic diseases such as bronchial asthma. The role of β_1 integrins and its regulation by cytokines and other inflammatory mediators during eosinophil adhesion to endothelium, ECM proteins, and transendothelial migration has been well-documented *(23,24)*. The interactions of VLA-4 with alternatively spliced fibronectin containing CS-1 to design receptor blockers that bind to the VLA-4 integrin receptor have been utilized in targeting small-molecule inhibitors. Evaluation of these analogs in animal models of disease indicate that VLA-4 blockade has the potential to achieve dramatic in vivo effects in a variety of chronic inflammatory disorders *(19–21)*.

3.3.3. Antibodies Against α_4 Integrin Prevent Immune-Cell Infiltration of the CNS and Reverse Progression of Experimental Autoimmune Encephalomyelitis (EAE)

Infiltration of circulating immune cells into the CNS, resulting in edema, myelin damage, and paralysis, has been documented *(25)*. The role for the adhesion molecule $\alpha_4\beta_1$ integrin in this process has been demonstrated. When administered to animals with EAE, antibodies against α_4 integrin prevented the adhesion of lymphocytes and monocytes to inflamed endothelium within blood vessels of the CNS, and prevented immune-cell infiltration. Even when administered to animals after the onset of paralysis, anti-α_4 integrin reversed all clinical signs of disease. MRI analysis of these animals showed that antibody treatment reduced edema and reduced permeability of the blood–brain barrier to Gd-DPTA, and histological analysis demonstrated that treatment prevented the destruction of myelin. Remarkably, anti-α_4 integrin reversed the accumulation of lymphocytes and monocytes within the CNS, and did not affect the level of the cells in the circulation. These results suggest that the active disease process requires an ongoing recruitment of circulating cells into the CNS, and that anti-α_4 integrin prevents this recruitment and reverses disease progression.

3.3.4. Integrins in Other Diseases

3.3.4.1. INTEGRINS IN GI DISEASES

Inflammatory bowel disease (IBD), Crohn's disease, and ulcerative colitis (UC) are immunologically mediated illnesses. Using antibodies to the β family of integrins, isolated intestinal lamina mononuclear cells from IBD and the normal intestine express a pattern of integrins found on normal solid organs with more β_7 expression than IBD. Crohn's CD3+ cells express more β_1 than normal, supporting separate β integrin systems in GI diseases. However, β_1 and β_7 integrins in particular remain as a potential therapeutic target for GI inflammatory disease *(26)*.

3.3.4.2. $\alpha_5\beta_1$ INTEGRIN IN ANGIOGENESIS

Recent evidence suggested the role this integrin in the modulation of angiogenesis. Thus antagonist for $\alpha_5\beta_1$ may have potential utility in various angiogenesis-mediated disorders *(27)*.

3.3.4.3. $\alpha_5\beta_1$ Integrin and Bacterial Infection

Recent studies suggested a key role for $\alpha_5\beta_1$ integrin in mediating certain types of bacterial invasion into human host cells, leading to antibiotic resistance *(28)*.

3.4. β_2 Integrins

The leukocyte-restricted β_2 (CD18) integrins promote a variety of homotypic and heterotypic cell adhesion events required for normal and pathologic functioning of the immune system *(29)*. Several physiological processes including cell adhesion, activation, migration, and transmigration require direct contact between cells or ECM proteins via CAM receptors. To date, only three members of this integrin subfamily have been identified, including: CD11a/CD18 (LFA-1), CD11b/CD18 (Mac-1), and CD11c/CD18 (P150,95). In vitro studies have shown that LFA-1(CD11a/CD18) and Mac-1 on neutrophils can be differentially activated for distinct function *(29)*. In addition, investigations in vivo, including studies in CD11b-deficient mice, further underscore the biologic significance of the distinct contributions of LFA-1 and Mac-1 to neutrophil-dependent tissue injury.

3.5. β_3 Integrins

3.5.1. $\alpha IIb/\beta_3$ Integrin

3.5.1.1. Intravenous and Oral Platelet $\alpha IIb/\beta_3$-Receptor Antagonists: Potential Clinical Use

There is an urgent need for more efficacious antithrombotic drugs that are superior to aspirin or ticlopidine for the prevention and treatment of various cardiovascular and cerebrovascular thromboembolic disorders. The realization that the platelet integrin $\alpha IIb\beta_3$ is the final common pathway for platelet aggregation, regardless of the mechanism of action, has prompted the development of several small-molecule $\alpha IIb/\beta_3$-receptor antagonists for intravenous (iv) and/or oral antithrombotic utilities. Platelet $\alpha IIb/\beta_3$-receptor blockade represents a very promising therapeutic and diagnostic strategy of thromboembolic disorders. Clinical experiences (efficacy/safety) gained with injectable $\alpha IIb\beta_3$ antagonists will provide valuable insights into the potential of long-term chronic usage of oral $\alpha IIb/\beta_3$ antagonists. At this point, there are still many unanswered questions, and thorough studies are needed to determine the safety and efficacy of this mechanism either alone or in combination with antiplatelet/anticoagulant therapies.

The clinical utility of Abciximab (ReoPro, c7E3 Fab) based on several trials involving coronary-artery intervention procedures *(30–32)*. The potent, rapid, and sustained blockade of platelet GPIIb/IIIa receptors and perhaps its $\alpha v\beta_3$

blockade may be the key aspect that contributes to the dramatic early antithrombotic benefits. Early benefits were maintained for more than 3 yr in-patients who received 12-hr Abciximab treatment in the EPIC trial. These unique pharmacological characteristics may also provide benefits in other thrombotic conditions such as stroke, unstable angina, and acute myocardial infarction (AMI). Coronary Intervention: Epic (high-risk abrupt closure), Epilog (broad entry criteria), Capture (refractory unstable angina [UA]), Epistent (stent), and Rapport (direct angioplasty). Integrilin is a cyclic heptapeptide KGD analog. Impact II (coronary intervention—broad entry criteria) and Pursuit (UA—chest pain <24 h ischemic ECG changes) both demonstrated significant clinical benefits *(33)*. Tirofiban: the Restore (Coronary intervention—high risk of abrupt closure per clinical and anatomic criteria), Prism and Prism plus trials (UA, chest pain 24 and 12 h) demonstrated significant clinical benefits. Lamifiban: the Paragon trial demonstrated significant clinical benefits *(34)*. Studies with Lamifiban in Canada were stopped because of lack of efficacy and nuisance bleeding.

3.6. Chronic Therapy With Platelet GPIIb/IIIa Antagonists

3.6.1. Orally Active GPIIb/IIIa Antagonists

A high level of platelet antagonism has been required when GPIIb/IIIa antagonists have been employed for acute therapy of coronary artery disease. However, the requirements for chronic therapy using orally active agents are only now being determined. Interaction with aspirin and other antiplatelet and anticoagulant drugs lead to shifts in the dose-response curves for both efficacy and unwanted side effects, such as increased bleeding time *(36–38)*. More recently, both Xemilofiban (EXCITE) and Orbofiban (OUPIS) sponsored by Searle and Sibrafiban (SYMPHONY) sponsored by Roche were withdrawn because of a disappointing outcome. This raises many serious questions regarding the potential of oral GPIIb/IIIa antagonists *(39,40)*.

3.6.2. Issues in Clinical Development

These include thrombocytopenia, monitoring, bleeding risk, and drug interactions *(41,42)*.

3.6.3. The Role of Platelet Integrin GPIIb/IIIa-Receptor Antagonists in the Rapid Diagnosis of Thromboembolic Events

The role of the platelet integrin GPIIb/IIIa receptor and its potential utility as a radiodiagnostic agent in the rapid detection of thromboembolic events has been demonstrated *(43)*.

3.7. $\alpha_v\beta_3$ *Integrin*

3.7.1. The Role of Integrin $\alpha_v\beta_3$ and Matrix Proteins in Vascular Remodeling Via Endothelial and Smooth-Muscle-Cell Actions

Vascular remodeling processes play a key role in the pathological mechanisms of atherosclerosis and restenosis. In response to vascular injury such as by PTCA, matrix proteins such as osteopontin and vitronectin are rapidly upregulated *(44)*. Osteopontin stimulates smooth-muscle cell (SMC) migration through its action on the integrin $\alpha_v\beta_3$, and thereby contributes to neointima formation and restenosis *(45,46)*. In addition, the matrix protein osteopontin and vitronectin induce angiogenesis, which may support neointima formation and arteriosclerosis *(47)*. Thus, specific matrix proteins—via selected integrins and especially $\alpha_v\beta_3$—may be important targets for selective antagonists aimed at blocking the pathological processes of restenosis *(44)*.

3.8. Cellular and Integrin-Based Assays

3.8.1. Antiplatelet Efficacy Assays

3.8.1.1. LIGHT TRANSMITTANCE AGGREGOMETRY ASSAY

Venous blood was obtained from healthy nonsmokers and non-fasted human donors (35–45 yr old, males and females) who were drug- and aspirin-free for at least 2 wk prior to blood collection, as previously described *(5,6)*. Briefly, blood was collected into citrated Vacutainer tubes. The blood was centrifuged for 10 min at 150g in a Sorvall RT6000 Tabletop Centrifuge with H-1000 B rotor) at room temperature, and platelet-rich plasma (PRP) was removed. The remaining blood was centrifuged for 10 min at 1,500g at room temperature, and platelet-poor plasma (PPP) was removed. Samples were assayed on a PAP-4 Platelet Profiler, using PPP as the blank (100% transmittance). Two hundred microliters of PRP (2×10^8 platelets/mL) were added to each micro test tube, and transmittance was set to 0%. Twenty microliters of platelet agonist, ADP (10 μM final concentration) was added to each tube, and the aggregation profiles were plotted (percentage transmittance vs time). Twenty microliters of antiplatelet agent were added at different concentrations ranging from 0.001–100 μM for 8 min prior to the addition of adenosine diphosphate (ADP). Results were expressed as the percentage of inhibition of agonist-induced platelet aggregation or IC$_{50}$ (μM).

3.8.1.2. PLATELET ^{125}I-FIBRINOGEN-BINDING ASSAY

Human PRP (h-PRP) was applied to a size-exclusion sepharose column to prepare human-gel-purified platelets (h-GPP). Aliquots of h-GPP (2×10^8 platelets/mL) along with 1 mM calcium chloride were added to removable

96-well plates, ^{125}I-fibrinogen (26.5 µCi/mg) was added, and the h-GPP were activated by addition of ADP, epinephrine, and sodium arachidonate at 100 µ*M* each. The ^{125}I-fibrinogen bound to the activated platelets were separated from the free form by centrifugation, and then counted on a gamma counter. Nonspecific binding (caused by entrapment of ^{125}I-fibrinogen), either in the presence or absence of a test agent, was shown (in the absence of agonists) to be in the range of 4–6% of total ^{125}I-fibrinogen binding to agonist-activated platelets.

3.8.2. Integrin-Based Assays

3.8.2.1. 293/β$_3$-FIBRINOGEN ADHESION

In this assay, an α$_v$β$_3$-transefected 293/β$_3$ cell line was used. The adhesion of this cell line to fibrinogen was shown to be dependent on the α$_v$β$_3$, as shown by the total inhibition by an α$_v$β$_3$ MAb. The method briefly involves the use of enzyme-linked immunosorbent assay (ELISA) plate wells, which were coated with fibrinogen at 25 µg/well and stored at 4°C until use. On the day of the assay, wells were washed twice with phosphate-buffered saline (PBS) without cations, and the wells were blocked with 5% BSA made in PBS for 2 h. The 293/β$_3$ cells at 30–70% confluence were harvested and brought up to 1×10^6 cells/mL. On a 96-well polypropylene plate, 65 µL of buffer was added followed by 5 µL of test agent at different concentrations. Then, 130 µL of cells was added and incubated at 37°C, 5% CO$_2$ for 15 min. After the incubation, non-adhered cells were removed. Cells were lysed with 100 m*M* potassium phosphate, 0.2% Triton X-100, pH 7.8 solution, and 5 µL was assayed for β-galactosidase using a Galactolight luminescence assay. Luminescence values were converted to β-galactosidase using a standard curve, nonspecific was subtracted, the percentage of inhibition was calculated for each test agent concentration, and IC50 was computed.

3.8.2.2. SK-BR-3 CELL-VITRONECTIN (α$_v$β$_5$- MEDIATED) ADHESION ASSAY

An α$_v$β$_5$ expressing SK- breast cancer cell line (SK-BR-3, ATCC, Rockville, MD) was used. The adhesion of this SK-BR-3 cell line to vitronectin was determined to be an α$_v$β$_5$-mediated adhesion, as evident from the total blockade by α$_v$β$_5$ MAb (*23*). The method briefly involves the use of a Costar plate coated with 100 µL of vitronectin (0.25 µg per well) overnight at 4°C. Following overnight coating, each well was washed twice with 200 µL PBS, and nonspecific binding was blocked by adding 200 µL of PBS + 5% BSA per well for 1 h at room temperature. Cells were labeled with 2 µ*M* calcein-AM (Molecular Probes) for 30 min at 37°C humidified incubator. Cells (1×10^6 cells/mL) were pre-incubated with either 150 µL of test compounds or medium, gently mixed, then incubated for 15 min at room temperature. Test agent-treated SK-BR-3 cells were added to the assay plate in duplicate and incubated for 60 min on a shaker at room temperature. Plates were covered with foil to prevent photobleaching of the dye from labeled cells. Following the washing of unattached cells, 100 μL of media was added to each well, and the fluorescence was read on a Cytofluor 2300, Ex = 485 nm and EM = 530 nm.

3.8.2.3. PURIFIED $\alpha_5\beta_1$-RECEPTOR-BIOTINYLATED FIBRONECTIN-BINDING ASSAY

Purified receptor $\alpha_5\beta_1$ obtained from human placenta was coated onto Costar high-capacity binding plates overnight at 4°C. Coating solution was discarded, and plates were washed once with buffer. Wells were then blocked with 200 μL buffer containing 1% BSA. After washing once with buffer, 100 μL of biotinylated fibronectin (2 nM) was added, plus 11 μL of either test agent or buffer containing 1.0% BSA to each well and incubated for 1 h at room temperature. The plate was then washed twice with buffer and incubated for 1 h at room temperature with 100 μL anti-biotin alkaline phosphatase. Plates were washed twice with buffer and incubated for 1 h with 100 μL alkaline phosphatase substrate. Color was developed at room temperature for approx 45 min, and the reaction was stopped by adding 2 N NaOH. Developed color was read at 405 nm.

3.8.3. Functional Assays

Integrin-mediated intracellular signaling can be studied using integrin-transfected cells or other cell systems and specific blocking antibody or small-molecule ligand for the integrin of interest. Additionally, integrin-mediated cell migration or proliferation can be studied using classical migration or proliferation assays.

4. Immunoglobulin (Ig)

ICAMs and VCAMs are members of the Ig superfamily. Most of the effort in targeting the Ig superfamily is focused on the development of specific MAbs and/or anti-sense oligonucleotide and small molecules that may specifically block gene transcriptional factors. Strategies for designing small molecular weight inhibitors for the Ig superfamily are somewhat more difficult. However, with current advances in molecular modeling and crystal structure information, it might be possible to develop cyclic peptides and peptidomimetics Ig antagonist.

Several studies with MAbs to ICAM-1 demonstrated anti-inflammatory properties with tremendous therapeutic potential in liver and kidney transplantation as well as in rheumatoid arthritis (*48,49*). In contrast to current immunosuppressants, which demonstrated efficacy in organ transplantation along with major adverse effects, the use of anti-CAM as a strategy may be proven to be effective and safer.

4.1. Role of PECAM-1 in Regulating Transendothelial Migration of PMNs in Disease States

PMNs adhere to the inflamed vascular endothelium, and eventually undergo transendothelial migration. This latter process is largely regulated by PECAM-1, which is expressed on platelets, leukocytes and at the intercellular junctions of endothelial cells. Specific antibodies that neutralize PECAM-1 selectively block PMN migration and markedly attenuate injury to ischemic-reperfused myocardium and the coronary endothelium. Intravital microscopy confirms that the protective mechanism of PECAM-1 blockade is by the inhibition of their transendothelial migration *(50)*.

4.2. Soluble Adhesion Molecules as Surrogate Markers

CAMs are well-recognized as adhesive receptors to facilitate adhesion, migration, and transmigration of circulating cells into damaged vascular tissues. Recent studies have demonstrated that expression of ICAM-1 on human athersclerotic plaques and treatment with an anti-ICAM-1 MAb resulted in a significant reduction of myocardial infarct size in experimental myocardial/ischemia reperfusion injury models *(51,52)*. Soluble isoforms of these CAMs are believed to be shed from the surface of activated cells, which can be quantified in peripheral blood. Increased serum concentrations of soluble CAMs have been observed in a variety of diseases *(53,54)*. Recent studies have suggested the prognostic and diagnostic potential for various soluble adhesion molecules in various vascular and cardiovascular diseases. *See* **Fig. 2** for diagrammatic sketch of soluble immunoglobulins.

4.3. Human Soluble VCAM-1, ICAM-1, or PECAM Assays

These assays involve the simultaneous reaction of sVCAM-1 present in the sample or standard to two antibodies directed against different epitopes on the sVCAM-1 molecule. One antibody is coated onto the walls of the microtiter wells, and the other is conjugated to the enzyme HRP. Any sVCAM-1 present forms a bridge between the two antibodies. The same concept applies to sICAM-1 or PECAM.

After removal of unbound material by aspiration and washing, the amount of conjugate bound to the well is detected by reaction with a substrate that is specific for the enzyme that yields a colored product proportional to the amount of conjugate (and thus sVCAM-1 in the sample). The colored product can be quantified photometrically.

By analyzing standards of known sVCAM-1 concentration coincident with samples and plotting a curve of signal vs concentration, the concentration of unknowns can be determined.

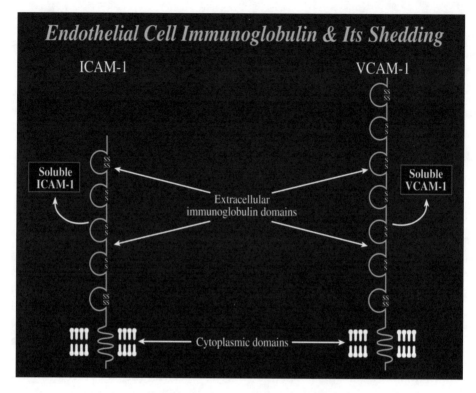

Fig. 2. Diagrammatic sketch of soluble immunoglobulins.

5. Assay Procedure Summary

1. For most samples (serum, plasma, or cell-culture fluids), a dilution of 1 in 50 should be adequate.
2. Add 100 µL diluted anti-VCAM-1-HRP conjugate to each well.
3. Add 100 µL standard, diluted sample, or diluted parameter control to each well with sufficient force to ensure mixing. Shaking or tapping is not recommended.
4. Cover the plate with a plate sealer provided and incubate at room temperature for 1.5 h.
5. Aspirate or decant contents from each well and wash by adding 300 µL or wash buffer per well. Repeat the process 5× for a total of six washes. After the last wash, aspirate or decant the contents and remove any remaining wash buffer by tapping the inverted plate firmly on clean paper toweling.
6. Immediately after decanting, add 100 µL substrate to each well.
7. Cover the plate with a plate sealer provided and incubate at room temperature for 30 min.
8. Add 100 µL or Stop Solution to each well. The Stop Solution should be added to the wells in the same order as the substrate.

9. Determine the optical density (OD) of each well within 30 min using a microtiter-plate reader or Photometer set at 450 nm with a correction wavelength of 620 nm. The photometer or plate reader should be blanked according to the manufacturer's instructions. If the wavelength correction facility is not available, read plates at 450 nm and then separately at 620 nm. Subtract the OD_{620} from the OD_{450}.

6. Conclusion

It is very clear that several members in the CAM superfamilies—particularly the integrin family—will serve as potential therapeutic and diagnostic strategies for a number of diseases with unresolved medical needs. The selection of a certain CAM that is associated with specific pathophysiological aspect of certain disease processes, as well as the ease of achieving a small anti-CAM molecules, will determine the ultimate success in the discovery and development of therapeutic and diagnostic drugs.

References

1. Cox, D., Aoki, T., Seki, J., Motoyama, Y., and Yoshida, K. (1994) The pharmacology of the integrins. *Med. Res. Rev.* **14(2),** 195–228.
2. Albelda, S. M. and Buck, C. A. (1990) Integrins and other cell adhesion molecules. *FASEB J.* **4,** 2868–2880.
3. Cook, N. S., Kottirsch, G., and Zerwes, H. (1994) Platelet glycoprotein IIb/IIIa antagonists. *Drugs Future* **19(2),** 135–159.
4. Gold, H., Gimple, L. W., Yasuda, T., et al. (1990) Pharmacodynamic study of F(ab′)2 fragments of murine monoclonal antibody 7E3 directed against human platelet glycoprotein IIb/IIIa in patients with unstable angina pectoris. *J. Clin. Invest.* **86,** 651–659.
5. Mousa, S. A., Bozarth, J. M., Forsythe, M. S., et al. (1993) Anti-platelet efficacy and specificity of DMP 728, a novel platelet GPIIb/IIIa receptor antagonist. *Cardiology* **83,** 374–382.
6. Mousa, S. A., Bozarth, J. M., Forsythe, M. S., et al. (1994) Antiplatelet and antithrombotic efficacy of DMP 728, a novel platelet GPIIb/IIIa receptor antagonist. *Circulation* **89(1),** 3–12.
7. Mousa, S. A. and Topol, E. (1997) Novel antiplatelet therapies: Recent advances, in *the development of platelet GPIIb/IIIa receptor antagonists. Current Review of Interventional Cardiology*, 3rd ed. (Serruys, P. W. and Holmes, D., eds.), Current Medicine, Philadelphia, PA, **13,** 114–129.
8. Brooks, P. C., Clark, R. A. F., and Cheresh, D. A. (1994) Requirement of vascular integrin $\alpha_v\beta_3$ for angiogenesis. *Science* **264,** 569–571.
9. Brooks, P. C., Montgomery, A. M. P., Rosenfield, M., et al. (1994) Integrin $\alpha v\beta_3$ antagonists promote tumor regression by inducing apoptosis of angiogenic blood vessels. *Cell* **79,** 1157–1164.
10. Brandley, B., Swiedler, S., and Rabbins, P. (1990) Carbohydrate ligands for the LEC cell adhesion molecules. *Cell* **63,** 861–863.

11. Lasky, L. A., Singer, M., Dowbenko, D., et al. (1992) An endothelial ligand for L-selectin is a novel mucin-like molecule. *Cell* **69,** 927–938.

12. Lasky, L. A. (1992) Selectins: interproteins of cell-specific carboyhdrate information during inflammation. *Science* **258,** 964–968.

13. Phillips, M. L., Nudelman, E., Gaeta, F. A., et al. (1990) ELAM-1 mediate cell adhesion by recognition of a carbohydrate ligand, sialyl-Lex. *Science* **250,** 1130–1132.

14. Weyrich, A. S., Ma, X.-L., Leter, D. J., Albertine, K. H., and Lefer, A. M. (1993) In vivo neutralization of P-selectin protects feline heart and endothelium in myocardial ischemia and reperfusion injury. *J. Clin. Investig.* **91,** 2620–2629.

15. Mulligan, M. S., Paulson, J. C., De Frees, S., et al. (1993) Protective effects of oligo-saccharides in P-selectin-dependent lung injury. *Nature* **364,** 149–151.

16. Hullinger, T. G., DeGraaf, G. L., Hartman, J. C., and Shebuski, R. J. (1995) The effect of P-selectin blockade on neointimal lesion development in a primate carotid injury model. *FASEB J.* **9,** 4897.

17. Paulson, J. C. (1992) Selectin/carbohydrate-mediated adhesion of leukocytes, in *Adhesion: Its role in inflammatory disease* (Harlan, J. M. and Liu, D. Y., eds.), W.H. Freeman and Company, pp. 19–42.

18. Topol, E. J., Califf, R. M., Weisman, H. F., et al. (1994) Randomised tiral of coronary intervention with antibody against platelet IIb/IIIa integrin for reduction of clinical restenosis: results at six months. *Lancet* **343,** 881–886.

19. Hamann, A., Andrew, D. P., Jablonski-Westrich, D., Holzmann, B., and Butcher, E. C. (1994) Role of α_4-integrins in lymphocyte homing to mucosal tissues in vivo. *J. Immunol.* **152,** 3282–3293.

20. Issekutz, T. B. (1991) Inhibition of in vivo lymphocyte migration to inflammation and homing to lymphoid tissues by TA-2 monoclonal antibody. *J. Immunol.* **147,** 4178–4184.

21. Elices, M. J., Osborn, L., Takada, Y., et al. (1990) VCAM-1 on activated endothelium interacts with leukocyte integrin VLA-4 at asite distinct from the VLA-4/fibronectin binding site. *Cell* **60,** 577–578.

22. Berlin, C., Berg, E. L., Briskin, M. J., Andrew, D. P., et al. (1994) $\alpha_4\beta_7$ integrin mediates lymphocyte binding to the mucosal vascular addressin MAdCAM-1. *Cell* **74,** 185–195.

23. Yednock, T. A., Cannon, C., Fritz, L. C., Sanchez-Madrid, F., Steinman, L., and Karin, N. (1992) Prevention of experimental autoimmune encephalomyelitis by antibodies against $\alpha_4\beta_1$ integrin. *Nature* **356,** 63–66.

24. Springer, T. A. (1994) Traffic signals for lymphocyte recirculation and leukocyte emigration. The multistep paradigm. *Cell* **76,** 301–314.

25. Cannella, B. and Raine, C. S. (1995) The adhesion molecule and cytokine profile of multiple sclerosis lesions. *Ann. Neurol.* **37,** 424–435.

26. Cerf-Bensussan, N., Jarry, A., Lisowska-Grospierre, B., et al. (1987) A monoclonal (HML-1) defining a novel membrane molecule present on human intestinal lymphocytes. *Eur. J. Immunol.* **17,** 1279–1285.

27. Varner, J. and Mousa, S. A. (1998) Antagonists of vascular cell integrin $\alpha_5\beta_1$ inhibi angiogenesis. *Circulation* **98 (Suppl. 1),** 1795, 4166.

28. Cue, D., Southern, S., Southern, P., Jadhav, P. K., Lorelli, W., Smallheer, J., et al. (2000) A nonpeptide integrin antagonist can inhibit epithelial cell ingestion of streptococcus pyogenes by blocking formation of integrin $\alpha_5\beta_1$-fibronectin-M1 protein complex. *Proc. Natl. Acad. Sci. USA* **97(6)**, 2858–2863.

29. Figdor, C. G. and Kooyk, Y. V. (1992) Regulation of cell adhesion. (Harlan, J. M. and Liu, D. Y., eds.), W.H. Freeman and Company, pp. 151–182.

30. Tcheng, J. E., Ellis, S. G., George, B. S., et al. (1994) Pharmacodynamics of chimeric glycoprotein IIb/IIIa integrin antiplatelet antibody Fab 7E3 in high-risk coronary angioplasty. *Circulation* **90**, 1757–1764.

31. EPIC Investigators (1994) Use of a monoclonal antibody directed against the platelet glycoprotein IIb/IIIa receptor in high-risk coronary angioplasty. *N. Engl. J. Med.* **330**, 956–961.

32. Kleiman, N. S., Ohman, E., Califf, R. M., et al. (1993) Profound inhibition of platelet aggregation with monoclonal antibody 73E Fab after thrombolytic therapy: results of the Thrombolysis and Angioplasty in Myocardial Infarction (TAMI) 8 Pilot Study. *J. Am. Coll. Cardiol.* **22**, 381–389.

33. Tcheng, J. E., Harrington, R. A., Kottke-Marchant, K., et al. (1995) Multicenter, randomized, double-blind, placebo-controlled trial of the platelet integrin glycoprotein IIb/IIIa blocker, Integrilin in elective coronary intervention. IMPACT Investigators. *Circulation* **91(8)**, 215–217.

34. Peerlinck, K., De Lepeleire, I., Goldberg, M., et al. (1993) MK383 (L-700462), a selective nonpeptide platelet glycoprotein IIb/IIIa antagonist, is active in man. *Circulation* **88(4 pt 1)**, 1512–1517.

35. Théroux, P., Kouz, S., Knudtson, M. L., et al. (1994) A randomized double-blind controlled trial with the non-peptide platelet GPIIb/IIIa antagonist RO 44-9883 in unstable angina [abstract]. *Circulation* **90**, 1–232.

36. Kottke-Marchant, K., Simpfendorfer, C., Lowrie, M., Burns, D., and Anders, R. J. (1995) Sustained but variable inhibition of platelet aggregation with Xemilofiban, an oral GPIIb/IIIa receptor antagonist, in patients with unstable angina. *Circulation* **92 (8 Suppl.)**, 1–488.

37. Muller, T. H., Weisenberger, H., Brickl, R., Narjes, H., Himmelsbach, F., and Krause (1997) Profound and sustained inhibition of platelet aggregation by Fradafiban, nonpeptide platelet glycoprotein IIb/IIIa antagonist, and its orally active rodrug, Lefradafiban, in men. *Circulation* **96(4)**, 1130–1138.

38. Cannon, C. P., McCabe, C. H., Borzak, S., Henry, T. D., Tischler, M. D., Mueller, H. S., et al. (1998) Randomized trial of an oral platelet glycoprotein IIb/IIIa antagonist, sibrafiban, in patients after an acute coronary syndrome: results of the TIMI 12 trial. Thrombolysis in myocardial infarction. *Circulation* **97(4)**, 340–349.

39. Mousa, S. A. and Wityak, J. (1998) Orally active Isoxazoline GPIIb/IIIa antagonists. *Cardiovasc. Drug Rev.* **16(1)**, 48–61.

40. Harrington, R. A., Graffagnino, C., Armstrong, P. W., Joseph, D., Card, T. L., et al. (1998) Dose-finding and tolerability of a new oral platelet GPIIb/IIIa inhibitor, SB 214857, in patients with coronary artery and cerebrovascular disease: the APLAUD results. *Circulation* **98 (17 Suppl.)**, I-251, P1303.

41. Vorchheimer, D. A. and Fuster, V. (1998) Oral platelet glycoprotein IIb/IIIa receptor antagonists: the present challenge is safety [editorial; comment]. *Circulation* **97(4)**, 312–314.

42. Quinn, M. and Fitzgerald, D. J. (1998) Long-term administration of glycoprotein IIb/IIIa antagonists. *Am. Heart J.* **135 (5 Pt. 2 Suppl.)**, S113–S118.

43. Mousa, S., Bozarth, J., Edward, S., Carroll, T., and Barrett, J. (1998) Novel Technetium-99m labelled platelet GPIIb/IIIa receptor antagonists for imaging venous and arterial thrombosis. *Coron. Artery Dis.* **9(2/3)**, 1–11.

44. Srivasata, S., Reilly, T., Shwartz, R., Holmes, D., and Mousa, S. (1996) Selective $\alpha v \beta_3$ integrin blockade limits neointima hyperplasia and lumen stenosis in stented coronary artery injury in pig. *Circulation* **94(8)**, I–41, 0231 (abstract).

45. Yue, T.-L., McKenna, P. J., Ohlstein, E. H., et al. (1994) Osteopontin-stimulated vascular smooth muscle cell migration is mediated by β_3 integrin. *Exp. Cell Res.* **214**, 459–464.

46. Liaw, L., Skiner, M. P., Raines, E. W., et al. (1995) The adhesive and migratory effects of osteopontin are mediated via distinct cell surface integrins. *J. Clin. Invest.* **95**, 713–724.

47. Zee, R., Passeri, J., Barry, J., Cheresh, D., and Isner, J. (1996) A neutralizing antibody to the alpha v Beta 3 integrin reduces neointimal thickening in a balloon-injured iliac artery. *Circulation* **94(8)**, 1505 [abstract].

48. Flavin, T., Rothlein, R., Faanes, R., Ivens, K., and Starnes, V. A. (1991) Monoclonal antibody against intercellular adhesion molecule (ICAM)-1 prolongs cardiac allograft survival in cynomologus monkey. *Transplant Proc.* **23**, 533–534.

49. Haug, C. E., Colvin, R. B., Delmonico, F. L., et al. (1993) A phase I trial of immunosuppression with anti-ICAM-1 (CD54) mAb in renal allograft recipient. *Transplantation* **55(4)**, 766–773.

50. Rosenblum, W. I., Nelson, G. H., Wormley, B., Werner, P., Wang, J., and Shih, C. Y. (1996) Role of platelet-endothelial cell adhesion molecule (PECAM) in platelet adhesion/aggregation over injured but not denuded endothelium in vivo and ex vivo. *Stroke* **27**, 709–711.

51. Yamazald, T., Seko, Y., Tamatani, T., et al. (1993) Expression of intracellular adhesion molecule-1 in rat heart with ischemia/reperfusion and limitation of infarct size with antibodies against cell adhesion molecules. *Am. J. Pathol.* **143**, 410–418.

52. Simpson, P. J., Todd, R. F., Micelson, J. K., et al. (1990) sustained limitation of myocardial reperfusion injury by a monoclonal antibody that alter leukocyte function. *Circulation* **81**, 226–237.

53. Newman, W., Dawson, B. L., Carson, C. W., et al. (1993) Soluble E-selectins is found in supernatants of activated endothelial cells and is elevated in serum of patients with septic shock. *J. Immunol.* **150**, 644–654.

54. Gearing, A. J. H. and Newman, W. (1993) Circulating adhesion molecules in disease. *Immunol. Today* **14(10)**, 506–512.

12

Development and Applications of Animal Models of Thrombosis

Ronald J. Shebuski, Larry R. Bush, Alison Gagnon,
Liguo Chi, and Robert J. Leadley, Jr.

1. Introduction

Of more than 2 million deaths in the United States each year (from all causes), nearly 1 million are caused by cardiovascular disease (CVD). CVD claims more lives each year than the next seven leading causes combined. The prevalence of CVD in the United States is indicated by the statistics: 50 million people with high blood pressure, 12.5 million people with coronary heart disease (CHD) (7.2 million with myocardial infarction [MI]; 6.3 million with angina pectoris), 4.4 million with stroke, 4.6 million with congestive heart failure, and 2.8 million suffering from other CVD diseases.

In 1997, there were 60.2 million physician office visits and 4.5 million hospital emergency room (ER) visits with the principal diagnosis of CVD. An estimated 1.1 million Americans each year will have a new or recurrent coronary attack, defined as acute coronary syndromes (ACS) or CHD. Of these, 650,000 are first attacks and 450,000 are recurrent. More than 40% of people who experience a heart attack will die. CHD accounts for 50% of all segments of cardiovascular disease, and represents the largest market opportunity for the development of novel diagnostics and therapeutics.

It is well-known that ACS such as unstable angina (UA) and non-Q-wave AMI involve the participation and interaction of blood platelets and procoagulant proteins to form a thrombus or blood clot *(1)*. Thrombi are often precipitated by acute rupture of an underlying atherosclerotic plaque in which the thin fibrous cap of the atherosclerotic lesion ruptures, exposing surfaces and cells that activate platelets and the coagulation cascade in an attempt to repair the

From: *Methods in Molecular Medicine, vol. 93: Anticoagulants, Antiplatelets, and Thrombolytics*
Edited by: S. A. Mousa © Humana Press Inc., Totowa, NJ

damage. Plaque rupture is now widely recognized as the primary cause of acute thrombus formation, and complete occlusion of the vessel may result in irreversible ischemic damage to the cardiac tissue supplied downstream from the obstruction. Angiography often reveals incomplete occlusion of the vessel, but has a substantial atherosclerotic lesion (>90%) and is thus at extremely high risk of complete blockage and eventual acute myocardial infarction (AMI). These patients may also experience periodic episodes of platelet-dependent unstable angina.

During the past two decades, great advances have been made in the pharmacological treatment and prevention of thrombotic disorders (e.g., tissue-plasminogen activators (tPAs), platelet GPIIb/IIIa antagonists, adenosine diphosphate (ADP)-receptor antagonists such as clopidogrel, low molecular weight heparins [LMWHs], and direct thrombin inhibitors). New research is leading to the next generation of antithrombotic compounds such as direct coagulation FVIIa inhibitors, tissue-factor pathway inhibitors (TFPIs), gene therapy, and orally active direct thrombin inhibitors and coagulation Factor Xa (FXa) inhibitors.

The development and application of animal models of thrombosis have played a crucial role in discovering and validating novel drug targets, selecting new agents for clinical evaluation, and providing dosing and safety information for clinical trials. These models have also provided valuable information regarding the mechanisms of these new agents and the interactions between antithrombotic agents that work by different mechanisms. Animal models have contributed greatly to the discovery of currently available antithrombotic agents, and will play a primary role in the discovery and characterization of the novel antithrombotic agents that will provide safe and effective pharmacological treatment for life-threatening thrombotic diseases.

Several excellent reviews covering the different theoretical and technical aspects of thrombosis and thrombolysis models have been published previously *(2–7)*. These reviews, along with more specialized reviews of models of atherosclerosis *(8)*, restenosis *(9)*, and stroke *(10)*, provide comprehensive information regarding the details of many models and provide the pathological rationale for using specific models for specific diseases. In addition, the advantages and disadvantages of each model of thrombosis and thrombolysis are described in these reviews. This chapter focuses on the use of thrombosis models in the drug discovery process, with a focus on the practical application of these models. Examples from studies evaluating therapeutic approaches that target various antithrombotic mechanisms will be presented to demonstrate the current use of thrombosis models in drug discovery. Important issues in evaluating novel antithrombotic compounds are also addressed. Evidence demonstrating the clinical relevance of preclinical data derived from animal models of thrombosis is also presented. Finally, a summary of the use of genetic models of thrombosis/hemostasis and their current and potential use in drug discovery is also discussed.

2. Development and Application of Small Animal Models of Thrombosis in the Discovery of Novel Antithrombotic Agents

Although each occurrence of thrombotic disease may reveal somewhat unique etiology, the general understanding of the pathophysiology of thrombosis has not changed dramatically since the observation of Virchow in 1856 *(11)*. Thus, the components of Virchow's triad—namely vessel injury, hypercoagulability of the blood, and obstruction of blood flow—remain the predominant factors believed to be responsible for thrombotic episodes. Many models of thrombotic disease have been introduced that focus on one, two, or all of these factors in combination. Indeed, the ability to isolate one factor and study the mechanisms by which that factor contributes to thrombosis is a strong argument for performing in vitro experiments in which individual components (e.g., coagulation enzymes or platelets) can be studied in detail. However, these in vitro results are often difficult to correlate with in vivo results because they cannot mimic the myriad of hemodynamic and localized cellular and molecular interactions that occur during the generation, propagation, and lysis of thrombi in vivo. In addition, the potential side effects, caused either to the expected pharmacology of the drug (e.g., bleeding diatheses) or by an unexpected effect (e.g., hypotension or thrombocytopenia) require the evaluation of novel antithrombotic agents in animal models of thrombosis prior to testing in humans.

The modern drug discovery process generally consists of target identification, high-throughput screening, and/or chemical optimization by rational, molecular modeling-aided drug design, and the evaluation of select compounds in animal models of disease. Throughout the process, a decision tree, flowchart, or testing funnel is employed to winnow from the thousands of compounds a diminishingly smaller portion, which receives greater attention and undergoes intensified evaluation, notably in vivo testing. New technologies in combinatorial chemistry are capable of generating huge numbers of compounds that can be evaluated quickly for in vitro activity against the targeted mechanism by automated high-throughput screening. In vitro analysis initially provides potency and selectivity data for the desired target and eliminates the vast majority of compounds from further testing. Antithrombotic agents that meet the specified potency and selectivity criteria are evaluated further in human plasma using in vitro clotting assays such as activated partial thromboplastin time (aPTT) or prothrombin time (PT)—or, in the case of antiplatelet agents—by platelet aggregation tests. These tests are often referred to as "functional" tests because they monitor clot formation or platelet aggregation, as opposed to isolated enzyme activity or receptor binding. The compounds that meet predetermined potency criteria in these functional assays are then evaluated for in vitro anti-coagulant activity using plasma obtained from the species that will be used for efficacy testing in vivo. As discussed in detail here, some compounds have demonstrated marked species-specificity *(12)*, so it is important to evaluate the activity in vitro using plasma from the chosen species prior to evaluating the compounds in animal models in vivo.

If the in vitro functional assay results using rodent plasma are acceptable, rodents are usually chosen for primary in vivo evaluation of compounds. Several factors make rodents desirable for primary evaluation of compounds. First, their small size decreases the amount of compound required for testing, and the lower cost of acquisition and housing minimizes the investment. Second, the ease of handling and the ability to perform multiple experiments simultaneously increases efficiency, providing important information quickly in order to decide which compounds will be advanced to the next stage. Also, many animal models of thrombosis have been developed for rodents, so there are many detailed techniques as well as a large body of data in the scientific literature to help guide the investigator and reduce the number of experiments needed to provide useful information. Finally, the primary evaluation of new compounds in rats can also include a preliminary evaluation of the hemodynamic effects of the drug. Measurements of heart rate and blood pressure are relatively easy to obtain, and can be very useful in quickly eliminating a compound or a series of compounds from further evaluation.

2.1. Ferric Chloride-Induced Carotid-Artery Thrombosis

Rodents have been used extensively in the primary evaluation of novel coagulation Factor Xa (FXa) inhibitors. RPR120844 and RPR208566 were initially evaluated for efficacy in the carotid-artery ferric chloride-induced thrombosis model *(13,14)*. This model elicits acute thrombus formation by chemical damage to the vessel wall via topical administration of $FeCl_3$.

2.2. Venous Thrombosis

For antithrombotic efficacy on the venous side, several compounds were evaluated using methods that induce stasis of blood in the inferior vena cava (IVC) *(15,16)*. In this model, a section of the IVC is isolated and ligated so that the stasis in this region promotes thrombus generation. Thrombus formation can be accelerated by administering a thrombogenic substance such as FXa or tissue factor (TF) directly into the stasis region.

2.3. Arteriovenous Shunt Model

An arteriovenous shunt model, which results in the formation of a "mixed" thrombus (platelet and fibrin-dependent), has been utilized by numerous investigators. A polyethylene tube of varying diameter and length, containing a thread or other thrombogenic surface, is placed in-line between the carotid artery and the jugular vein *(15–22)* in rats or rabbits. After a specified time, the thrombus is removed and weighed, or the protein content of the thrombus is determined. All of these models use thrombus mass as a primary end point, and some of the models provide a flow readout that indicates the time required to produce a completely occlusive thrombus (e.g., time-to-occlusion). The flow parameter requires specialized equipment and added experimental preparation time, so these factors should be carefully considered when selecting and optimizing a model.

2.4. Disseminated Intravascular Coagulation

Another model that is also used widely in rats and mice is a model of systemic thrombosis or disseminated intravascular coagulation (DIC), which is induced by TF, endotoxin (lipopolysaccharide), or FXa *(16,23,24)*. After systemic administration of the thrombogenic stimulus, this model can be performed with or without mechanical vena caval stasis. When stasis is used, the major parameter is the thrombus mass, but when stasis is not used, the readouts are fibrin degradation products, fibrinogen, platelet count, PT, and aPTT, among others. As shown by the many and varied parameters, when used without stenosis, the postexperimental analysis can be time-consuming and technically demanding. Although rodents are useful as a primary efficacy model, limitations such as the ability to withdraw multiple blood samples over the course of the experiment and the difference in activity of at least some FXa inhibitors in human compared to rat plasma in vitro require that compounds be characterized further in more advanced in vivo models of thrombosis.

2.5. Wessler Rabbit Model

Generally, after initial evaluation in rodent models proves that a compound is efficacious, other models of thrombosis using larger animals are employed to confirm and extend the rodent results. For the evaluation of novel FXa inhibitors, rabbit models have been extensively used. The Wessler model *(25)* is relatively simple and highly reproducible, and, most importantly, rabbit and human FXa appear to have similar binding affinity to the FXa enzyme substrate and to small-molecule inhibitors of FXa *(12)*. Further evidence supporting the use of rabbits to characterize FXa inhibitors is that the FXa cleavage site resulting in the formation of meizothrombin is identical in rabbit and human prothrombin *(26)*. Another advantage of rabbit over the rat models is that multiple blood samples can be obtained from the rabbit without compromising the hemodynamic system. Most models of venous thrombosis in rabbits are modifications of the Wessler model, in which a stasis is produced in the jugular vein and a thrombogenic substance, such as thrombin or thromboplastin, is placed in the stasis "pouch" (either before the initiation of stasis by infusing the substance intravenously, or by injecting the thrombogenic substance directly into the "pouch" via a side-branch vessel after the stasis is employed). These Wessler-type rabbit models have been used to characterize novel FXa inhibitors *(16,27)*. FXa inhibitors have also been shown to be effective in this model when endothelial damage in the stasis region is produced chemically, resulting in a surface that promotes thrombus formation and growth *(28)*. In addition, a rabbit model of arteriovenous shunt thrombosis has also been used extensively to evaluate the antithrombotic efficacy of FXa inhibitors *(17,29–32)*. Wong et al. *(31)* used the arteriovenous shunt model to demonstrate that the in vitro potency of FXa inhibitors is significantly correlated with their antithrombotic efficacy in vivo. These data provided important information regarding the contribution of selective FXa inhibition to the antithrombotic effect of drugs evaluated in this model.

2.6. Thrombin-Induced Rabbit Femoral-Artery Thrombosis

Localized thrombosis can also be produced in rabbit peripheral blood vessels such as the femoral artery by injection of thrombin, calcium chloride, and fresh blood via a side branch *(33)*.

Either femoral artery is isolated distal to the inguinal ligament and traumatized distally from the lateral circumflex artery by rubbing the artery with the jaws of forceps. An electromagnetic flow probe is placed distal to the lateral circumflex artery to monitor femoral-artery blood flow (FABF) (**Fig. 1**). The superficial epigastric artery is cannulated for induction of the thrombus and subsequent infusion of thrombolytic agents. Localized thrombi distal to the lateral circumflex artery with snares approx 1 cm apart are induced by the sequential injection of thrombin, $CaCl_2$ (1.25 mmol), and a volume of blood sufficient to distend the artery. After 30 min, the snares are released and FABF is monitored for 30 mm to confirm total obstruction of flow by the thrombus.

These models are not appropriate for evaluating drugs for their ability to inhibit original thrombosis. However, the model is particularly appropriate for evaluating thrombolytic agents and adjunctive therapies—e.g., for their ability to hasten and/or enhance lysis or prevent acute reocclusion after discontinuing administration of a thrombolytic agent.

3. Development and Application of Large Animal Models of Thrombosis in the Discovery of Novel Antithrombotic Agents

More advanced experimental models, which are reserved for compounds that have successfully met the efficacy and safety criteria established for rodent and

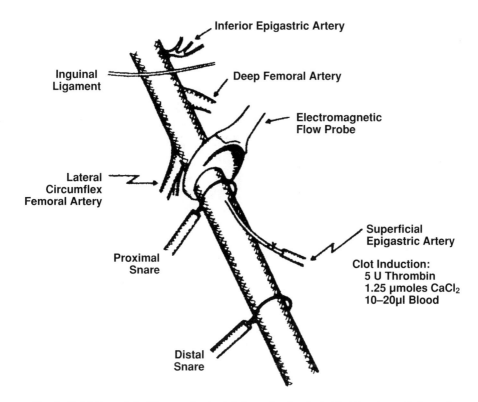

Fig. 1. Rabbit model of femoral arterial thrombosis. A clot is introduced into an isolated segment of femoral artery by injection of thrombin, $CaCl_2$, and whole blood. After aging for 1 h, t-PA is infused. Reperfusion is assessed by restoration of blood flow.

rabbit models, include canine, porcine, and nonhuman primate thrombosis models. These models are obviously more costly, have a slower turnaround time to achieve statistically significant results, and require careful design considerations in order to minimize the number of animals used.

3.1. Folts Coronary Thrombosis Model

In 1976 Folts and colleagues *(34)* described a model of repetitive thrombus formation, or cyclic flow reductions (CFRs), in stenosed coronary arteries of open-chest, anesthetized dogs **(Fig. 2)**. This model is also applicable to the rabbit femoral or carotid artery *(35)*. Using this model, several groups have described the antithrombotic effects of a variety of drugs, primarily prostaglandin-inhibitory, prostacyclin-mimetics, or fibrinogen-receptor antagonists *(36–42)*. The combination of two thrombogenic stimuli leads to the development of CFRs in this model: severe, concentric stenosis and focal, intimal injury. With few exceptions, CFRs will not develop unless both stimuli exist.

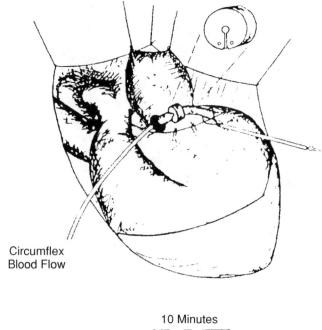

Circumflex
Blood Flow

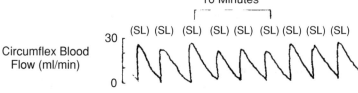

10 Minutes

(SL) (SL) (SL) (SL) (SL) (SL) (SL) (SL) (SL)

Circumflex Blood
Flow (ml/min)

30

0

Fig. 2. Technique for monitoring platelet aggregation in the partially obstructed left circumflex coronary artery of the dog. Elecetromagnetic flow probes measure blood flow iii nil/mm. Partial obstruction of the coronary artery with a plastic Lexan cylinder results in episodic cyclical reductions in coronary blood flow that are caused by platelet-dependent thrombus formation. Every 2–3 mm the thrombus must he mechanically shaken loose (SL) to restore blood.

The rheological conditions required to produce turbulence and stasis upon vessel narrowing dictate that lumenal diameter must be reduced by at least 50%. Two- to 3-mm long constrictors are cut from Lexan® rods readily available from local plastics distributors. One center hole of varying diameter(s) and two smaller collar holes are drilled, into which the prongs of snap-ring pliers fit to spread the constrictor's slit in the top-central portion to apply or remove them. Other plastics will suffice, but Lexan is ideal because of its strength and resiliency. Both circumflex and left anterior descending (LAD) coronary arteries have been used in this model. Aside from personal preferences, we know of no physiologic basis for preferring one to the other.

Because of the prominent autoregulation of the coronary circulation, it is difficult to evaluate the severity of a stenosis on the basis of changes in basal coronary blood flow (CBF). However, the robust reactive hyperemia (RH) characteristic of the coronary circulation provides a powerful tool with which to gauge the severity of the stenosis. With gradual narrowing, basal CBF will remain unchanged or decline negligibly, whereas the RH will begin to decline more quickly as the vasodilatory reserve of downstream vessels is progressively exhausted. Reduction of lumenal diameter to this degree is required if one wishes to produce CFRs in a high percentage (e.g., >90%) of dogs. It is also critical if one wishes to compare two or more drugs in this model and draw meaningful conclusions about drug effects. Inasmuch as the severity of the stenosis is an important component of the thrombogenic stimulus, then comparable and uniform degrees of constriction between treatment groups are required, preferably those in which basal CBF is reduced between 10% and 25% and the RH is abolished, or nearly so. It is important to apply these criteria when one is investigating a drug that possesses vasodilatory effects or one with a pharmacologic profile that is not completely known. Without exhaustion of the vasodilatory reserve (as evidenced by abolition of the RH), elimination of CFRs could result (at least partly) from coronary vasodilation. One difficulty in using the RH or basal-flow reduction immediately after placing a constrictor on the coronary artery is that CBF starts to decline quickly as platelets accumulate at the site of stenosis and intimal injury. Thus, one needs to evaluate the degree of flow reduction immediately after constricting the artery. Delaying this assessment will result in an overestimation of the stenosis severity because of the accumulation of platelets on the vessel lining. Alternatively, the degree of stenosis can be ascertained by applying the constrictor before denuding the artery, in which case the constrictor (or constrictors) must be removed and reapplied.

After damaging and stenosing the coronary artery sufficiently, CBF starts declining immediately, reaching zero within 4–12 min and remaining there until blood flow is restored by manually shaking loose the thrombus ("SL"; *see* **Fig. 2**, *bottom*). This is usually accomplished by either flicking the Lexan constrictor or sliding the constrictor up and down the artery to mechanically dislodge the thrombus. Spontaneous flow restorations occur in three circumstances: i) nonsevere conditions (e.g., minimal stenosis or de-endothelialization); ii) waning CFRs (which can occur as late as 30–45 mm after establishing CFRs); and/or iii) administration of a partially effective antithrombotic agent.

Although the influence of blood pressure on the rate of formation of occlusive thrombi or their stability has not been studied systematically, one might predict that higher arterial pressures would increase the deceleration of CBF to zero by enhancing platelet aggregation through increased shear forces and increased delivery of platelets to the growing thrombus. Higher arterial pressure also might increase the propensity for spontaneous flow restorations before an occlusive thrombus is formed, because of greater stress on the nascent, unconsolidated thrombus.

Several groups have histologically examined the coronary arteries harvested from dogs undergoing CFRs usually when CBF is declining or has ceased. Extensive intimal injury, including de-endothelialization with adherent platelets and/or microthrombi, is consistently observed. Arteries harvested when CBF is zero invariably reveal a platelet-rich thrombus filling the stenotic segment *(34,36,40,43)*. These histological observations, coupled with the pattern of gradual, progressive declines in CBF and abrupt increases thereof (whether spontaneous or deliberate) provide further evidence that CFRs are caused primarily by platelet thrombi, not vasoconstriction.

Although the primary cause of CFRs is platelet aggregation, it is possible that local vasospasm and/or vasoconstriction downstream from the site of thrombosis are induced by vasoactive mediators released by activated and/or aggregating platelets. Experimental evidence supporting vasoconstriction just downstream from the stenosis during CFRs has been demonstrated *(44)*.

Further evidence for platelet-dependent thrombus formation in the etiology of CFRs is derived from the pharmacological profile of this model. In general, platelet-inhibitory agents consistently abolish or attenuate CFRs, whereas vasodilators (e.g., nitroglycerin, calcium entry blockers, and papaverine) affect them negligibly *(45)*. Aspirin was the first described inhibitor of CFRs *(34)*. However, in subsequent studies, its effects on CFRs were found to be variable and dose-dependent *(39)*. Variability in the response to aspirin may be related to the severity of the stenosis, as further tightening of the constrictor after an effective dose of aspirin or ibuprofen usually restores CFRs.

Prostacyclin, a powerful antiaggregatory and potent coronary vasodilatory product of endothelial arachidonic acid metabolism, is extremely efficacious and potent in abolishing CFRs. Notably, different drug classes can be compared, as evidenced by the wide range of percentages of responders *(43)*.

Advances in platelet physiology and pharmacology have identified a new class of antiplatelet agents that block the platelet membrane glycoprotein IIb/IIIa (GPIIb/IIIa) receptor and thus fibrinogen binding. Fibrinogen binding between platelets is an obligate event in aggregation and is initiated by blood-borne platelet agonists such as adenosine diphosphate (ADP), serotonin, thrombin, epinephrine, and collagen *(46)*. The tripeptide sequence Arg-Gly-Asp (RGD), which occurs twice in the $A\alpha$-chain of fibrinogen, is believed to mediate, at least in part, the binding of fibrinogen to the GP IIb/IIIa complex.

Early experimental results with GPIIb/IIIa antagonists in studies by Coller et al. *(47)* and Bush *(41)* and Shebuski *(42,48)* demonstrated that fibrinogen-receptor antagonists are as effective as prostacyclin as anti-aggregatory and antithrombotic agents and do not possess the hemodynamic liabilities associated with prostaglandin-based compounds. Monoclonal antibodies (MAbs) directed against the platelet fibrinogen-receptor (abciximab) are essentially irreversible, whereas RGD- (tirofiban) or KGD- (eptifibatide)-based fibrinogen receptor antagonists are reversible, their effects dissipating within hours after discontinuation of an iv infusion.

The prominence of platelet aggregation vis-à-vis coagulation mechanisms in the Folts model is evidenced by the lack of effect of heparin and thrombin inhibitors reported by most investigators *(34,39)*. However, heparin and MCI-9038, a thrombin inhibitor, were reported to abolish CFRs in about two-thirds of dogs with recently (30 mm) established CFRs, but not in those extant after 3 h *(49)*. The explanation for the differential effects of heparin is not immediately apparent. It may be related to the severity of the stenosis used. The apparent discrepancy in observations could be related to inhibition of thrombin-stimulated platelet activation and/or aggregation.

One attractive feature of the Folts model is its amenability to dose-response studies. Unlike other models in which the thrombotic processes are dynamic, occurring over a period of several minutes to hours, CFRs in the Folts model are repetitive and remarkably unchanging. In the many dogs that received either no intervention or vehicle 1 h after initiating CFRs, flow patterns remained unchanged for at least another hour *(40)*. Thus, one can evaluate several doses of an investigational drug in a single dog. We and others have exploited this to determine potencies, an important basis of comparison between drugs with similar mechanisms of action, thus underscoring another feature of the model: its amenability to quantification of drug response. Two methods for quantifying drug effects in this model have been described.

Aiken et al. *(36)* first described a four-point scoring scheme to evaluate and compare different doses or drugs, ranging from 0 (no effect on CFRs) to 3 (fully effective; complete abolition of CFRs). Intermediate scores of 1 and 2 were respectively applied when the CFR frequency was slowed (but occlusive thrombi still occurred) and when non-occlusive, spontaneously embolizing thrombi were observed. One advantage of this system is the provision of a single number for each evaluation period. A disadvantage is that agents that decrease systemic blood pressure (e.g., prostacyclin) will also decrease coronary perfusion pressure; the coronary flow pattern will be affected, making the scoring system somewhat more subjective.

Another method of quantifying CFRs, described by Bush et al. *(40)*, addresses the frequency—expressed on a per hour basis—and severity—based on the average nadir of CBF before a flow restoration. This system is less subjective, but it produces two values per evaluation period, and combinations of the two in an effort to provide a single parameter are awkward. In practical terms, both methods for quantifying CFRs described here provide similar answers. The important point for both is consistency in scoring. This end is best served by well-defined and communicated criteria.

To date, the Folts model has been used only to evaluate antithrombotic drugs (**Table 1**). No description of this model for the evaluation of thrombolytic drugs or adjunctive agents has been made. However, preliminary data reveal these thrombi to be resistant to doses of thrombolytic agents that lyse thrombi in the other models *(50)*. Of all the models described in this chapter, the thrombi in this model are probably the most platelet-rich, and possess relatively less fibrin than—for example—the copper coil or wire models. However, it may be erroneous to conclude that these thrombi are devoid of fibrin, as the fibrinogen that links platelets during aggregation via the GPIIb/IIIa receptor is theoretically capable of undergoing fibrin formation.

Several investigators have shown that the same combination of severe vessel narrowing and de-endothelialization results in CFRs in arteries other than the coronary. We have elicited CFRs in femoral arteries in anesthetized dogs with similar degrees of vessel narrowing and deliberate denudation of the artery (unpublished observation). Folts et al. *(38)* have demonstrated that CFRs can be produced in conscious dogs with chronically implanted Lexan® coronary constrictors and flow probes. CFRs were prevented in the interim between implantation and acute study by the administration of aspirin. Al-Wathiqui *(51)* and Gallagher *(52)* and colleagues have demonstrated that progressive carotid or coronary arterial narrowing with ameroid constrictors will result in CFRs in a period of days to weeks after surgical implantation. These dogs apparently did not undergo deliberate vessel denudation at the time of implantation. Perhaps focal inflammation developed in the intervening week(s) between surgery and the development of CFRs in these animals. Alternatively, there was sufficient intimal vessel injury during implantation of the ameroid constrictors to induce development of CFRs at a later time. CFRs have also been elicited in the renal *(53)* and carotid *(54)* arteries of cynomolgus monkeys.

Eidt et al. *(55)* showed that conscious dogs equipped with the same constrictors over segments of the LAD showing endothelial injury undergo repetitive CFRs in response to exercise, but not ventricular pacing. The frequency and severity of CFRs varied more in this model. Some CFRs were nonocclusive. CFRs of most dogs eventually deteriorated to persistent no- or low-flow states. Unlike the open-chest preparation, flow restorations observed in this model occurred spontaneously. Also, the severity of the stenosis produced by Eidt et al. *(55)* was not as great as that produced by most practitioners of the Folts model, as reflected by the ability of CBF to increase above control levels initially during exercise.

Table 1
Animal Models of Thrombosis and their Clinical Correlates

Compound	Preclinical animal model	Preclinical results	References	Clinical indication	Clinical result	References
Recombinant t-PA (Activase)	Rabbit pulmonary-artery thrombosis	Lysis of preformed pulmonary thrombus	Matsuo et al., 1981	AMI thrombolysis	Improved recanalization	Collen et al., 1984
Abciximab (ReoPro)	Canine coronary CFR (Folts et al., 1991)	Significant inhibition of platelet-dependent thrombosis	Coller et al., 1986.	High-risk coronary angioplasty	Reduction in death, MI, refractory ischemia, or unplanned revascularization	EPIC Investigators, 1994
Tirofiban (Aggrestat)	Canine coronary CFR (Folts et al., 1991)	Significant inhibition of platelet-dependent thrombus	Lynch et al., 1995	Unstable angina	Reduction in death, MI, refractory ischemia	PRISM Investigators, 1998
Eptifibitide (Integrilin)	TPA-induced coronary thrombolysis	Significant improvement in lysis of occlusive thrombus	Nicolini et 1994	Acute myocardial infarction—thrombolysis with tPA	Improvement in incidence and speed of reperfusion	Ohman et al., 1997
Enoxaparin (Lovenox)	Canine coronary CFR (Folts et al., 1991)	Significant inhibition of platelet-dependent	Leadley et al., 1998	Unstable Angina	Significant decrease in death, MI, and need for revascularization at 30 d	Cohen et al., 1998
Hirudin (Refludan)	Rabbit jugular vein thrombus growth	Inhibition of thrombus growth compared to standard heparin	Agnelli et al., 1990	Deep venous thrombosis after total hip replacement	Significantly decreased rate of DVT	Eriksson et al., 1997
	Porcine deep-caroitid artery injury	Prevented mural thrombosis	Heras et al., 1990	Unstable angina or AMI	Superior to heparin in reducing endpoints of death, MI, and refractory angina	OASIS-2, 1999
Argatroban	Canine coronary-artery electrolytic-injury (TPA-induced thrombolysis)	Accelerated reperfusion and prevented reocclusion	Fitzgerald et al., 1989	Unstable angina	No episodes of MI during drug infusion	Gold et al., 1993

In summary, the Folts model of platelet-dependent thrombus formation is a well-established method to determine the pharmacology of antithrombotic agents. It represents an excellent choice for initial evaluation of antiplatelet activity in vivo, regardless of the artery used. Qualitatively, the thrombogenic stimuli in the Folts model and those responsible for unstable angina may be similar, since involvement by platelets has clearly been demonstrated in the model and is strongly suspect clinically. However, it should be remembered that flow restorations in the Folts model require vigorous shaking. In contrast, unstable angina is not believed to involve persistent, total thrombotic coronary occlusion. On the basis of the model's pharmacological profile, the thrombi in this model also do not appear to resemble those usually responsible for AMI, as the former appear to be unresponsive to thrombolytic agents. The preliminary observations that either streptokinase (SK) or tissue plasminogen activator (t-PA) do not lyse thrombi in the Folts model contrasts with the 50–75% response rate to thrombolytic therapy in patients with evolving MI *(50)*. However, it is tempting to speculate that the platelet-rich thrombi produced in this model are more like thrombi in those patients whose coronary arteries are not reopened by even early intervention and/or high doses of t-PA *(56)*, and thus could represent a model of "thrombolytic-resistant" coronary thrombosis.

3.2. Copper Coil-Induced Canine Arterial Thrombosis

Blair et al. *(57)* reported on the ability of spiral wires constructed of aluminum-magnesium alloy inserted into the coronary circulation of dogs to produce slowly developing occlusive thrombi. In this early description of the technique, the spiral was inserted through the coronary-vessel wall in open-chest dogs. Several years later, Kordenat et al. *(58)* described a modification of this model, and the salient feature was insertion of the thrombogenic coils via the left carotid artery under fluoroscopic guidance in closed-chest dogs. Subsequent studies by Cercek et al. *(59)* and Bergmann *(60)* and colleagues used this basic experimental method for producing arterial thrombi to evaluate thrombolysis and the utility of reperfusion.

As described by Kordenat et al. *(58)* and Bergmann et al. *(60)*, a thrombogenic coil is advanced via the left carotid artery into a coronary artery with the aid of a hollow guiding catheter and a smaller inner catheter or guide wire in closed-chest dogs. Occlusive thrombosis, heralded by electrocardiographic signs of ischemia and confirmed by the development of a filling defect distal to the coil, occurs in a period of minutes to hours, depending on the composition (alloy) and size of the coil. Ventricular fibrillation (VF) occurs in approximately one of five dogs that undergo coronary thrombosis. Although some of these dogs can be converted to sinus rhythm by DC countershock, most die. There is no firm evidence that anti-arrhythmic agents effectively prevent or attenuate the frequency of VF. Another disadvantage of the model is the requirement for expensive fluoroscopic equipment to insert the coil into the coronary circulation. Not all investigators have such equipment at their disposal.

A femoral arterial version of this model in anesthetized dogs was described by Bush and colleagues (*61*). It uses the same thrombogenic coils, but does not require fluoroscopy. With Doppler flow probes placed directly on the femoral artery just proximal to the site of thrombosis, it allows the exact moment of thrombosis and thrombolysis to be detected, and the extent of blood-flow restoration after lysis to be monitored continuously and accurately (**Fig. 3**). One attractive feature of this model is the ability to perform the procedure in smaller dogs, which saves expensive thrombolytic agents or investigational adjunctive drugs. Moreover, use of the femoral artery enables the model to be adapted to smaller animals such as rabbits (*62*).

Of the four models discussed in this chapter, this model may be the least attractive from the standpoint of the thrombogenic stimulus resembling the human pathophysiology of MI. However, it may be no less relevant to the human situation than the other three in its degree of thrombogenicity and response to thrombolytic agents. A particularly attractive feature of the model is the uniform time to original thrombus formation, thrombolysis, and reocclusion (*60–62*).

In the femoral artery model, thrombotic occlusion consistently occurs within 10–12 min after insertion, following a flow pattern that suggests gradual platelet accumulation, and leading in turn to a progressively narrowing stenosis within the coil. Occasionally, spontaneous flow restorations similar to those seen in the Folts and electrical stimulation models precede total occlusion, but this occurs rarely (in approx 10% of dogs).

Thrombi produced in the coil model are considered to be relatively platelet-poor and fibrin-rich, on the basis of the model's pharmacologic profile. Clinically relevant doses of t-PA and SK lyse these thrombi (*60,63,64*), and heparin prolongs (but does not prevent) original thrombosis (*58,65*). However, histological examination of thrombi removed from copper coils 15 mm after occlusive thrombus formation reveals a platelet-rich thrombus that also contains red blood cells and fibrin (*61*).

The model's amenability to thrombolytic agents and the inability of several anti-platelet agents—which abolish CFRs in the Folts model—to prevent or delay thrombosis support this notion. Another interpretation, however, is that these models differ in their degree of thrombogenicity, rather than having qualitatively different thrombogenic stimuli. Echistatin, the RDG-containing snake venom peptide with no known anticoagulant effects, prevented original thrombosis in four of five dogs (*41*).

Certain methodological factors can greatly influence the nature of thrombi in this model. The speed with which the copper coil is inserted to its destina-

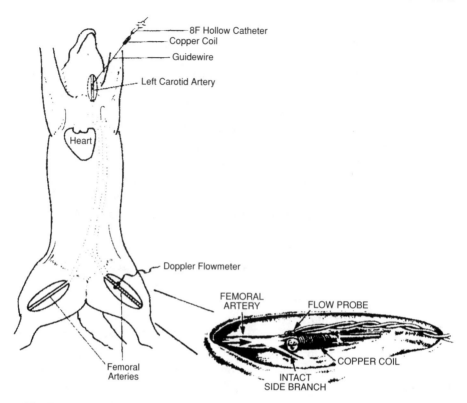

Fig. 3. Schematic diagram of the canine femoral artery copper coil model of thrombolysis. A thrombogenic copper coil is advanced to either femoral artery via the left carotid artery. By virtue of the favorable anatomical angles of attachment, a hollow polyurethane catheter advanced down the left carotid artery nearly always enters the descending aorta, and with further advancement, into either femoral artery without fluoroscopic guidance. A flexible, Teflon-coated guidewire is then inserted through the hollow catheter and the latter is removed. A copper coil is then slipped over the guidewire and advanced to the femoral artery (*see inset*). Femoral artery flow velocity is measured directly and continuously with a Doppler flow probe placed just proximal to the thrombogenic coil and distal to a prominent sidebranch, which is left patent to dissipate any dead space between the coil and the next proximal sidebranch. Femoral artery blood flow declines progressively to total occlusion over the next 10–12 mm after coil insertion.

tion may contribute significantly to the differences in the relative contribution by platelets between the femoral and coronary models, and thus to different results between investigators. We have inserted copper coils into the LAD (under fluoroscopic guidance) and femoral arteries *(61)*. Moreover, we have observed more varied and shorter average times to occlusion in the coronary model. Sometimes a filling defect is observed immediately after coil placement, presumably because of "snow-plowing" by the coil of clotted blood on the guidewire during its passage to the coronary artery. Golino et al. *(63)*, who inserted copper coils into coronary arteries of dogs under fluoroscopy, reported occlusion times ranging from 0 to 12 min, with an average of 2 ± 1 min; compare this with the longer and more consistent 10–12 min observed in the femoral-artery model *(61)*.

Another technical aspect worth noting is the geometry and composition of the coil. Kordenat and Kezdi *(6)* observed times to occlusion exceeding 2 h, with shorter coils containing fewer spirals. Aluminum and magnesium alloys appear to be less thrombogenic than copper coils, as signs of infarction did not appear until 24–48 h after placement of coils or spirals constructed of these metals *(57,58)*.

Because the coils fit snugly against the vessel lining and the wall of the coil possesses some thickness, strictly speaking, a stenosis is produced. However, experience in our laboratory suggests that it is minor, as blood flow immediately after coil insertion usually is decreased slightly *(61)*. The coil lumen narrows quickly with progressive thrombus formation. The extent to which vessel-wall injury immediately subjacent to the coil contributes to thrombus formation is unknown. Intimal injury of the artery proximal to the coil as a result of insertion probably occurs; its contribution to thrombosis and/or thrombolysis is unknown.

The original description of this model for the study of thrombolytic agents and their influence on myocardial injury was by Bergmann et al. *(64)*, who demonstrated that timely reperfusion with intracoronary SK salvaged myocardium and metabolic function. Subsequent studies from that group with this model demonstrated the ability of t-PA to lyse thrombi *(60)*. Bush et al. *(61)* and van der Werf et al. *(65)* have demonstrated a dose-response with t-PA and pro-urokinase, respectively, in this model.

In contrast to the Folts model, the copper coil model has been used almost exclusively for the evaluation of either thrombolytic agents or adjunctive drugs *(59,60,62–66)*. However, we have evaluated several potential antiplatelet and anticoagulant agents for their ability to prevent or delay original thrombosis after coil insertion. In our laboratory, heparin doubled the time to occlusive thrombosis, but the only agent that delayed thrombus formation significantly was the RGD-containing snake venom, echistatin *(41)*. In these studies, the peptide was infused via a proximal femoral artery catheter at a rate calculated to achieve a plasma concentration of about 0.2 μM. Neither aspirin (25 mg/kg p.o. every 12 h starting 24 h before the acute study) nor a selective TXA_2-receptor antagonist extended the time to original thrombosis significantly. Heparin (100 U/kg plus 1.5 U/kg/min) doubled the time to thrombus formation but did not prevent it. MCI-9038, a synthetic, selective thrombin inhibitor, was variably effective in delaying original thrombosis, but very effective in preventing reocclusion after t-PA induced thrombolysis (66). Although echistatin was more effective than MC-9038 in delaying or preventing original thrombosis, the opposite order of efficacy held for reocclusion after discontinuing t-PA. These observations led us to believe that the thrombogenic stimulus responsible for original occlusion and reocclusion after thrombolysis differ qualitatively or quantitatively. L-670,596 a potent TXA_2-receptor antagonist, with or without ketanserin, a selective serotonin$_2$-receptor antagonist, did not significantly delay reocclusion after stopping t-PA (66). Different results were observed by Golino et al. (63), who reported that the combination of a serotonin$_2$-receptor antagonist and TXA_2-receptor antagonist (but neither agent alone) delayed reocclusion after t-PA-induced thrombolysis in dogs with coronary thrombosis induced by copper coils.

3.3. Thrombin-Induced Clot Formation in the Canine Coronary Artery

A canine model of thrombin-induced clot formation was developed by Gold et al. (67) in which localized coronary thrombosis was produced in the LAD. This is a variation of the technique described by Collen et al. (68) who used radioactively labeled fibrinogen to monitor the occurrence and extent of thrombolysis of rabbit jugular-vein clots. The vessel was intentionally de-endothelialized by external compression with blunt forceps. Snare occluders were then placed proximal and distal to the damaged site, and thrombin (10 U) was injected into the isolated LAD segment in a small volume via a previously isolated side branch. Autologous blood (0.3–0.4 mL) mixed with calcium chloride (0.05 M) was also injected into the isolated LAD segment, producing a stasis-type red clot superimposed on an injured blood vessel. The snares were released 2–5 min later, and total occlusion was confirmed by selective coronary angiography.

This model of coronary-artery thrombosis relies on the conversion of fibrinogen to fibrin by thrombin. The fibrin-rich thrombus contains platelets, but at no greater concentration than in a similar volume of whole blood. Once the thrombus is formed, it is allowed to age for 1–2 h, after which a thrombolytic agent can be administered to lyse the thrombus and restore blood flow.

In the initial study described by Gold et al. (67) in 1984, recombinant t-PA was characterized for its ability to lyse 2-h-old thrombi. Then, tPA was infused at doses of 4.3, 10, and 25 µg/kg/min (iv) and resulted in reperfusion times of 40, 31, and 13 min, respectively. Thus, in this model of canine coronary thrombosis, t-PA exhibited dose-dependent coronary thrombolysis. Furthermore, it is possible to study the effect of different doses of t-PA on parameters of systemic fibrinolytic activation, such as fibrinogen, plasminogen, and α_2-antiplasmin, as well as to evaluate myocardial infarct size. For example, Kopia et al. *(69)* demonstrated that SK elicited dose-dependent thrombolysis in this model.

Subsequently, Gold et al. *(70,71)* modified the model to study reperfusion as well as acute reocclusion. Clinically, reocclusion is a persistent problem after effective coronary thrombolysis, which is reported to occur in 15–45% of patients *(72)*. Thus, an animal model of coronary reperfusion and reocclusion would be important from the standpoint of evaluating adjunctive therapies to t-PA to hasten and/or increase the response rate to thrombolysis and to prevent acute reocclusion.

The model of thrombin-induced clot formation in the canine coronary artery was modified so that a controlled high-grade stenosis was produced with an external constrictor. Blood flow was monitored with an electromagnetic flow probe. In this model of clot formation with superimposed stenosis, reperfusion in response to t-PA occurs with subsequent reocclusion *(70)*. The MAb against the human GPIIb/IIIa receptor developed by Coller et al. *(73)* and tested in combination with t-PA in the canine thrombosis model hastened t-PA-induced thrombolysis and prevented acute reocclusion *(70,74)*. These actions in vivo were accompanied by the abolition of ADP-induced platelet aggregation and markedly prolonged bleeding time.

3.4. Injury-Induced (Electrolytic) Arterial Thrombosis in the Canine

A novel technique for inducing arterial thrombosis was introduced by Salazar *(75)* in which anodal current was delivered to the intravascular lumen of a coronary artery in the dog via a stainless-steel electrode. The electrode was positioned under fluoroscopic control, which somewhat complicated the procedure. Subsequently, Romson et al. *(76)* modified the procedure so that the electrode was placed directly into the coronary artery of an open-chest, anesthetized dog. This technique then allows one to produce a thrombus in the anesthetized animal or to close the chest after inserting the electrode and allow the animal to recover, after which thrombosis can be elicited later in the conscious animal. The advantage of this modification is that it allows induction of thrombus formation without the need for fluoroscopy.

The stimulation electrode is constructed from a 25- or 26-gauge stainless-steel hypodermic needle tip, which is attached to a 30-gauge Teflon-insulated silver-coated copper wire. Anodal current is delivered to the electrode via either a 9-V nickel cadmium battery with the anode connected in series to a 250,000-ohm potentiometer or with a Grass stimulator connected to a Grass constant current unit and a stimulus isolation unit. The cathode in both cases is placed into a subcutaneous (sc) site completing the circuit. The anodal current can be adjusted to deliver 50–200 μA. Anodal stimulation results in focal endothelial disruption, which in turn induces platelet adhesion and aggregation at the damaged site. This process is then followed by further platelet aggregation and consolidation, with the growing thrombus entrapping red blood cells.

A modification of the method of Romson et al. *(76)* involves placement onto the coronary artery of an external, adjustable occluder *(77)* to produce a fixed stenosis on the coronary artery. A flow probe to record CBF is placed on the proximal portion of the artery followed by the stimulation electrode, with the clamp being placed most distally **(Fig. 4)**. The degree of stenosis can then be controlled by adjusting the clamp. The resulting stenosis is produced in an effort to mimic the human pathophysiology of atherosclerotic coronary-artery disease, in which thrombolytic therapy restores CBF through a coronary artery with residual narrowing as a result of atherosclerotic plaque formation.

Another modification of the electrical stimulation model that merits discussion is described by Benedict et al. *(78)*. They discontinued anodal current when mean distal coronary flow velocity (measured with Doppler flowmetry) increased by approx 50%, reflecting disruption of normal axial flow by the growing thrombus. Occlusive thrombosis occurred within 1 h after stopping the current (2 h after starting the current). In these studies, coronary sinus plasma levels of serotonin—an index of intravascular platelet aggregation—were increased approx 20-fold just before occlusive thrombus formation. The results of these studies agree with others in showing that either proximal flow velocity or electromagnetically measured CBF decline trivially over the majority of the time period in which the thrombus is growing. The largest declines in (volume) flow occur over a small and terminal fraction of the period between initial vessel perturbation and final occlusion. During that interval, coronary lumenal area decreases rapidly and to a critical degree, as platelets accrue at the growing thrombus. The studies by Benedict et al. *(78)* demonstrate that this final phase of thrombosis can occur independently of electrical stimulation. This variation of the model may be attractive to those who wish to produce occlusive thrombosis without continued electrical stimulation.

Regardless of whether electrical stimulation is continued until occlusive thrombosis, there is another component to this model that has upside and downside potential—the opportunity for coronary vasoconstriction to occur. Although the incidence of Prinzmetal's angina is low, it is widely suspected that vasospasm superimposes on a primarily thrombotic event in unstable angina and MI. In studies by Van der Giessen et al. *(79)*, nifedipine was reported to increase the extent of CBF after plasmin-induced thrombolysis in a porcine model of electrically induced coronary thrombosis. In their model, the anodal stimulation was applied circumferentially to the exterior surface of the LAD, and an external constrictor was not used.

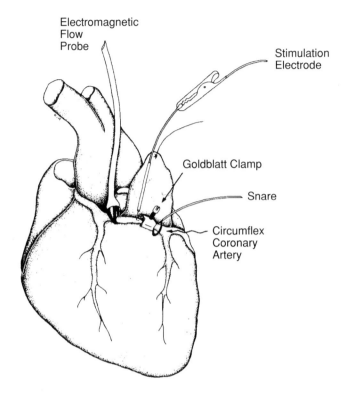

Fig. 4. Model of coronary artery thrombosis in the dog. Electrical injury to the intimal surface of the artery leads to occlusive thrombus formation. The thrombus is formed in the presence of a flow-limiting stenosis induced by a Goldblatt clamp. Upon spontaneous occlusion, heparin is administered and the clot is aged for 1 h before initiating the t-PA infusion.

Depending on the hypothesis being tested, the experimenter can leave intact or minimize this potential through the use or disuse of an external constrictor. As in the Folts and Gold coronary thrombo(ly)sis models, blood pressure must be taken into account or maintained within acceptable limits, since, in the presence of a critical stenosis, autoregulation no longer exists. Under these conditions, CBF is highly dependent on driving pressure (arterial pressure).

Numerous experimental studies evaluating anticoagulants, antithrombotic, and/or thrombolytic drugs have been performed using this model. In the initial report by Romson et al. *(76)*, the cyclooxygenase inhibitor ibuprofen was evaluated. Comparison of myocardial infarct size, thrombus weight, arrhythmia development, and scanning electron microscopy (SEM) of drug-treated and control animals indicated that ibuprofen protected against the deleterious effects of coronary-artery thrombosis in the conscious dog. Subsequent studies in the same model and laboratory evaluated the antithrombotic potential of various TXA$_2$ synthetase inhibitors, such as U 63557a, CGS 13080, OKY 1581, and dazoxiben. When the TXA$_2$ synthetase inhibitors were administered before induction of the current, OKY 1581 *(80)* and CGS 13080 *(81)* reduced the incidence of coronary thrombosis, whereas U 63557A *(82)* and dazoxiben *(83)* were ineffective and partially effective, respectively. The differences in efficacy noted among the TXA$_2$ synthetase inhibitors were ascribed to differences in potency and duration of action.

Other investigators have used this model to study the prevention of original coronary thrombosis in the dog. Fitzgerald et al. *(84)* studied the combination of the TXA$_2$ synthetase inhibitor, U 63557A, alone or in combination with L-636,499, an endoperoxide/thromboxane-receptor antagonist. U 63557A alone did not prevent coronary thrombosis when administered before current application, whereas the combination of U 63557A and L-636,499 was highly effective. These data suggest that prostaglandin endoperoxides may modulate the effects of TXA$_2$ synthetase inhibitors and that this response may be blocked by concurrent administration of an endoperoxide/thromboxane-receptor antagonist. The murine MAb to platelet GPIIb/IIIa (7E3) was studied in this model for its ability to prevent thrombus formation. At a dose of 0.8 mg/kg (iv), the 7E3 MAb completely prevented original thrombus formation *(85)*.

In addition to evaluation of antithrombotic (e.g., antiplatelet) agents, the electrical injury model is useful for studying anticoagulant FXa inhibitors, such as YM 60628 *(86)*, and thrombolytic drugs. When evaluating thrombolytic agents, the thrombus is allowed to form without drug intervention and then aged for various periods. Schumaker et al. *(77)* demonstrated that intracoronary streptokinase was an effective thrombolytic drug in the model, the thrombolytic effectiveness being augmented by the concurrent administration of heparin and prostacyclin, or by a TXA$_2$ synthetase inhibitor *(77)*. In other studies reported by Shebuski et al. *(87)*, the TXA$_2$ receptor antagonist, BM 13.177, hastened t-PA-induced thrombolysis and prevented acute thrombotic reocclusion. Van der Giessen et al. *(88)* subsequently demonstrated that BM 13.177 prevented original thrombus formation in 75% of pigs undergoing electrical stimulation as described here *(79)*; aspirin was ineffective in this porcine model. These and other studies underscore the potential for adjunctive therapy to hasten thrombolysis and/or prevent reocclusion, both contributing to greater salvage of ischemic myocardium.

Like the copper coil model, the electrical stimulation model has been used to produce experimental myocardial infarction (MI). Patterson et al. *(89)* have used this technique to produce coronary thrombosis in the left circumflex coronary artery (which supplies blood flow to the posterior LV wall in dogs) in dogs with a previous anterior wall infarct to mimic sudden cardiac death that occurs in people during a second (recurrent) MI or ischemic event.

This model has also been modified to demonstrate the efficacy of adjuncts to thrombolytic therapy *(91–94)*. In this case, the thrombus is allowed to extend until it completely occludes the vessel. Usually, the thrombus is allowed to stabilize, or "age," to mimic the clinical setting in which a time lag exists between the thrombotic event and the pharmacological intervention. At the end of the stabilization period, thrombolytic agents such as t-PA or streptokinase are administered in conjunction with the novel antithrombotic agent to lyse the thrombus and maintain vessel patency. The incidence and times of reperfusion and reocclusion are the major end points. These studies have established that recombinant tick anticoagulant peptide (rTAP), a potent and selective FXa inhibitor derived from the soft tick *(95)*, promotes rapid and prolonged reperfusion at doses that produce relatively minor elevations in PT, aPTT, and template bleeding time.

4. Extracorporeal Thrombosis Models

These models employ passing blood over a section of damaged vessel (or other selected substrates) and recording the thrombus accumulation on the damaged vessel histologically or by scintigraphic detection of radiolabeled platelets or fibrin *(97)*. This model is interesting because the results can be directly compared to the in vivo deep arterial injury model *(96)* results and to results from a similar extracorporeal model used in humans *(98,99)*. Dangus et al. *(98)* used this model to characterize the antithrombotic efficacy of abciximab, a MAb-based platelet glycoprotein IIb/IIIa inhibitor, after administration to patients undergoing percutaneous coronary intervention. They demonstrated that abciximab reduces both the platelet and fibrin components of the thrombus, thereby providing further insight into the unique long-term effectiveness of short-term administration of this drug. Orvim et al. *(99)* also used this model in humans to evaluate the antithrombotic efficacy of rTAP, but instead of evaluating the compound after administration of rTAP to the patient, the drug was mixed with the blood immediately as it flowed into the extracorporeal circuit prior to flowing over the thrombogenic surface. By changing the thrombogenic surface, they were able to determine that rTAP was more effective at inhibiting thrombus formation on a TF-coated surface compared to a collagen-coated surface. These results suggest that optimal antithrombotic efficacy requires an antiplatelet approach along with an anticoagulant. Although this model does not completely represent pathological intravascular thrombus formation, this "human model" of thrombosis may be very useful in developing new drugs because it directly evaluates the ex vivo antithrombotic effect of a drug in flowing human blood.

4.1. Arteriovenous Shunt Model in Baboons

Because of similarities between human and nonhuman primate blood clotting *(100)*, nonhuman primate thrombosis models are believed to be the best models to evaluate novel thrombotic agents prior to administration of the drug to humans in clinical trials. A well-established model of thrombosis in baboons has been used to evaluate numerous antithrombotic approaches. Briefly, a thrombogenic segment is placed in an exteriorized chronic arteriovenous shunt, blood is pumped at a specified shear rate through the segment, and the thrombus is quantified by deposition of radiolabeled platelets or fibrin on the segment *(101)*. Also, the segments can be easily removed and replaced with fresh segments so that a time-course or dose-response for the drug effect can be determined.

This model was used to evaluate SR90107A/ORG31540, a synthetic pentasaccharide that is a selective, antithrombin-III-dependent FXa inhibitor that has recently entered the marketplace *(102)*, and DX-9065a, a novel small molecule direct inhibitor of FXa that is currently in clinical development (103). A multi-compartment segment was placed in the shunt for these experiments. For the SR90107A/ORG31540 experiments, the components consisted of a collagen-coated segment followed by two sections of expanded polytetrafluoroethylene tubing. SR90107A/ORG31540 dose-dependently inhibited platelet and fibrin deposition on the expanded chambers, but had little effect on the collagen-coated segment, which generates a platelet-dependent thrombus. In experiments evaluating DX-9065a, a two-compartment model was used. The first compartment consisted of a tubular segment of knitted Dacron vascular graft followed by the second compartment composed of expanded polytetrafluoroethylene tubing. The vascular graft is believed to generate arterial-like thrombi, and the expanded compartment generates a venous-type thrombus. Intravenous and oral administration of DX-9065a significantly inhibited thrombus formation in the venous-type chamber, but had no significant antithrombotic effect in the arterial-type chamber. These results suggest that selective inhibition of FXa results in specific inhibition of fibrin formation and that optimal antithrombotic therapy with FXa inhibitors may require antiplatelet treatment as well. These studies have provided efficacy and safety data that supported the initiation of clinical studies with these agents *(104,105)*.

In a separate study, platelet deposition on Dacron vascular grafts was examined in baboons during and after a 2-h iv infusion of rTAP *(106)*. Platelet deposition was inhibited during the infusion and also for an additional 2 h and 53 h after termination of low-dose (10 μg/kg/min) and high-dose (25 μg/kg/min) rTAP, respectively. These data suggest that the thrombus can be passivated for long periods of time with only brief inhibition of FXa, again providing important data for designing clinical studies to evaluate novel FXa inhibitors.

The porcine and nonhuman primate models used to evaluate compounds for efficacy in vivo are complex and resource-intensive, especially when considering veterinary care and husbandry. In addition, the training and expertise required to perform the important work of large animal pharmacology in drug discovery is diminishing as universities focus more on molecular and cellular physiology and less on integrative physiology. Thus, these more complex models are not performed "in-house" and are usually contracted to experts at academic or contractual research centers. This is especially true for smaller biotech companies that do not have the facilities and personnel for performing such studies. The requirement for outsourcing such studies creates a new role for the pharmaceutical industry investigator in thrombosis—namely, the role of collaboration manager. The challenges of managing a collaboration are not trivial and include contract negotiations, agreement on protocols, overseeing the study, and deciding who, how, and when to present the results of this work, which is usually proprietary. Once these issues are resolved, these collaborations can yield very interesting results that provide scientific rationale and opinion leader support for specific pharmacological approaches to the treatment of thrombotic diseases.

4.2. Venous Thrombosis

Animal models of venous thrombosis have been developed in cats *(107)* and baboons *(108,109)*. These models rely primarily on stasis in which blood flow is interrupted for varying periods of time to induce clot formation. The effect of inflammatory mediators such as P-selectin have been determined in venous thrombosis models and led to the conclusion that P-selectin is not only a prothrombotic molecule but also possesses pro-inflammatory actions. Pharmacological antagonism of P-selectin results in resolution of venous thrombi and decreased inflammatory-cell infiltration *(107–109)*.

5. Notes

5.1. The Use of Positive Controls in Models of Thrombosis

Clearly, there are many antithrombotic agents that can be used to compare and contrast the antithrombotic efficacy and safety of novel agents. The classic antithrombotic agents are heparin, warfarin, and aspirin. However, new and more selective agents such as hirudin, low molecular weight heparins (LMWHs), and clopidogrel are commercially available that will either replace or augment these older treatments. Novel antithrombotic agents should certainly be demanded to demonstrate better efficacy than currently available therapy in animal models of thrombosis. This should be demonstrated by performing dose-response experiments that include maximally effective doses of each compound in the model. At the maximally effective dose, parameters such as aPTT, PT, template bleeding time, or other, more sensitive measurements of systemic hypocoagulability or bleeding should be compared. A good example of this approach is a study by Schumacher et al. *(110)*, who compared the antithrombotic efficacy of argatroban and dalteparin in arterial and venous models of thrombosis. Consideration of potency and safety compared to other agents should be taken into account when advancing a drug through the testing funnel.

The early in vivo evaluation of compounds that demonstrate acceptable in vitro potency and selectivity requires evaluation of each compound alone in order to demonstrate antithrombotic efficacy. However, to provide adequate dosing, safety and efficacy information to colleagues in clinical development, it is no longer such a simple question as to what does this new agent do by itself? Now the question is: What does this new agent do when administered with aspirin, heparin, LMWHs (which one?), GPIIb/IIIa antagonists (again, which one?), clopidogrel, thrombolytics, or combinations of these agents? The antithrombotic landscape is becoming complicated by so many agents from which to choose that it will become increasingly difficult to design preclinical experiments that mimic the clinical setting in which poly-antithrombotic therapy is required for optimal efficacy and safety. Thus, secondary and tertiary preclinical experiments will need to be carefully designed in order to answer these specific, important questions.

5.2. Evaluation of Bleeding Tendency of Novel Antithrombotics in Animal Models of Thrombosis

Although the clinical relevance of animal models of thrombosis has been well-established in terms of efficacy, the preclinical tests for evaluating safety— e.g., bleeding tendency, have not been as predictable. The difficulty in predicting major bleeding, such as intracranial hemorrhage, resulting from antithrombotic or thrombolytic therapy stems from the complexity and lack of understanding of the mechanisms involved in this disorder. Predictors of anticoagulant-related intracranial hemorrhages are advanced age, hypertension, intensity, and duration of treatment, head trauma, and prior neurologic disease *(111,112)*. These risk factors are clearly difficult, if not impossible, to simulate in laboratory animals. Thus, more general tests of anticoagulation and primary hemostasis have been employed.

Coagulation assays provide an index of the systemic hypocoagulability of the blood after administration of antithrombotic agents. However, the sensitivity and specificity of these assays varies from compound-to-compound, so these assays do not provide a consistent safety measure across all mechanisms of inhibition. Thus, many laboratories have attempted to develop procedures that provide an indication of bleeding risk by evaluating primary hemostasis after generating controlled incisions in anesthetized animals. Some of the tests used in evaluating FXa inhibitors include template bleeding time, tail transection bleeding time, cuticle bleeding time, and evaluation of clinical parameters such as hemoglobin and hematocrit. Unfortunately, template bleeding tests, even when performed in humans, have not been good predictors of major bleeding events in clinical trials *(113–115)*. However, these tests have demonstrated relative advantages of certain mechanisms and agents over others *(18,20)*. For example, hirudin, a direct thrombin inhibitor, appears to have a narrow therapeutic window when used as an adjunct to thrombolysis in clinical trials, producing unacceptable major bleeding when administered at 0.6 mg/kg, iv bolus, plus 0.2 mg/kg/h *(116,117)*. When the dose of hirudin was adjusted to avoid major bleeding (0.1 mg/kg and 0.1 mg/kg/h), no significant therapeutic advantage over heparin was observed. If the relative improvement in the ratio between efficacy and bleeding observed preclinically with Xa inhibitors compared to thrombin inhibitors such as hirudin is supported in future clinical trials, this will establish an important safety advantage for FXa inhibitors and provide valuable information for evaluating the safety of new antithrombotic agents in preclinical experiments.

5.3. Selection of Model Based on Species-Dependent Pharmacology/Physiology

Species selection for animal models of disease is often limited by the unique physiology of a particular disease target in different species or by the species specificity of the pharmacological agent for the target. For example, it was discovered relatively early in the development of platelet GPIIb/IIIa antagonists that these compounds were of limited use in rats *(118)* and that there was a dramatic species-dependent variation in the response of platelets to GPIIb/IIIa antagonists *(119–121)*. This discovery led to the widespread use of larger animals (particularly in dogs, whose platelet response to GPIIb/IIIa antagonists resembles humans) in the evaluation of GPIIb/IIIa antagonists. Of course, the larger animals required more compound for evaluation, which created a resource problem for medicinal chemists. This was especially problematic for companies that generated compounds by combinatorial parallel synthetic chemistry in which many compounds can be made, but usually in very small quantities. However, some pharmacologists devised clever experiments that partially overcame this problem. Cook et al. *(122)* administered a GPIIb/IIIa antagonist orally and intravenously to rats, and then mixed the platelet-rich plasma (PRP) from the treated rats with platelet-rich plasma from untreated dogs. The mixture was then evaluated in an agonist-induced platelet aggregation assay, and the resulting inhibition of canine platelet aggregation (rat platelets were relatively unresponsive to this GPIIb/IIIa antagonist) was a result of the drug present in the plasma obtained from the rat. Using this method, only a small amount of drug is required to determine the relative bioavailability in rats. However, the animal models chosen for efficacy in this report (guinea pigs and dogs) were selected based on their favorable platelet response to the GPIIb/IIIa antagonist.

Similarly for inhibitors of FXa, there are significant variations in the activity of certain compounds against FXa purified from plasma of different species and in plasma-based clotting assays using plasma from different species. DX-9065 is much more potent against human FXa (Ki = 78 nm) than against rabbit (Ki = 102 nm) and rat (Ki = 1980 nm) FXa *(12)*. Likewise, in the PT assay, DX-9065a was very potent in human plasma (concentration required to double PT, PT × 2, was 0.52 μM) and in squirrel monkey plasma (PT × 2 = 0.46 μM), but was much less potent in rabbit, dog, and rat plasma (PT × 2 = 1.5, 6.5, and 22.2 μM, respectively). Other FXa inhibitors have also demonstrated these species-dependent differences in activity *(123–125)*. These differences in potency in vitro can be dramatic; however, in vivo efficacy can still be demonstrated in species that exhibit limited sensitivity to these inhibitors in vitro *(19,20)*. In any case, the investigator must be aware of these differences so that appropriate human doses can be extrapolated from the laboratory animal studies.

Although in many cases the exact mechanism for the species-dependent differences in response to certain therapeutic agents remains unclear, these differences must be examined to determine the appropriate species to be used for preclinical pharmacological evaluation of each agent. This evaluation can routinely be performed by in vitro coagulation or platelet aggregation tests prior to evaluation in animal models.

5.4. Selection of Model Based on Pharmacokinetics

Much debate surrounds the issue as to which species most resembles humans in terms of gastrointestinal (GI) absorption, clearance, and metabolism of therapeutic agents. Differences in GI anatomy, physiology, and biochemistry between humans and commonly used laboratory animals suggest that no single animal can precisely mimic the GI characteristics of humans *(126)*. Because of resource issues (mainly compound availability) and animal care and use considerations, small rodents, such as rats, are usually considered for primary in vivo evaluation of pharmacokinetics for novel agents. However, there is great uncertainty about moving a compound into clinical trials based on oral bioavailability data derived from rat experiments alone. Usually, larger animals such as dogs or nonhuman primates, which have similar GI morphology compared to humans, are the next step in the evaluation of pharmacokinetics of new agents. The pharmacokinetic characteristics of the FXa inhibitor, YM-60828, have been studied extensively in a variety of laboratory animals. YM-60828 demonstrated species-dependent pharmacokinetics, with oral bioavailability estimates of approx 4%, 33%, 7%, and 20% in rats, guinea pigs, beagle dogs, and squirrel monkeys, respectively *(86)*. Although these results suggest that YM-60828 has somewhat limited bioavailability, evaluating the pharmacokinetic profile of novel agents in a number of species *(13,30,86,127)* is a well-established approach used to identify compounds for advancement to human testing. That is, acceptable bioavailability in a number of species suggests that a compound will be bioavailable in humans. Which of the laboratory species adequately represents the bioavailability of a specific compound in humans can only be determined after appropriate pharmacokinetic evaluation in humans. Nevertheless, preclinical pharmacokinetic data are important in selecting the appropriate animal model for testing the antithrombotic efficacy of compounds because the ultimate proof-of-concept experiment is to demonstrate efficacy by the intended route of administration.

5.5. Clinical Relevance of Data Derived From Animal Models of Thrombosis

Animal models of thrombosis have played a crucial role in the discovery and development of a number of compounds that are now successfully being used for the treatment and prevention of thrombotic diseases. The influential preclinical results using novel antithrombotics in a variety of laboratory animal experiments are listed in **Table 1**, along with the early clinical trials and results for each compound. This table intentionally omits many compounds that were tested in animal models of thrombosis, but failed to succeed in clinical trials or, for other reasons, did not become approved drugs. However, these negative outcomes would not have been predicted by animal models of thrombosis because the failures were generally caused by other shortcomings of the drugs (e.g., toxicity, narrow therapeutic window, or undesirable pharmacokinetics or pharmacodynamics), which are not always clearly presented in the scientific literature because of proprietary restrictions in this highly competitive field.

Nonetheless, it is clear that animal models have supplied valuable information for investigators who are responsible for evaluating these drugs in humans, providing pharmacodynamic, pharmacokinetic, and safety data that can be used to design safe and effective clinical trials.

5.6. Genetic Models of Hemostasis and Thrombosis

Recent advances in genetic molecular biology have provided tools that allow scientists to design genetically altered animals that are deficient in certain proteins involved in thrombosis and hemostasis (so-called "knockouts" or "nulls") *(128,129)*. These animals have been extremely useful for identifying and validating novel targets for therapeutic intervention. That is, by examining the phenotype (e.g., spontaneous bleeding, platelet defect, or prolonged bleeding after surgical incision) of a specific knockout strain, scientists can identify the role of the knocked-out protein. If the phenotype is favorable (e.g., not lethal), pharmacological agents can be designed to mimic the knockout. More recently, novel gene medicine approaches have also benefited greatly from the availability of these models, as discussed here. The following section briefly summarizes some of the major findings in thrombosis and hemostasis using genetically altered mice, and concludes with an example of how these models have been used in the drug discovery process.

Mouse knockout models of virtually all of the known hemostatic factors have been reported (**Table 2**). The majority of these gene knockouts result in mice that develop normally, are born in the expected Mendelian ratios, and are viable as defined by the ability to survive to adulthood. Although seemingly normal, these knockout mice display alterations in hemostatic regulation, especially when challenged. Deletion of FVIII, FIX, vWF, and the β_3-integrin *(130–133)* all result in mice that bleed upon surgical challenge, and despite some minor differences in bleeding susceptibility, these mouse knockout models mirror the human disease states quite well (hemophilia A, hemophilia B, von Willebrand's disease, and Glanzmann's thrombasthenia, respectively). In addition, deletion of some hemostatic factors results in fragile mice with severe deficiencies in their ability to regulate blood loss. Prenatally, these mice appear to develop normally, but are unable to survive the perinatal period because of severe hemorrhage, in most cases because of the trauma of birth.

Genetic knockouts have also been useful in dissecting the role of individual signaling proteins in platelet activation. Deletion of the β_3-integrin *(133)* or of $G_{\alpha q}q$ *(134)* results in dramatic impairment of agonist-induced platelet aggregation. Alteration of the protein coding region in the β_3-integrin carboxy-tail, β_3-DiY, at sites that are believed to be phosphorylated upon platelet activation, also results in unstable platelet aggregation *(135)*. Deletion of various receptors such as thromboxane A_2, P-selectin, P2Y1, and PAR-3 demonstrate diminished responses to some agonists, and other platelet responses are intact *(136–139)*. Deletion of PAR-3, another thrombin receptor in mice, has little effect on hemostasis. This indicated the presence of yet another thrombin receptor in platelets and led to the identification of PAR-4 *(139)*.

Since knockouts of prothrombotic factors yield mice with bleeding tendencies, it follows that deletion of factors in the fibrinolytic pathway results in increased thrombotic susceptibility in mice. Plasminogen *(140,141)*, t-PA, urokinase-type plasminogen activator (u-PA), and the combined t-PA/u-PA knockout *(142)* result in mice that demonstrate impaired fibrinolysis, susceptibility for thrombosis, vascular occlusion, and tissue damage caused by fibrin deposition. Interestingly, as a result of fibrin formation in the heart, these mice

Table 2
Genetic Models of Thrombosis and Hemostasis

Knock-out	Viable	Embryonic development/survival	References
Coagulation			
Protein C	No	Normal	Jalbert et al., 1998
		Perinatal death	
Fibrinogen	Yes	Normal	Suh et al., 1995
		Perinatal death	
Fibrinogen-QAGVD	Yes	Normal	Holmback et al., 1996
fV	No	Partial embyronic loss	Cui et al., 1996
		Perinatal death	
FVII	Yes	Normal	Rosen, et al., 1997
		Perinatal death	
fVIII	Yes	Normal	Bi et al., 1996
fIX	Yes	Normal	Wang, et al., 1997
fXI	Yes	Normal	Gailani et al., 1997
Tissue Factor	No	Lethal	Toomey et al., 1996
			Bugge et al., 1996
			Carmeliet et al., 1996
TFPI	No	Lethal	Huang et al., 1997
vWF	Yes	Normal	Denis, et al., 1998
Prothrombin	No	Partial embryonic loss	Xue et al., 1998
		Perinatal death	Sun et al., 1998
Fibrinolytic			
u-Pa and t-PA	Yes	Normal	Carmeliet et al., 1994
		Growth retardation	
uPAR	Yes	Normal	Dewerchin et al., 1996
			Bugge et al., 1995a
Plasminogen	Yes	Normal	Bugge et al., 1995b
		Growth retardation	Ploplis, et al., 1995
PA-I	Yes	Normal	Carmeliet et al., 1993
thrombomodulin	No	Lethal	Healy et al., 1995
Platelet			
β_3	Yes	Normal	Hodivala-Dilke et al., 1999
		Partial embryonic loss	
β_3-DiYF	Yes	Normal	Law et al., 1999
P-Selectin	Yes	Normal	Subramaniam et al., 1996
PAR-1	Yes	Normal	Connolly et al., 1996
		Partial embryonic loss	
PAR-3	Yes	Normal	Kahn et al., 1998
$G_{\alpha q}$	Yes	Normal	Offermans et al., 1997
		Perinatal death	
TXA_2 receptor	Yes	Normal	Thomas et al., 1998
NF-E2	Yes	Normal	Shivdasani et al., 1995
		Perinatal death	
P2Y1	Yes	Normal	Leon, et al.

may provide a good model of MI and heart failure caused by thrombosis *(143)*. Intriguingly, mice deficient in PAI-1, the primary inhibitor of plasminogen activator, demonstrate no spontaneous bleeding and a greater resistance to venous thrombosis as a result of a mild fibrinolytic state *(144)*, suggesting that inhibition of PAI-1 might be a promising approach for novel antithrombotic agents.

In addition to their role in the regulation of hemostasis, several of these genes are important in embryonic development. For example, deletion of tissue factor (TF) *(145–147)*, tissue-factor pathway inhibitor (TFPI) *(148)*, or thrombomodulin *(149)* results in an embryonic lethal phenotype. These and other *(150,151)*, hemostatic factors also appear to contribute to vascular integrity in the developing embryo. These data suggest that initiation of coagulation and generation of thrombin is important at a critical stage of embryonic development, yet other factors must contribute because some of these embryos are able to progress and survive to birth.

Clearly, genetically altered mice have provided valuable insight into the roles of specific hemostatic factors in physiology and pathophysiology. The results of these studies have provided a rationale and impetus for attacking certain targets pharmacologically. These types of models have also provided excellent model systems for studying novel treatments for human diseases. For example, these models provided exceptional systems for studying gene therapy for hemophilia. Specifically, the deletion of FIX, generated by specific deletions in the FIX gene and its promoter, results in mice that mimic the human phenotype of hemophilia B *(152)*. When these mice are treated with adenoviral-mediated transfer of human FIX, the bleeding diathesis is fully corrected *(153)*. Similarly, selectively bred dogs that have a characteristic point mutation in the sequence encoding the catalytic domain of FIX also have a severe hemophilia B that is phenotypically similar to the human disease *(154)*. When adeno-associated virus-mediated canine FIX gene was administered to these dogs intramuscularly, therapeutic levels of FIX were measured for up to 17 mo *(155)*. Clinically relevant partial recovery of whole-blood clotting time and APTT was also observed during this prolonged period. These data provided support for initiating the first study of adeno-associated virus-mediated FIX gene transfer in humans *(156)*. Preliminary results from this clinical study provided evidence for expression of FIX in the three hemophilia patients studied and also provided favorable safety data to substantiate studying this therapy at higher doses. Although it is likely that there are differences between the human disease and animal models of hemophilia (or other diseases), it is clear that these experiments have provided pharmacological, pharmacokinetic, and safety data that were extremely useful in developing this approach and designing safe clinical trials.

Gene therapy approaches to rescuing patients with bleeding diatheses are more advanced than gene therapy for thrombotic indications. However, promising preclinical data indicates that local overexpression of thrombomodulin *(157)* or t-PA *(158)* inhibits thrombus formation in a rabbit model of arterial thrombosis. Similarly, local gene transfer of TFPI prevented thrombus formation in balloon-injured porcine carotid arteries *(159)*. These, and other studies *(160)* suggest that novel gene therapy approaches will also be effective for thrombotic indications, but these treatments must be carefully optimized for pharmacokinetics, safety, and efficacy in laboratory animal studies prior to administration to humans.

References

1. Yeghiazarians, Y., Braunstein, J. B., Askari, A., and Stone, P. (2000) Unstable angina pectoris. *N. Engl. J. Med.* **342,** 101–114.
2. Anderson, H. V. and Willerson, J. T. (1994) Experimental models of thrombosis, in *Thrombosis and Hemorrhage* (Loscalzo, J. and Schafer, A. I., eds.), Blackwell Scientific, Boston, pp. 385–393.
3. Badimon, L. (1997) Models to study thrombotic disorders. *Thromb. Haemostasis* **78,** 667–671.
4. Bush, L. R. and Shebuski, R. J. (1990) In vivo models of arterial thrombosis and thrombolysis. *FASEB J.* **4,** 3087–3098.
5. Chi, L., Rebello, S., and Lucchesi, B. R. (1999) In vivo models of thrombosis, in *Handbook of Experimental Pharmacology, Vol. 132, Antithrombotics.* Springer-Verlag, Berlin, pp. 101–127.
6. Gold, H. K., Yasuda, T., Jang, I.-K., Guerrero, J. L., Fallon, J. T., Leinbach, R. C., et al. (1991) Animal models for arterial thrombolysis and prevention of reocclusion. *Circulation* **83,** IV-26–IV-40.
7. Leadley, R. J., Jr., Chi, L., Rebello, S. S., and Gagnon, A. (2000) Contribution of in vivo models of thrombosis to the discovery and development of novel antithrombotic agents. *J. Pharmacol. Toxicol. Methods* Mar-Apr;**43(2),** 101–116
8. Bocan, T. M. A. (1998) Animal models of atherosclerosis and interpretation of drug intervention studies. *Current Pharmaceutical Design* **4,** 37–52.
9. Johnson, G. J., Griggs, T. R., and Badimon, L. (1999) The utility of animal models in the preclinical study of interventions to prevent human coronary artery restenosis: analysis and recommendations. *Thromb. Haemostasis* **81,** 835–843.
10. Hunter, A. J., Green, A. R., and Cross, A. J. (1995) Animal models of acute ischaemic stroke: can they predict clinically successful neuroprotective drugs? *Trends Pharmacol. Sci.* **16,** 123–128.
11. Virchow, R. (1856) I. Über die Verstopfung der Lungenarterie, in *Gesammelte Abhandlungen zur wissenschaftlichen Medicin.* Meidinger Sohn, Frankfurt, p. 221.
12. Hara, T., Yokoyama, A., Morishima, Y., and Kunitada, S. (1995) Species differences in anticoagulant and anti-Xa activity of DX-9065a, a highly selective factor Xa inhibitor. *Thromb. Res.* **80,** 99–104.

13. Leadley, R. J., Jr., Morgan, S., Bentley, R., Bostwick, J., Kasiewski, C., Chu, V., et al. (1999) Pharmacodynamic activity and antithrombotic efficacy of RPR120844, a novel inhibitor of coagulation factor Xa. *J. Cardiovasc. Pharmacol.* **34,** 791–799.

14. Heran, C., Morgan, S., Kasiewski, C., Bostwick, J., Bentley, R., Klein, S., et al. (2000) Antithrombotic efficacy of RPR208566, a novel factor Xa inhibitor, in a rat model of carotid artery thrombosis. *Eur. J. Pharmacol.* **389,** 201–207.

15. Sato, K., Kawasaki, T., Hisamichi, N., Taniuchi, Y., Hirayama, F., Koshio, H., et al. (1998) Antithrombotic effects of YM-60828, a newly synthesized factor Xa inhibitor, in rat thrombosis models and its effects on bleeding time. *Br. J. Pharmacol.* **123,** 92–96.

16. Herbert, J. M., Bernat, A., Dol, F., Herault, J. P., Crepon, B., and Lormeau, J. C. (1996) DX 9065A, a novel, synthetic selective and orally active inhibitor of factor Xa: in vitro and in vivo studies. *The Journal of Pharmacology and Experimental Therapeutics* **276,** 1030–1038.

17. Wiley, M. R., Weir, L. C., Briggs, S., Bryan, N. A., Buben, J., Campbell, C., et al. (2000) Structure-based design of potent, amidine-derived inhibitors of factor Xa: evaluation of selectivity, anticoagulant activity, and antithrombotic activity. *J. Med. Chem.* **43,** 883–899.

18. Sato, K., Kawasaki, T., Taniuchi, Y., Hirayama, F., Koshio, H., and Matsumoto, Y. (1997) YM-60828, a novel factor Xa inhibitor: separation of its antithrombotic effects from its prolongation of bleeding time. *Eur. J. Pharmacol.* **339,** 141–146.

19. Sato, K., Taniuchi, Y., Kawasaki, T., Hirayama, F., Koshio, H., and Matsumoto, Y. (1998) Relationship between the antithrombotic effect of YM-75466, a novel factor Xa inhibitor, and coagulation parameters in rats. *Eur. J. Pharmacol.* **347,** 231–236.

20. Morishima, Y., Tanabe, K., Terada, Y., Hara, T., and Kunitada, S. (1997) Antithrombotic and hemorrhagic effects of DX9065a, a direct and selective factor Xa inhibitor: comparison with a direct thrombin inhibitor and antithrombin III-dependent anticoagulants. *Thromb. Haemostasis* **78,** 1366–1371.

21. Wong, P. C., Crain, E. J., Nguan, O., Watson, C. A., and Racanelli, A. (1996) Antithrombotic actions of selective inhibitors of blood coagulation factor Xa in rat models of thrombosis. *Thromb. Res.* **83,** 117–126.

22. Wong, A. G., Gunn, A. C., Ku, P., Hollenbach, S. J., and Sinha, U. (1997) Relative efficacy of active site-blocked factors IXa, Xa in models of rabbit venous and arterio-venous thrombosis. *Thromb. Haemostasis* **77(6),** 1143–1147.

23. Yamazaki, M., Asakura, H., Aoshima, K., Saito, M., Jokaji, H., Uotani, C., et al. (1994) Effects of DX-9065a, an orally active, newly synthesized and specific inhibitor of factor Xa, against experimental disseminated intravascular coagulation in rats. *Thromb. Haemostasis* **72,** 393–396.

24. Sato, K., Kaku, S., Hirayama, F., Koshio, H., Matsumoto, Y., Kawasaki, T., et al. (1998b) Antithrombotic effect of YM-75466 is separated from its effect on bleeding time and coagulation time. *Eur. J. Pharmacol.* **352,** 59–63.

25. Wessler, S. (1952) Studies in intravascular coagulation. I. Coagulation changes in isolated venous segments. *J. Clin. Invest.* **31,** 1011–1014.

26. Seifert, D., Mitchell, T. J., Wang, Z., Knabb, R. M., Barbera, F., Reilley, T. M., et al. (1999) Prothrombin activation in rabbits. *Thromb. Res.* **93,** 101–112.

27. Vlasuk, G. P., Ramjit, D., Fujita, T., Dunwiddie, C. T., Nutt, E. M., Smith, D. E., et al. (1991) Comparison of the in vivo anticoagulant properties of standard heparin and the highly selective Factor Xa inhibitors antistasin and tick anticoagulant peptide (TAP) in a rabbit model of venous thrombosis. *Thromb. Haemostasis* **65,** 257–262.

28. Bostwick, J. S., Bentley, R., Morgan, S., Brown, K., Chu, V., Ewing, W. R., et al. (1999) RPR120844, a novel, specific inhibitor of coagulation factor Xa, inhibits venous thrombus formation in the rabbit. *Thromb. Haemostasis* **81,** 157–160.

29. Quan, M. L., Liauw, A. Y., Ellis, C. D., Pruitt, J. R., Carini, D. J., Bostrom, L. L., et al. (1999a) Design and synthesis of isoxazoline derivatives as factor Xa inhibitors. 1 *J. Med. Chem.* **42,** 2752–2759.

30. Quan, M. L., Ellis, C. D., Liauw, A. Y., Alexander, R. S., Knabb, R. M., Lam, G., et al. (1999b) Design and synthesis of isoxazoline derivatives as factor Xa inhibitors. 2 *J. Med. Chem.* **42,** 2760–2773.

31. Wong, P. C., Quan, M. L., Crain, E. J., Watson, C. A., Wexler, R. R., and Knabb, R. M. (2000) Nonpeptide factor Xa inhibitors: I. Studies with SF303 and SK549, a new class of potent antithrombotics. *J. Pharmacol. Exp. Ther.* **292,** 351–357.

32. Sinha, U., Ku, P., Malinowski, J., Zhu, B. Y., Scarborough, R. M., Marlowe, C. K., et al. (2000) Antithrombotic and hemostatic capacity of factor Xa versus thrombin inhibitors in models of venous and arteriovenous thrombosis. *Eur. J. Pharmacol.* **395,** 51–59.

33. Shebuski, R. J., Storer, B. L., and Fujita, T. (1988) Effect of thromboxane synthetase inhibition on the thrombolytic action of tissue-type plasminogen activator in a rabbit model of peripheral arterial thrombosis. *Thromb. Res.* **52,** 381–392.

34. Folts, J. D., Crowell, E. B., and Rowe, G. G. (1976) Platelet aggregation in partially obstructed vessels and its elimination with aspirin. *Circulation* **54,** 365–370.

35. Golino, P., Ragni, M., Cirillo, P., D'Andrea, D., Scognamiglio, A., Ravera, A., et al. (1998) Antithrombotic effects of recombinant human, active site-blocked factor VIIa in a rabbit model fo recurrent arterial thrombosis. *Circ. Res.* **82,** 39–46.

36. Aiken, J. W., Gorman, R. R., and Shebuski, R. J. (1979) Prevention of blockage of partially obstructed coronary arteries with prostacyclin correlates with inhibition of platelet aggregation. *Prostaglandins* **17,** 483–494.

37. Uchida, Y., Yoshimoto, N., and Murao, S. (1975) Cyclic reductions in coronary blood pressure and flow induced by coronary artery constriction. *Jpn. Heart J.* **16,** 454–464.

38. Folts, J. D., Gallagher, K., and Rowe, G. G. (1982) Blood flow reductions in stenosed canine coronary arteries: vasospasm or platelet aggregation. *Circulation* **65,** 248–255.

39. Aiken, J. W., Shebuski, R. J., Miller, O. V., and Gorman, R. R. (1981) Endogenous prostacyclin contributes to the efficacy of a thromboxane synthetase inhibitor for preventing coronary artery thrombosis. *J. Pharmacol. Exp. Ther.* **219,** 299–308.

40. Bush, L. R., Campbell, W. B., Buja, L. M., Tilton, G. D., and Willerson, J. T. (1984) Effects of the selective thromboxane synthetase inhibitor dazoxiben on variations in coronary blood flow in stenosed canine coronary arteries. *Circulation* **69,** 1161–1170.

41. Bush, L. R., Holahan, M. A., Kanovsky, S. M., Mellott, M. J., Garsky, V. J. and Gould, R. J. (1989) Antithrombotic profile of echistatin, a snake venom peptide and platelet fibrinogen receptor antagonist in the dog. *Circulation* **80,** 11–23.

42. Shebuski, R. J., Ramjit, D. R., Bencen, G. H., and Polokoff, M. A. (1989) Characterization and platelet inhibitory activity of bitistatin, a potent RGD-containing peptide from the venom of the viper, *Bitis arietans. J. Biol. Chem.* **264,** 21,550–21,556.

43. Bush, L. R. and Patrick, D. (1986) The role of the endothelium in arterial thrombosis and the influence of antithrombotic therapy. *Drug Dev. Res.* **7,** 319–340.

44. Golino, P., Ashton, J. H., Buja, L. M., Rosolowsky, M., Taylor, A. L., McNatt, J., et al. (1989) Local platelet activation causes vasoconstriction of large epicardial canine coronary arteries in vivo. Thromboxane A_2 and serotonin are possible mediators. *Circulation* **79,** 154–166.

45. Bush, L. R., Campbell, W. B., Kern, K., Tilton, G. D., Apprill, P., Ashton, J., et al. (1984) The effects of alpha$_2$-adrenergic and serotonergic receptor antagonists on cyclic blood flow alterations in stenosed canine coronary arteries. *Circ. Res.* **55,** 642–652.

46. Bennett, J. S. and Vilaire, G. (1979) Exposure of platelet fibrinogen receptors by ADP and epinephrine. *J. Clin. Invest.* **64,** 1393–1401.

47. Coller, B. S. and Scudder, L. E. (1985) Inhibition of dog platelet function by in vivo infusion of F(ab')$_2$ fragments of a monoclonal antibody to the platelet glycoprotein IIb/IIIa receptor. *Blood* **66,** 1456–1459.

48. Shebuski, R. J., Berry, D. E., Bennett, D. B., Romoff, T., Storer, B. L., Au, F., and Samanen, J. (1989) Demonstration of Ac-ArgGly-Asp-Ser-NH$_2$ as an antiaggregatory agent in the dog by intracoronary administration. *Thromb. Haemostasis* **61,** 183–188.

49. Eidt, J. E, Allison, P., Noble, S., Ashton, J., Golino, P, McNatt, J., et al. (1989) Thrombin is an important mediator of platelet aggregation in stenosed canine coronary arteries with endothelial injury. *J. Clin. Invest.* **84,** 18–27.

50. Smith, J. M. and Shebuski, R. J. (1988) Lack of an inhibitory effect of tissue plasminogen activator (tPA) on platelet aggregation in vivo. *FASEB J.* **2,** A1164.

51. Al-Wathiqui, M. H., Hartman, J. C., Brooks, H. L., Gross, G. J., and Warltier, D. C. (1988) Cyclical carotid artery flow reduction in conscious dogs: effect of a new thromboxane receptor antagonist. *Am. Heart J.* **116,** 1482–1487.

52. Gallagher, K. P., Folts, J. D., and Rowe, G. G. (1978) Comparison of coronary arteriograms with direct measurements of stenosed coronary arteries in dogs. *Am. Heart J.* **95,** 338–347.

53. Schumacher, W. A., Heran, C. L., Goldenberg, H. J., Harris, D. N., and Ogletree, M. L. (1989) Magnitude of thromboxane receptor antagonism necessary for antithrombotic activity in monkeys. *Am. J. Physiol.* **256,** H726–H734.

54. Coller, B. S., Folts, J. D., Scudder, L. E., and Smith, S. R. (1986) Antithrombotic effect of a monoclonal antibody to the platelet glycoprotein IIb/IIIa receptor in an experimental animal model. *Blood* **68,** 783–786.

55. Eidt, J. F., Ashton, J., Golino, P., McNatt, J., Buja, L. M. and Willerson, J. T. (1989) Treadmill exercise promotes cyclic alterations in coronary blood flow in dogs with coronary artery stenoses and endothelial injury. *J. Clin. Invest.* **84,** 517–526.

56. O'Neill, W. W., Topol, E. J., and Pitt, B. (1988) Coronary thrombolysis for evolving myocardial infarction. *Prog. Cardiovasc. Dis.* **30,** 465–483.

57. Blair, E., Nygren, E., and Cowley, R. A. (1964) A spiral wire technique for producing gradually occlusive coronary thrombosis. *J. Thorac. Cardiovasc. Surg.* **48,** 476–485.

58. Kordenat, R. K. and Kezdi, P. (1972) Experimental intracoronary thrombosis and selective in situ lysis by catheter technique. *Am. J. Heart* **83,** 360–364.

59. Romson, J. L., Haack, D. W., and Lucchesi, B. R. (1980) Electrical induction of coronary artery thrombosis in the ambulatory canine: a model for in vivo evaluation of antithrombotic agents. *Thromb. Res.* **17,** 841–853.

60. Bergmann, S. R., Fox, K. A. A., Ter-Pogossian, M. M., Sobel, B. E., and Collen, D. (1983) Clot-selective coronary thrombolysis with tissue-type plasminogen activator. *Science* **220,** 1181–1183.

61. Bush, L. R., Mellott, M. J., Kanovsky, S. M., Holahan, M. A., and Patrick, D. H. (1989) A model of femoral artery thrombolysis in dogs. *Fibrinolysis* **3,** 107–114.

62. Marsh-Leidy, E., Stern, A. M., Friedman, P A., and Bush, L. R. (1990) Enhanced thrombolysis by a factor XIIIa inhibitor in a rabbit model of femoral artery thrombosis. *Thromb. Res.* **59,** 15–26.

63. Golino, P, Ashton, J. H., Glas-Greenwalt, P, McNatt, J., Buja, L. M., and Willerson, J. T. (1988) Mediation of reocclusion by thromboxane A_2 and serotonin after thrombolysis with tissue-type plasminogen activator in a canine preparation of coronary thrombosis. *Circulation* **77,** 678–684.

64. Bergmann, S. R., Lerch, R. A., Ludbrook, P A., Welch, M. J., Ter-Pogossian, M. M., and Sobel, B. E. (1982) Temporal dependence of beneficial effects of coronary thrombolysis characterized by positron tomography. *Am. J. Med.* **73,** 573–581.

65. Van der Werf, F., Jang, I. K., and Cohen, D. (1987) Thrombolysis with recombinant human single chain urokinase-type plasminogen activator (rscu-PA): dose-response in dogs with coronary artery thrombosis. *J. Cardiovasc. Pharmacol.* **9,** 91–93.

66. Mellott, M. J., Connolly, T. M., York, S. J., and Bush, L. R. (1990) Prevention of reocclusion by MCI-9038, a thrombin inhibitor, following t-PA induced thrombolysis in a canine model of femoral arterial thrombolysis. *Thromb. Haemostasis* **64,** 526–534.

67. Gold, H. K., Fallon, J. T., Yasuda, T., Leinbach, R. C., Khaw, B. A., Newell, J. B., et al. (1984) Coronary thrombolysis with recombinant human tissue-type plasminogen activator. *Circulation* **70,** 700–707.

68. Collen, D., Stassen, J. M., and Verstraete, M. (1983) Thrombolysis with human extrinsic (tissue-type) plasminogen activator in rabbits with experimental jugular vein thrombosis. *J. Clin. Invest.* **71,** 368–376.

69. Kopia, G. A., Kopaciewicz, L. J., and Ruffolo, R. R. (1988) Coronary thrombolysis with intravenous streptokinase in the anesthetized dog: a dose-response study. *J. Pharmacol. Exp. Ther.* **244,** 956–962.

70. Gold, H. K., Coller, B. S., Yasuda, T., Saito, T., Fallon, J. T., Guerrero, J. L., et al. (1988) Rapid and sustained coronary artery recanalization with combined bolus injection of recombinant tissue-type plasminogen activator and monoclonal antiplatelet Gp IIb/IIIa antibody in a canine preparation. *Circulation* **77,** 670–677.

71. Gold, H. K., Leinbach, R. C., Garabedian, H. D., Yasuda, T., Johns, J. A., Grossbard, E. B., et al. (1986) Acute coronary reocclusion after thrombolysis with recombinant human tissue-type plasminogen activator: prevention by a maintenance infusion. *Circulation* **73,** 347–352.

72. Goldberg, R. K., Levine, S., and Fenster, P. E. (1985) Management of patients after thrombolytic therapy for acute myocardial infarction. *Clin. Cardiol.* **8,** 455–459.

73. Coller, B. S., Peerschke, E. I., Scudder, L. E., and Sullivan, C. A. (1983) A murine monoclonal antibody that completely blocks the binding of fibrinogen to platelets produces a thrombasthenic-like state in normal platelets and binds to glycoproteins IIb and/or IIIa. *J. Clin. Invest.* **72,** 325–338.

74. Yasuda, T., Gold, H. K., Fallon, J. T., Leinbach, R. C., Guerrero, J. L., Scudder, L. E., et al. (1988) Monoclonal antibody against the platelet glycoprotein (GP) IIb/IIIa receptor prevents coronary artery reocclusion after reperfusion with recombinant tissue type plasminogen activator. *J. Clin. Invest.* **81,** 1284–1291.

75. Salazar, A. E. (1961) Experimental myocardial infarction, induction of coronary thrombosis in the intact closed-chest dog. *Circ. Res.* **9,** 135–136.

76. Romson, J. L., Haack, D. W., and Lucchesi, B. R. (1980) Electrical induction of coronary artery thrombosis in the ambulatory canine: a model for in vivo evaluation of antithrombotic agents. *Thromb. Res.* **17,** 841–853.

77. Schumacher, W. A., Lee, E. C., and Lucchesi, B. R. (1985) Augmentation of streptokinase-induced thrombolysis by heparin and prostacyclin. *J. Cardiovasc. Pharmacol.* **7,** 739–746.

78. Benedict, C. R., Matthew, B., Rex, K. A., Cartwright, J., Jr., and Sordahl, L. A. (1986) Correlation of plasma serotonin changes with platelet aggregation in an in vivo dog model of spontaneous occlusive coronary thrombus formation. *Circ. Res.* **58,** 58–67.

79. Van der Giessen, W. J., Harmsen, E., de Tombe, P. P., Hugenholtz, P. G., and Verdouw, P D. (1988) coronary thrombolysis with and without nifedipine in pigs. *Basic Res. Cardiol.* **83,** 258–267

80. Shea, M. J., Driscoll, E. M., Romson, J. L., Pitt, B., and Lucchesi, B. R. (1984) Effects of OKY 1581, a thromboxane synthetase inhibitor, on coronary thrombosis in the conscious dog. *Eur. J. Pharmacol.* **105,** 285–291.

81. Simpson, P. J., Smith, J. B., Jr., Rosenthal, G., and Lucchesi, B. R. (1986) Reduction in the incidence of thrombosis by the thromboxane synthetase inhibitor CGS 13080 in a canine model of coronary artery injury. *J. Pharmacol. Exp. Ther.* **238,** 497–501.

82. Hook, B. G., Schumacher, W. A., Lee, D. L., Jolly, S. R., and Lucchesi, B. R. (1985) Experimental coronary artery thrombosis in the absence of thromboxane A_2 synthesis: evidence for alternate pathways for coronary thrombosis. *J. Cardiovasc. Pharmacol.* **7,** 174–181.

83. Schumacher, W. A. and Lucchesi, B. R. (1983) Effect of the thromboxane synthetase inhibitor UK 37,248 (Dazoxiben) upon platelet aggregation, coronary artery thrombosis and vascular reactivity. *J. Pharmacol. Exp. Ther.* **227,** 790–796.

84. FitzGerald, D. J., Fragetta, J., and FitzGerald, G. A. (1988) Prostaglandin endoperoxides modulate the response to thromboxane synthetase inhibition during coronary thrombosis. *J. Clin. Invest.* **82,** 1708–1713.

85. Mickelson, J. K., Simpson, P J., and Lucchesi, B. R. (1989) Antiplatelet monoclonal $F(ab)_2$ antibody directed against the platelet. GPIIb/IIIa receptor complex prevents coronary artery thrombosis in the canine heart. *J. Mol. Cell. Cardiol.* **21,** 393–405.

86. Kawasaki, T., Sato, K., Sakai, Y., Hirayama, F., Koshio, H., Taniuchi, Y., et al. (1998) Comparative studies of an orally-active factor Xa inhibitor, YM-60828, with other antithrombotic agents in a rat model of arterial thrombosis. *Thromb. Haemostasis* **79,** 410–416.

87. Shebuski, R. J., Smith, J. M., Storer, B. L., Granett, J. R., and Bugelski, P. J. (1988) Influence of selective endoperoxide/thromboxane A_2 receptor antagonism with sulotroban on lysis time and reocclusion rate after tissue plasminogen activator-induced coronary thrombolysis in the dog. *J. Pharmacol. Exp. Ther.* **246,** 790–796.

88. Van der Giessen, W. J., Zijlstra, F. J., Berk, L., and Verdouw, P D. (1988) The effect of the thromboxane receptor antagonist BM 13,177 on experimentally induced coronary artery thrombosis in the pig. *Eur. J. Pharmacol.* **147,** 241–248.

89. Patterson, E., Eller, B. T., Abrams, G. D., Vasiliades, J., and Lucchesi, B. R. (1983) Ventricular fibrillation in a conscious canine preparation of sudden coronary death. Prevention by short- and long-term amiodarone administration. *Circulation* **68,** 857–864.

90. Rebello, S. S., Blank, H. S., Rote, W. E., Vlasuk, G. P., and Lucchesi, B. R. (1997) Antithrombotic efficacy of a recombinant nematode anticoagulant peptide (rNAP5) in canine models of thrombosis after single subcutaneous administration. *J. Pharmacol. Exp. Ther.* **283,** 91–99.

91. Sitko, G. R., Ramjit, D. R., Stabilito, I. I., Lehman, D., Lynch, J. J., and Vlasuk, G. P. (1992) Conjunctive enhancement of enzymatic thrombolysis and prevention of thrombotic reocclusion with the selective Factor Xa inhibitor, tick anticoagulant peptide. *Circulation* **85,** 805–815.

92. Lynch, J. J., Jr., Sitko, G. R., Mellott, M. J., Nutt, E. M., Lehman, E. D., Friedman, P. A., et al. (1994) Maintenance of canine coronary artery patency following thrombolysis with front loaded plus low dose maintenance conjunctive therapy. A comparison of factor Xa versus thrombin inhibition. *Cardiovasc. Res.* **28,** 78–85.

93. Nicolini, F. A., Lee, P., Rios, G., Kottke-Marchant, K., and Topol, E. J. (1994) Combination of platelet fibrinogen receptor antagonist and direct thrombin inhibitor at low doses markedly improves thrombolysis. *Circulation* **89,** 1802–1809.

94. Lefkovits, J., Malycky, J. L., Rao, J. S., Hart, C. E., Plow, E. F., Topol, E. J., et al. (1996) Selective inhibition of Factor Xa is more efficient than Factor VIIa-Tissue Factor complex at facilitating coronary thrombolysis in the canine model. *J. Am. Coll. Cardiol.* **28,** 1858–1865.

95. Waxman, L., Smith, D. E., Arcuri, K. E., and Vlasuk, G. P. (1990) Tick anticoagulant peptide is a novel inhibitor of blood coagulation factor Xa. *Science* **248,** 593–596.

96. Wysokinski, W., McBane, R., Chesebro, J. H., and Owen, W. G. (1996) Reversibility of platelet thrombosis in vivo. *Thromb. Haemostasis* **76,** 1108–1113.

97. Badimon, L. and Badimon, J. J. (1989) Mechanism of arterial thrombosis in non-parallel streamlines: Platelet thrombi grow on the apex of stenotic severely injured vessel wall. *J. Clin. Investig.* **84,** 1134–1144.

98. Dangas, G., Badimon, J. J., Coller, B. S., Fallon, J. T., Sharma, S. K., Hayes, R. M., et al. (1998) Administration of abciximab during percutaneous coronary intervention reduces both ex vivo platelet thrombus formation and fibrin deposition. *Arterioscler. Thromb. Vasc. Biol.* **18,** 1342–1349.

99. Ørvim, U., Brastad, R. M., Vlasuk, G. P., and Sakariassen, K. S. (1995) Effect of selective Factor Xa inhibition on arterial thrombus formation triggered by tissue factor/factor VIIa or collagen in an ex vivo model of shear-dependent human thrombogenesis. *Arterioscler. Thromb. Vasc. Biol.* **15,** 2188–2194.

100. Todd, M. E., McDevitt, E. L., and Goldsmith, E. I. (1972) Blood-clotting mechanisms of nonhuman primates: choice of the baboon model to simulate man. *J. Med. Primatol.* **1,** 132–141.

101. Harker, L. A., Kelly, A. B., and Hanson, S. R. (1991) Experimental arterial thrombosis in nonhuman primates. *Circulation* **83,** IV-41–IV-55.

102. Cadroy, Y., Hanson, S. R., and Harker, L. A. (1993) Antithrombotic effects of synthetic pentasaccharide with high affinity for plasma antithrombin III in nonhuman primates. *Thromb. Haemostasis* **70,** 631–635.

103. Yokoyama, T., Kelly, A. B., Marzec, U. M., Hanson, S. R., Kunitada, S., and Harker, L. A. (1995) Antithrombotic effects of orally active synthetic antagonist of activated factor X in nonhuman primates. *Circulation* **92,** 485–491.

104. Vuillemenot, A., Schiele, F., Meneveau, N., Claudel, S., Donat, F., Fontecave, S., et al. (1999) Efficacy of a synthetic pentasaccharide, a pure factor Xa inhibitor, as an antithrombotic agent—A pilot study in the setting of coronary angioplasty. *Thromb. Haemostasis* **81,** 214–220.

105. Murayama, N., Tanaka, M., Kunitada, S., Yamada, H., Inoue, T., and Terada, Y. (1999) Tolerability, pharmacokinetics, and pharmacodynamics of DX-9065a, a new synthetic potent anticoagulant and specific factor Xa inhibitor, in healthy male volunteers. *Clin. Pharmacol. Ther.* **66,** 258–264.

106. Kotze, H. F., Lamprecht, S., Badenhorst, P. N., Roodt, J. P., and van Wyk, V. (1997) Transient interruption of arterial thrombosis by inhibition of factor Xa results in long-term antithrombotic effects in baboons. *Thromb. Haemostasis* **77,** 1137–1142.

107. Eppehimer, M. J. and Schaub, R. G. (2000) P-selectin-dependent inhibition of thrombosis during venous stasis. *Arterioscler. Thromb. Vasc. Biol.* **20(11),** 2483–2488.

108. Wakefield, T. W., Strieter, R. M., Schaub, R., Myers, D. D., Prince, M. R., Wrobleski, S. K., et al. (2000) Venous thrombosis prophylaxis by inflammatory inhibition without anticoagulation therapy. *J. Vasc. Surg.* **31(2),** 309–324.

109. Myers, D. D., Jr., Schaub, R., Wrobleski, S. K., Londy, F. J., 3rd, Fex, B. A., Chapman, A. M., et al. (2001) P-selectin antagonism causes dose-dependent venous thrombosis inhibition. *Thromb. Haemostasis* **85(3),** 423–429.

110. Schumacher, W. A., Heran, C. L., and Steinbacher, T. E. (1996) Low-molecular-weight heparin (Fragmin) and thrombin active-site inhibitor (argatroban) compared in experimental arterial and venous thrombosis and bleeding time. *J. Card. Pharmacol.* **28,** 19–25.

111. Stieg, P. E. and Kase, C. S. (1998) Intracranial hemorrhage: diagnosis and emergency management. *Neurol. Clin.* **16,** 373–390.

112. Sloan, M. A. and Gore, J. M. (1992) Ischemic stroke and intracranial hemorrhage following thrombolytic therapy for acute myocardial infarction: a risk-benefit analysis. *Am. J. Cardiol.* **69,** 21A–38A.

113. Bernardi, M. M., Califf, R. M., Kleiman, N., Ellis, S. G., and Topol, E. J. (1993) Lack of usefulness of prolonged bleeding times in predicting hemorrhagic events in patients receiving the 7E3 glycoprotein IIb/IIIa platelet antibody. *Am. J. Cardiol.* **72,** 1121–1125.

114. Bick, R. L. (1995) Laboratory evaluation of platelet dysfunction. *Clin. Lab. Med.* **15,** 1–38.

115. Rodgers, R. P. C. and Levin, J. (1990) A critical reappraisal of the bleeding time. *Sem. Thromb. Hemost.* **16,** 1–20.

116. Antman, E. M. and TIMI 9B Investigators (1996) Hirudin in acute myocardial infarction: Thrombolysis and thrombin inhibition in myocardial infarction (TIMI) 9B trial. *Circulation* **4,** 911–921.

117. Global Use of Strategies to Open Occluded Coronary Arteries (GUSTO) IIb/IIIa Investigators (1996) A comparison of recombinant hirudin with heparin for the treatment of acute coronary syndromes. *N. Engl. J. Med.* **335,** 775–782.

118. Cox, D., Motoyama, Y., Seki, J., Aoki, T., Dohi, M., and Yoshida, K. (1992) Pentamadine: a non-peptide GPIIb/IIIa antagonist—in vitro studies on platelets from humans and other species. *Thromb. Haemostasis* **68,** 731–736.

119. Bostwick, J. S., Kasiewski, C. J., Chu, V., Klein, S. I., Sabatino, R. D., Perrone, M. H., et al. (1996) Anti-thrombotic activity of RG13965, a novel platelet fibrinogen receptor antagonist. *Thromb. Res.* **82,** 495–507.

120. Cook, N. S., Zerwes, H.-G., Tapparelli, C., Powling, M., Singh, J., Metternich, R., et al. (1993) Platelet aggregation and fibrinogen binding in human, rhesus monkey, guinea-pig, hamster and rat blood: activation by ADP and thrombin receptor peptide and inhibition by glycoprotein IIb/IIIa antagonists. *Thromb. Haemostasis* **70,** 531–539.

121. Panzer-Knodle, S., Taite, B. B., Mehrotra, D. V., Nicholson, N. S., and Feigen, L. P. (1993) Species variation in the effect of glycoprotein IIb/IIIa antagonists on inhibition of platelet aggregation. *J. Pharmacol. Toxicol. Methods* **30,** 47–53.

122. Cook, J. J., Holahan, M. A., Lyle, E. A., Ramjit, D. R., Sitko, G. R., Stranieri, M. T., et al. (1996) Nonpeptide glycoprotein IIb/IIIa inhibitors. 8. Antiplatelet activity and oral antithrombotic efficacy of L-734,217. *J. Pharmacol. Exp. Ther.* **278,** 62–73.

123. Tidwell, R. R., Webster, W. P., Shaver, S. R., and Geratz, J. D. (1980) Strategies for anticoagulation with synthetic protease inhibitors. Xa inhibitors versus thrombin inhibitors. *Thromb. Res.* **19,** 339–349.

124. Nutt, E. M., Jain, D., Lenny, A. B., Schaffer, L., Siegl, P. K., and Dunwiddie, C. T. (1991) Purification and characterization of recombinant antistasin: a leech-derived inhibitor of coagulation factor Xa. *Arch. Biochem. Biophys.* **285,** 37–44.

125. Taniuchi, Y., Sakai, Y., Hisamichi, N., Kayama, M., Mano, Y., Sato, K., et al. (1998) Biochemical and pharmacological characterization of YM-60828, a newly synthesized and orally active inhibitor of human Factor Xa. *Thromb. Haemostasis* **79,** 543–548.

126. Kararli, T. T. (1995) Comparison of the gastrointestinal anatomy, physiology, and biochemistry of humans and commonly used laboratory animals. *Biopharm. Drug Dispos.* **16,** 351–380.

127. Sanderson, P. E. J., Cutrona, K. J., Dorsey, B. D., Dyer, D. L., McDonough, C. M., Naylor-Olsen, A. M., et al. (1998) L-374,087, an efficacious, orally bioavailable, pyridinone acetamide thrombin inhibitor. *Bioorg. Med. Chem. Lett.* **8,** 817–822.

128. Carmeliet, P. and Collen, D. (1999) New developments in the molecular biology of coagulation and fibrinolysis, in *Handbook of Experimental Pharmacology, Vol. 132, Antithrombotics.* Springer-Verlag, Berlin, pp. 41–76.

129. Pearson, J. M. and Ginsburg, D. (1999) Use of transgenic mice in the study of thrombosis and hemostasis, in *Handbook of Experimental Pharmacology, Vol. 132, Antithrombotics.* Springer-Verlag, Berlin, pp. 157–174.

130. Bi, L., Sarkar, R., Naas, T., Lawler, A. M., Pain, J., Shumaker, S. L., et al. (1996) Further characterization of Factor VIII-deficient mice created by gene targeting: RNA and protein studies. *Blood* **88,** 3446–3450.

131. Wang, L., Zoppè, M., Hackeng, T. M., Griffin, J. H., and Lee, K.-F. (1997) A factor IX-deficient mouse model for hemophilia B gene therapy. *Proc. Natl. Acad. Sci. USA* **94,** 11,563–11,566.

132. Denis, C., Methia, N., Frenette, P. S., Rayburn, H., Ullman-Cullere, M., Hynes, R. O., et al. (1998) A mouse model of severe von Willebrand disease: defects in hemostasis and thrombosis. *Proc. Natl. Acad. Sci. USA* **95,** 9524–9529.

133. Hodivala-Dilke, K. M., McHugh, K. P., Tsakiris, D. A., Rayburn, H., Crowley, D., Ullman-Culleré, M., et al. (1999) β_3-integrin-deficient mice are a model for Glanzmann thrombasthenia showing placental defects and reduced survival. *J. Clin. Invest.* **103,** 229–238.

134. Offermanns, S., Toombs, C. F., Hu, Y.-H., and Simon, M. I. (1997) Defective platelet activation in $G\alpha_q$-deficient mice. *Nature* **389,** 183–186. ,

135. Law, D. A., DeGuzman, F. R., Heiser, P., Ministri-Madrid, K., Killeen, N., and Phillips, D. R. (1999) Integrin cytoplasmic tyrosine motif is required for outside-in αIIbβ3 signalling and platelet function. *Nature* **401,** 808–811.

136. Thomas, D. W., Mannon, R. B., Mannon, P. J., Latour, A., Oliver, J. A., Hoffman, M., et al. (1998) Coagulation defects and altered hemodynamic responses in mice lacking receptors for thromboxane A_2. *J. Clin. Invest.* **102,** 1994–2001.

137. Subramaniam, M., Frenette, P. S., Saffaripour, S., Johnson, R. C., Hynes, R. O., and Wagner, D. D. (1996) Defects in hemostasis in P-selectin-deficient mice. *Blood* **87,** 1238–1242.

138. Leon, C., Hechler, B., Freund, M., Eckly, A., Vial, C., Ohlmann, P., et al. (1999) Defective platelet aggregation and increased resistance to thrombosis in puriner-gic P2Y$_1$ receptor-null mice. *J. Clin. Invest.* **104,** 1731–1737.

139. Kahn, M. L., Zheng, Y.-W., Huang, W., Bigornia, V., Zeng, D., Moff, S., et al. (1998) A dual thrombin receptor system for platelet activation. *Nature* **394,** 690–694.

140. Bugge, T. H., Suh, T. T., Flick, M. J., Daugherty, C. C., Romer, J., Solberg, H., et al. (1995) The receptor for urokinase-type plasminogen activator is not essential for mouse development or fertility. *J. Biol. Chem.* **270,** 16,886–16,894.

141. Ploplis, V. A., Carmeliet, P., Vazirzadeh, S., Van Vlaenderen, I., Moons, L., Plow, E. F., et al. (1995) Effects of disruption of the plasminogen gene on thrombosis, growth, and health in mice. *Circulation* **92,** 2585–2593.

142. Carmeliet, P., Schoonjans, L., Kieckens, L., Ream, B., Degen, J., Bronson, R., et al. (1994) Physiological consequences of loss of plasminogen activator gene function in mice. *Nature* **368,** 419–424.

143. Christie, P. D., Edelberg, J. M., Picard, M. H., Foulkes, A. S., Mamuya, W., Weiler-Guettler, H., et al. (1999) A murine model of myocardial thrombosis. *J. Clin. Invest.* **104,** 533–539.

144. Carmeliet, P., Stassen, J. M., Schoonjans, L., Ream, B., van den Oord, J. J., De Mol, M., et al. (1993) Plasminogen activator inhibitor-1 gene-deficient mice. *J. Clin. Invest.* **92,** 2756–2760.

145. Bugge, T. H., Xiao, Q., Kombrinck, K. W., Flick, M. J., Holmback, K., Danton, M. J. S., et al. (1996) Fatal embryonic bleeding events in mice lacking tissue factor, the cell-associated initiator of blood coagulation. *Proc. Natl. Acad. Sci. USA* **93,** 6258–6263.

146. Toomey, J. R., Kratzer, K. E., Lasky, N. M., Stanton, J. J., and Broze, G. J., Jr. (1996) Targeted disruption of the murine tissue factor gene results in embryonic lethality. *Blood* **88,** 1583–1587.

147. Carmeliet, P., Mackman, N., Moons, L., Luther, T., Gressens, P., Van Vlaenderen, I., et al. (1996) Role of tissue factor in embryonic blood vessel development. *Nature* **383,** 73–75.

148. Huang, Z.-F., Higuchi, D., Lasky, N., and Broze, G. J., Jr. (1997) Tissue factor pathway inhibitor gene disruption produces intrauterine lethality in mice. *Blood* **90,** 944–951.

149. Healy, A. M., Rayburn, H. B., Rosenberg, R. D., and Weiler, H. (1995) Absence of the blood-clotting regulator thrombomodulin causes embryonic lethality in mice before development of a functional cardiovascular system. *Proc. Natl. Acad. Sci. USA* **92,** 850–854.

150. Connolly, A. J., Ishihara, H., Kahn, M. L., Farese, R. V., Jr., and Coughlin, S. R. (1996) Role of the thrombin receptor in development and evidence for a second receptor. *Nature* **381,** 516–519.

151. Cui, J., O'Shea, K. S., Purkayastha, A., Saunders, T. L., and Ginsburg, D. (1996) Fatal haemorrhage and incomplete block to embryogenesis in mice lacking coagulation factor V. *Nature* **384,** 66–68.

152. Lin, H.-F., Maeda, N., Sithies, O., Straight, D. L., and Stafford, D. W. (1997) A coagulation factor IX-deficient mouse model for human hemophilia B. *Blood* **90,** 3962–3966.

153. Kung, J., Hagstrom, J., Cass, D., Tai, S., Lin, H. F., Stafford, D. W., and High, K. A. (1998) Human FIX corrects bleeding diathesis of mice with hemophilia B. *Blood* **91,** 784–790.

154. Evans, J. P., Brinkhous, K. M., Brayer, G. D., Reisner, H. M., and High, K. A. (1989) Canine hemophilia B resulting from a point mutation with unusual consequences. *Proc. Natl. Acad. Sci. USA* **86,** 10,095–10,099.

155. Herzog, R. W., Yang, E. Y., Couto, L. B., Hagstrom, J. N., Elwell, D., Fields, P. A., et al. (1999) Long-term correction of canine hemophilia B by gene transfer of blood coagulation factor IX mediated by adeno-associated viral vector. *Nat. Med.* **5,** 56–63.

156. Kay, M. A., Manno, C. S., Ragni, M. V., Larson, P. J., Couto, L. B., McClelland, A., et al. (2000) Evidence for gene transfer and expression of factor IX in haemophilia B patients with an AAV vector. *Nat. Genet.* **24,** 257–261.

157. Waugh, J. M., Yuksel, E., Li, J., Kuo, M. D., Kattash, M., Saxena, R., et al. (1999) Local overexpression of thrombomodulin for in vivo prevention of arterial thrombosis in a rabbit model. *Circ. Res.* **84,** 84–92.

158. Waugh, J. M., Kattash, M., Li, J., Yuksel, E., Kuo, M. D., Lussier, M., et al. (1999) Gene therapy to promote thromboresistance: local overexpression of tissue plasminogen activator to prevent arterial thrombosis in an in vivo rabbit model. *Proc. Natl. Acad. Sci. U.S.A.* **96(3),** 1065–1070.

159. Zoldhelyi, P., McNatt, J., Shelat, H. S., Yamamoto, Y., Chen, Z. Q., and Willerson, J. T. (2000) Thromboresistance of balloon-injured porcine carotid arteries after local gene transfer of human tissue factor pathway inhibitor. *Circulation* **101,** 289–295.

160. Vassalli, G. and Dichek, D. A. (1997) Gene therapy for arterial thrombosis. *Cardiovasc. Res.* **35,** 459–469.

13

A Survey of Venous Thrombosis Models

Walter P. Jeske, Omer Iqbal, Jawed Fareed, and Brigitte Kaiser

1. Introduction

Animal models have played a crucial role in the development of new antithrombotic drugs during the past few decades. Through the use of these animal models, the differentiation between the anticoagulant and antithrombotic effects was first recognized. Drugs that were unable to produce a prolongation of blood clotting time were found to produce antithrombotic effects in animal models, and a recognition that endogenous effects in the intact animal resulting from the metabolic transformation of the drug and/or release of antithrombotic substances was appreciated. Without the use of intact animal models, such an observation would not have been possible.

Antithrombotic and anticoagulant drugs are effective in the control of thrombogenesis at various levels. These drugs are also capable of producing hemorrhagic effects. These effects are not predictable using in vitro testing methods. The bleeding effects of a drug may be direct or indirect; thus, the use of animal models adds to the pharmacodynamic profiling of drugs to project safety-to-efficacy ratios.

The repeated administration of drugs can result in a cumulative response that may alter the pharmacokinetic and pharmacodynamic indices of a given agent. It is only through the use of animal models that such information can be generated. Furthermore, since antithrombotic drugs represent a diverse class of agents, their interactions with physiologically active endogenous proteins can only be studied using animal models.

Species variation plays an important role in thrombotic, hemostatic, and hemorrhagic responses. Although there is no set formula to determine the relevance of the results obtained with animal models to man, the use of animal

From: *Methods in Molecular Medicine, vol. 93: Anticoagulants, Antiplatelets, and Thrombolytics*
Edited by: S. A. Mousa © Humana Press Inc., Totowa, NJ

models can provide valuable information on the relative potency of drugs, their bioavailability after various routes of administration, and their pharmacokinetic behavior. Specific studies have provided data on the species relevance of the responses in different animal models to the projected human responses. Thus, the use of animal models in the evaluation of different drugs can provide useful data to compare different drugs within a class. Caution must be exercised in extrapolating such results to the human clinical condition.

The selection of animal models for the evaluation of antithrombotic effects depends on several factors. The interaction of a particular drug with the blood and vascular components and its metabolic transformation are important considerations. Thus, ex vivo analysis of blood, along with the other end points, can provide useful information on the effects of different drugs. Unlike the screening of other drugs such as the antibiotics, antithrombotic drugs require multi-parametric end point analysis. Thus, animal models are most useful in the evaluation of the effects of these drugs.

Finally, it should be emphasized that the pharmacopeial and in vitro potency evaluations of antithrombotic drugs do not necessarily reflect the in vivo safety/efficacy profile. Endogenous modulation, such as the release of tissue-factor pathway inhibitor (TFPI) by heparins, plays a very important role in the overall therapeutic index of many drugs. Such data can only be obtained using animal models. Therefore, it is important to design experiments in which several data points can be obtained. This information is of critical value in the evaluation of antithrombotic drugs, and cannot be substituted by other in vitro or tissue culture-based methods.

2. Animal Models of Thrombosis

In most animal models of thrombosis, healthy animals are challenged with thrombogenic (pathophysiological) stimuli and/or physical stimuli to produce thrombotic or occlusive conditions. These models are useful for the screening of antithrombotic drugs. A more comprehensive review of animal models used to study venous and arterial thrombosis, hemorrhagic tendencies, and restenosis has recently been published (1).

2.1. Stasis-Thrombosis Model

Since its introduction by Wessler (2), the rabbit model of jugular stasis thrombosis has been extensively used for the pharmacologic screening of antithrombotic agents. This model has also been adapted for use in rats (3). In the stasis thrombosis model, a hypercoagulable state is mimicked by administration of one of a number of thrombogenic challenges, including human serum (4–8), thromboplastin (9–12), activated prothrombin complex concentrates (11,13), factor Xa (FXa) (11,14), and recombinant relipidated tissue factor

(TF) *(15)*. This administration serves to produce a hypercoagulable state. Diminution of blood flow achieved by ligating the ends of the vessel segments serves to augment the prothrombotic environment. The thrombogenic environment produced in this model simulates venous thrombosis, in which both blood flow and the activation of coagulation play a role in the development of a thrombus.

The procedure for the modified stasis thrombosis model of Fareed *(16)* is outlined here. Male white New Zealand rabbits are anesthetized. A 2-cm segment of each jugular vein, including the bifurcation, is carefully isolated from the fascia. The right carotid artery is cannulated in order to obtain blood samples. The test agent can be administered either subcutaneously in the abdominal region, intravenously via the marginal ear vein, or orally using a nasogastric feeding tube. 7.5 U/kg FEIBA,® administered via the marginal ear vein as a thrombogenic stimulus, is allowed to circulate for exactly 20 s before the jugular vein segments are ligated to induce stasis. After 10 min of stasis time, the left vein segment is excised and opened, and the clot is graded on a scale from 0 to +4. The right jugular segment is removed after 20 min of stasis time, and the clots are graded using the scale. Controls are run by administration of vehicle in place of the antithrombotic agent.

Other more quantitative means of measuring clot formation have also been reported with this model. These include administering radiolabeled fibrinogen or platelets to the test animal prior to the experiment, thus allowing clot size to be quantitated by measuring the incorporation of ^{125}I-fibrinogen or ^{111}In labeled platelets into the thrombus. Although these techniques can remove the subjectivity associated with visually grading the clot size, they make the model more technically complex because of the requirement of using radiolabeled material and to the need to incorporate a method to detect the radioactivity. Measurement of the wet weight of the clot formed has also been used with this model. With either of these clot measurement techniques, careful surgical isolation of the jugular vein is required, as excessive mechanical manipulation of the exposed vessels often results in vasoconstriction. The vessel segments used in such experiments must be of a consistent size in order to obtain valid results.

The formation of a thrombus in the jugular vein of rabbits also lends itself to studying the modulation of the fibrinolytic system. Models have been described in which clots formed, as in the stasis thrombosis model, are lysed by administration of a lytic agent by intravenous (iv) bolus and/or by constant iv infusion *(17)*. After a set period of time, any remaining clot can be graded, as in the stasis thrombosis model.

Criticisms of this model often revolve around the complete lack of blood flow during the thrombogenic period. The degree to which this model mimics the pathologic state is controversial. During many pathologic conditions in which a thrombus is formed, a certain degree of blood flow remains through the affected site. However, this model does offer the advantage of allowing the coagulation system to be activated at a number of distinct points. The activation of the coagulation system in vivo is known to be multivariate with respect to various clinical disease states *(16)*. Therefore, this model can be used to determine the potency of a particular agent against a variety of potential thrombogenic triggers.

In addition to differences in the thrombogenic triggers, a number of other factors can affect thrombus formation in this model *(16)*. These include the effect of preparatory agents such as anesthetics on various hemostatic parameters, variations in the circulation time of the thrombogenic challenge, and the duration of stasis. Xylazine and ketamine have no known effects on the hemostatic system. When an antithrombotic agent is administered subcutaneously or orally, pharmacokinetic and bioavailability considerations become important in evaluating the observed antithrombotic activity. Plasma drug levels are influenced by the extent of drug absorption as well as the time needed for the absorption to occur. During long periods of absorption, drug absorption and drug metabolism may occur simultaneously. Thus, it is necessary to determine antithrombotic activity at the proper time-point in order to assure that maximal plasma drug concentrations have been achieved, particularly if agents with different absorption or metabolism profiles are to be compared.

Figure 1 illustrates the effect of intravenously administered heparin and low molecular weight heparin (LMWH) on thrombus formation in this model using an activated prothrombin complex concentrate as the thrombogenic trigger. Both agents were tested 5 min following administration. By using this route of administration and short circulation time, little clearance or metabolism of any of the agents is likely to have occurred. In this system, each agent produced a dose-dependent reduction in thrombus formation.

2.2. Models Based on Vessel-Wall Damage

The formation of a thrombus is not solely induced by a plasmatic hypercoagulable state. In the normal vasculature, the intact endothelium provides a non-thrombogenic surface over which the blood flows. The non-thrombogenic properties of the endothelium are in part caused by release of such agents as prostacyclin that prevents platelet aggregation, the presence of TFPI, and heparin-like glycosaminoglycans (GAGs), and the synthesis of fibrinolytic activators. Disruption of the endothelium limits the beneficial effects previously enumerated, and also exposes subendothelial TF and collagen that serve to activate the coagulation and platelet aggregation processes, respectively. Endothelial damage can be induced experimentally by physical means (clamp-

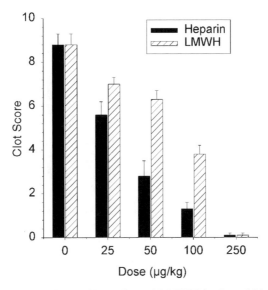

Fig. 1. Antithrombotic effect of heparin and LMWH in the rabbit stasis thrombosis model following intravenous administration. A stasis time of 10 min was utilized. The results represent the mean ±SEM of five rabbits per treatment group.

ing, catheter), chemical means (fluorescein isothiocyanate [FITC], Rose Bengal, ferrous chloride), thermal injury, or electrolytic injury.

2.2.1. Rat Jugular-Vein Clamping Model of Thrombosis

The process of thrombus formation following endothelial damage has been modeled in rats by Raake et al. *(18)*. Repeated clamping of the vessel wall using a hemostat produces damage to the endothelium that has been demonstrated histologically *(18,19)*.

In this model, male Sprague-Dawley rats are anesthetized, the skin on the neck is shaved, and an incision is made centrally above the trachea. The right jugular vein is isolated and covered with ultrasound transmission gel. A bi-directional Doppler probe is used to measure blood flow through the vessel. Because the carotid artery is located below the jugular vein, it is important to use a bi-directional Doppler probe so that only venous flow is measured. After recording the baseline blood flow, the jugular vein is clamped using a mosquito forceps for a period of 1 min. Following removal of the forceps, blood flow is measured for a period of 5 min with the Doppler probe. If measurable flow exists at the 5-min time-point, clamping is initiated again. This process is repeated until no flow can be measured 5 min post-clamping. The effectiveness of a particular antithrombotic agent is determined by the number of clampings required to cause vascular occlusion.

When high doses of an effective antithrombotic agent are used in this model, the maximal number of vessel clampings must be artificially limited. Beyond a certain point, excessive mechanical damage to the vessel leads to bleeding from the clamping site, thereby preventing an accurate determination of the time needed for thrombus formation. Because a maximal antithrombotic effect may not be determined, conventional potency designations such as ED_{50} cannot be used with this model. In setting up this model, it is essential to exercise caution in isolating the jugular vein, as excessive physical manipulation or the use of cautery result in a constriction of the vessel. Once constricted, blood flow through the jugular vein cannot be accurately measured by Doppler flow.

Unfractionated heparin (UFH), LMWH, the synthetic polyanion aprosulate, and a number of thrombin inhibitors have all been shown in the literature to dose-dependently increase the number of clampings required for vessel occlusion (*19,20*).

2.2.2. Catheter-Induced Thrombosis Models

Models that use a catheter to induce vessel-wall damage of both arteries and veins have been reported (*21–24*). Such models in the arterial system mimic potential injuries induced by angioplasty. In these models, the endothelium is damaged either by rubbing the catheter across the luminal surface of the vessel or by air desiccation. Inflation of the balloon and the induction of partial stasis in the area of damage produce additional injury. With this procedure, vessel-wall collagen, elastic tissues, and tissue thromboplastin are exposed to the circulating blood. Such models are typically carried out in rabbits or larger animals because of size considerations for both the vessel and the catheter.

In these models, the formation of thrombi has been detected in a number of ways. Measurement of flow by a distally placed flow meter or thermistor has been reported (*22*). A decrease in vessel temperature measured distally to the site of injury reflects a decrease in blood flow through the segment and the formation of a thrombus. Deposition of radiolabeled platelets at the site of injury and measurement of thrombus wet weight have also been used.

Figure 2 illustrates a typical flow measurement tracing obtained during and after induction of venous thrombus formation in the rabbit jugular vein. In this experiment, recombinant TFPI was administered at doses of either 10 or 20 µg/kg as an iv bolus. As observed in the figure, baseline blood flow was measured at approx 15 mL/min. Following vessel damage by repeated balloon inflation and gentle rubbing of the endothelium, a vessel clamp was placed to reduce blood flow nearly 90% relative to baseline. At this time, the test agent (TFPI) was

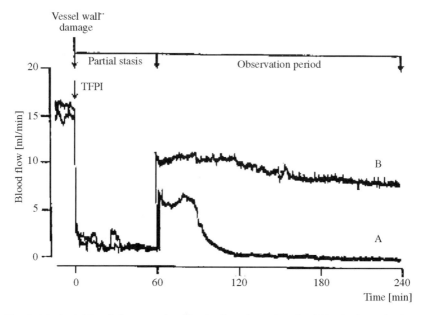

Fig. 2. Typical blood-flow tracings in the jugular vein of rabbits before, during and after the induction of venous thrombus formation. The effect of an iv bolus injection of TFPI on vascular patency is shown. Rabbits were administered either 10 (**A**) or 20 (**B**) µg/kg TFPI.

administered. A period of partial stasis was carried out for 60 min. Following removal of the vessel clamp, blood flow was observed to immediately increase. Flow was monitored for 3 h after removal of the clamp. At the lower dose of TFPI, full occlusion of the vessel was observed by 120 min post-damage, whereas at the higher dose of TFPI, flow was maintained for at least 240 min.

Platelets appear to play an important role in the formation of thrombi at sites in which the endothelium is damaged (*25*). Platelets may also play a key role in the initiation of the restenotic process following angioplasty (*26*). Therefore, these models provide an opportunity to evaluate the pharmacologic effects of agents that are capable of modulating either acute platelet function or the coagulation system that may be useful as adjunctive treatments in angioplasty. It has been demonstrated that platelets as well as the clotting system are activated by arterial intervention (*26,27*), and with this model, it has been shown that heparin and hirudin are both capable of inhibiting initial thrombosis. In addition, these models have also been used to evaluate the inhibition of rethrombosis following lysis of the initial clot (*22*).

2.2.3. Chemically Induced Thrombosis Models

The administration of a variety of chemicals either systemically or locally can result in damage to the endothelium, with subsequent generation of thrombus. Such compounds include ferric/ferrous chloride, fluorescein-labeled dextran, and Rose Bengal. Although typically used to induce arterial thrombosis, such agents may also be useful in inducing venous thrombosis.

In models employing ferric (ferrous) chloride *(28)*, the carotid artery of rats is isolated. A flow probe is placed proximal to the intended site of lesion, and a 3-mm disk of filter paper that has been soaked in ferric/ferrous chloride (35–50%) is placed on the artery. The application of ferric (ferrous) chloride results in a transmural vascular injury, leading to the formation of occlusive thrombi. This injury is believed to be a result of lipid peroxidation catalyzed by the ferric (ferrous) chloride. Thrombus formation, measured as a decrease in blood flow through the vessel, typically occurs within 30 min. Microscopic analysis of the thrombi has shown them to be predominantly platelet-rich clots. This model has been used to study the antithrombotic effects of direct thrombin inhibitors *(29–31)* and heparins.

Endothelial damage can also be induced by fluorescein or FITC-conjugated compounds. A model has been described in which FITC-dextran is administered intravenously to mice. Thrombus formation is induced upon exposure of the arterioles and venules of the ear to the light of a mercury lamp (excitation wavelength of 450–490 nm) *(32)*. The endothelial damage induced in this model is believed to be a result of the generation of singlet molecular oxygen produced by energy transfer from the excited dye *(33)*. Thrombus formation is measured using intravital fluorescence microscopy. This detection technique allows for a number of end points to be quantitated, including changes in luminal diameter resulting from thrombus formation, blood flow measurements, and extravasation of the FITC-dextran. This model offers the advantages of not requiring surgical manipulations that can cause hemodynamic or inflammatory changes—it allows repeated analysis of the same vessel segments over time and is applicable to the study of both arteriolar and venular thrombosis. The administration of Rose Bengal has been used similarly *(34)*.

2.2.4. Laser-Induced Thrombosis Model

The physiologic responses to injury in the arterial and venous systems vary, partly because of differences in blood-flow conditions that lead to different clot compositions. This model of thrombosis is based on the development of a platelet-rich thrombus following a laser-mediated thermal injury to the vascular wall of arterioles or venules *(36–38)*. This model was first described by Weichert et al. *(35)*. In this model, an intestinal loop of an anesthetized rat is

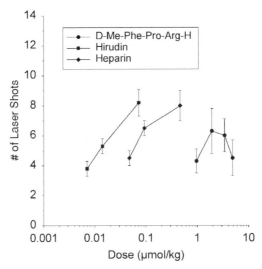

Fig. 3. Comparison of the antithrombotic effects of various thrombin inhibitors in the rat laser-induced thrombosis model. Each thrombin inhibitor was administered via the tail vein and allowed to circulate for 5 min prior to initiation of the laser injuries. (•)D-MePhe-Pro-Arg-H, (—■—) hirudin, (—♦—) heparin.

exposed through a hypogastric incision and spread on a microscope stage while being continuously irrigated with sterile physiologic saline. Vascular lesions are induced on small mesenteric arterioles with an argon laser beam (50 mW at microscope, 150-ms duration) directed through the optical path of the micro-scope. Exposure of the laser beam is controlled by means of a camera shutter, and laser shots are made every minute. Antithrombotic potency is evaluated in real time by microscopic evaluation of vascular occlusion. The number of laser injuries to induce a thrombus with a length of at least 1.5× the inner diameter of the vessel is taken as an end point.

The antithrombotic activity of several thrombin inhibitors has been compared to UFH using the laser-induced thrombosis model. Each inhibitor was admin-istered intravenously via one of the tail veins and allowed to circulate for 5 min prior to the initiation of the laser-induced lesions. Saline-treated control rats required an average of three laser shots to reach an end point. Each thrombin inhibitor produced a dose-dependent antithrombotic effect in this model **(Fig. 3)**. In comparing the dose of each agent required to extend the end point to six laser shots, hirudin was observed to be the most potent antithrombotic agent (0.08 μmol/kg), followed by heparin (0.154 μmol/kg). Consistent with the results obtained with these agents in the rabbit jugular-vein stasis thrombosis model, D-Me-Phe-Pro-Arg-H exhibited the weakest effects in the laser-induced thrombosis model (2 μmol/kg).

2.3.2. Vena-Caval Ligation Model

Vena-caval ligation models in rats have been used to study the antithrombotic activities of heparin, thrombin inhibitors, and antiplatelet agents *(39–41)*. One variation on this model is similar to the stasis-thrombosis model in rabbits in that dilute thromboplastin is administered to the rats prior to complete ligation of the vessel segment. After a defined time period, the vessel segment is opened, and the size of the resulting thrombus is determined by weight or protein content. Similar models have been reported in which copper or stainless-steel coils are placed in the vena cava, providing a thrombogenic surface on which a thrombus can form.

2.4. Disease Models

2.4.1. Microvascular Thrombosis in Trauma Models

Successful replantation of amputated extremities is dependent in large degree on maintaining the microcirculation. A number of models have been developed in which blood vessels are subjected to crush injury with or without vascular avulsion and subsequent anastomosis *(42–44)*.

In the model of Stockmans *(44)*, both femoral veins are dissected from the surrounding tissue. A trauma clamp, which has been adjusted to produce a pressure of 1500 g/mm,[2] is positioned parallel to the long axis of the vein. The anterior wall of the vessel is grasped between the walls of the trauma clamp, and the two endothelial surfaces are rubbed together for a period of 30 s as the clamp is rotated. Formation and dissolution of platelet-rich mural thrombi are monitored over a period of 35 min by transillumination of the vessel. By using both femoral veins, the effect of drug therapy can be compared to control in the same animal, minimizing intra-animal variations.

The models of Korompilias *(43)* and Fu *(42)* examine the formation of arterial thrombosis in rats and rabbits, respectively. In these models, either the rat femoral artery or the rabbit central ear artery is subjected to a standardized crush injury. The vessels are subsequently divided at the midpoint of the crushed area, and then anastomosed. Vessel patency is evaluated by milking the vessel at various time-points post-anastomosis. These models have been used to demonstrate the effectiveness of topical administration of LMWH in preventing thrombotic occlusion of the vessels. Such models effectively mimic the clinical situation, yet are limited by the necessity of a high degree of surgical skill to effectively anastomose the crushed arteries.

2.4.2. Cardiopulmonary Bypass Models

Cardiopulmonary bypass (CPB) models have been described in baboons *(45)*, swine *(46,47)*, and dogs *(48,49)*. In each model, the variables that can affect the hemostatic system such as anesthesia, shear stresses caused by the CPB pumps and the exposure of plasma components and blood cells to foreign surfaces (e.g., catheters or oxygenators) are comparable to that observed with human patients. With these models, it is possible to examine the potential usefulness of novel anticoagulants in preventing thrombosis under relatively harsh conditions in which both coagulation and platelet function are altered. The effectiveness of direct thrombin inhibitors *(45,48)*, LMWHs *(50)*, and heparinoids *(49)* has been compared to standard heparin. End points have included the measurement of plasmatic anticoagulant levels, the histological determination of microthrombi deposition in various organs, the formation of blood clots in the components of the extracorporeal circuit, and the deposition of radiolabeled platelets in various organs and on the components of the extracorporeal circuit. Therefore, these models can be used to evaluate the antithrombotic potential of new agents for use in CPB surgery and to assess the biocompatability of components used to maintain extracorporeal circulation.

3. Discussion

A wide range of animal models has been developed to mimic thrombotic, vascular, bleeding, and cardiovascular disorders. These animal models have provided useful information of the pathogenesis of hemostatic and thrombotic disorders, and have also served as crucial models to test the safety and efficacy of newer antithrombotic drugs. The information obtained from animal models remains indispensable, and has helped in the design of human clinical trials. The animal models have played a key role in the development of such newer drugs as the LMWHs, glycoprotein IIb/IIIa antagonists, and hirudin.

It is not possible to survey all of the animal models used in the investigation of antithrombotic drugs in a single manuscript. In this chapter, only the most commonly used animal models of venous thrombosis have been described. Since rats, rabbits, and monkeys have been used extensively and are available for the investigation of the pathogenesis of thrombosis and pharmacokinetic/pharmacodynamic modeling studies, these models have been included in this manuscript. Other animal models based on the use of such animals as the mouse, guinea pig, and hamster are not discussed. However, these and other species have been used by various investigators.

The original model of jugular-vein thrombosis described by Wessler remains the most practical and widely used model for testing antithrombotic drugs. Since its introduction, several modifications have been proposed, including the use of different thrombogenic challenges such as TF, prothrombin complexes, and purified clotting enzymes. The nature of the thrombogenic challenge is the primary determinant of the outcome, and has provided a basis for simulating multiple thrombogenic conditions. This model simulates both the decrease in blood flow and the activation of the coagulation system observed in deep venous thrombosis (DVT). The use of this model to investigate antiplatelet drugs is rather limited. The jugular-vein stasis thrombosis model can also be extended to other species. In particular, rats have often been used with this model. However, significant attenuation of the antithrombotic efficacy for various drugs has been noted in rats in comparison to the effects observed in rabbits.

In both rabbit and rat models, mechanical and physical damage of blood vessels has also been used to trigger thrombogenesis. These lesions eventually lead to occlusive processes and simulate human pathologic responses. Stasis and other induced impediments to flow have also been used in conjunction with these models. In both rats and rabbits, ligation has been used to simulate venous thrombosis. The laser-induced thrombosis model has also been developed to test the effects of drugs on the microcirculation of the arterial and venous systems. This model mimics the dynamic condition and allows the direct effect of a test agent to be readily evaluated. The thrombogenic trigger in this model involves both vascular and platelet components. Several other models in dogs have also been developed. These models are valuable in the study of antithrombotic drugs for cardiovascular indications.

The choice of relevant models to test new antithrombotic drugs depends on several factors such as the intended indication, sites of drug action, route of drug administration, and the nature of the data required. Thus, before choosing an animal model for scientific studies, a careful analysis of the study objectives should be conducted.

The nonhuman primates provide one of the most useful models for studying antithrombotic drugs in simulated conditions that mimic human diseases. The results obtained from the primates closely approximate human responses, and the data provide relevant information for developing new antithrombotic drugs in human trials. These primates exhibit significant phylogenetic similarities to humans, and the humoral and cellular sites mimic the human receptors. Some of the antibodies engineered for human antigens can be used to investigate the responses in primates. A classic example of this is the development of glycoprotein IIb/IIIa (GP IIb/IIIa) antagonists. The platelets from other species, such as the dog, rat, rabbit, guinea pig, and hamster, exhibit varying degrees of very low affinity to GP IIb/IIIa, whereas platelets from both the Cynomolgus and *Macaca mulatta* primates exhibit comparable responses to humans and can be used to investigate the antiplatelet effects of these inhibitors. Similarly, several occlusive disorders such as thrombotic and ischemic stroke can be studied in baboons, in which the pathophysiology of tissue damage mimics the human response. Primates have been used extensively for various studies. Because of the cost, many of these studies are not terminal. Primates are extremely useful in the study of human receptor-specific drugs because of their similarity to humans.

Bleeding is the most common side effect of anticoagulant and antithrombotic drugs. For methodologic reasons, bleeding models are difficult to develop. However, several animal models of bleeding have been used to profile the safety of antithrombotic drugs. The rabbit ear-bleeding model reported by Cade remains the most practical and widely used model. The rat-tail transection and template bleeding models have also been used. The pathophysiology of bleeding models is usually based on mechanical damage to the blood vessels. A model based on the endogenous modulation of the hemostatic system is not available at this time.

Microvascular hemorrhagic responses can be mimicked by inducing mechanical damage to rabbit mesenteric arteries. However, this method is difficult to standardize. Primates also provide a useful model for simulating the bleeding response. Gum-bleeding and ear-bleeding responses have been used to determine the bleeding effects of various agents. Standardization of the bleeding response has been a major problem, and a large number of primates are needed to obtain standardized, valid data. Regardless of the limitations of the bleeding models, it is important to profile the pharmacologic effects of the antithrombotic drugs using these models.

Despite their limitations, the animal models of bleeding and thrombosis have provided invaluable tools for investigating anticoagulant and antithrombotic drugs. These models provide crucial data on both direct and indirect (endogenous) effects of drugs. Furthermore, the endogenous modulation of drugs can be studied only in intact animals. Species variation, sex, age, and other physiologic parameters contribute to the variability of the data obtained, and should be evaluated with caution in animal studies.

Acknowledgments

The authors are grateful to Dr. Lee Cera and the staff of the Animal Research Facility of Loyola University Medical Center for their advice and critical input in the development of various animal models. The expert advice of Dr. Walenga in setting up the stasis thrombosis model is acknowledged. We are also thankful to Professor Breddin of the International Institute for Blood and Vascular Disorders for his assistance in setting up the laser-induced thrombosis model.

References

1. Jeske, W. P., Iqbal, O., Fareed, J., and Kaiser, B. (2003) A survey of animal models to develop novel antithrombotic agents, in *New Therapeutic Agents in Thrombosis*

and Thrombolysis, 2nd ed. (Sasahara, A. A. and Loscalzo, J., eds.), Marcel Dekker, Inc., New York, pp. 9–32.

2. Wessler, S., Reimer, S. M., and Sheps, M. C. (1959) Biologic assay of a thrombosis-inducing activity in human serum. *J. Appl. Physiol.* **14,** 943–946.

3. Meuleman, D. G., Hobbelen, P. M., Van Dinther, T. G., Vogel, G. M., Van Boeckel, C. A., and Moelker, H. C. (1991) Antifactor Xa activity and antithrombotic activity in rats of structural analogues of the minimum antithrombin III binding sequence: discovery of compounds with a longer duration of action than the natural pentasaccharide. *Semin. Thromb. Hemost.* **17 (Suppl. 1),** 112–117.

4. Carrie, D., Caranobe, C., Saivin, S., Houin, G., Petitou, M., Lormeau, J. C., et al. (1994) Pharmacokinetic and antithrombotic properties of two pentasaccharides with high affinity to antithrombin III in the rabbit: comparison with CY 216. *Blood* **84(8),** 2571–2577.

5. Bara, L., Bloch, M. F., and Samama, M. M. (1992) A comparative study of recombinant hirudin and standard heparin in the Wessler model. *Thromb. Res.* **68(2),** 167–174.

6. Saivin, S., Petitou, M., Lormeau, J. C., Dupouy, D., Sie, P., Caranobe, C., et al. (1992) Pharmacological properties of a low molecular weight butyryl heparin derivative (C4-CY 216) with long lasting effects. *Thromb. Haemostasis* **67(3),** 346–351.

7. Thomas, D. P., Gray, E., and Merton, R. E. (1990) Potentiation of the antithrombotic action of dermatan sulfate by small amounts of heparin. *Thromb. Haemostasis* **64(2),** 290–293.

8. Walenga, J. M., Fareed, J., Petitou, M., Samama, M., Lormeau, J. C., and Choay, J. (1986) Intravenous antithrombotic activity of a synthetic heparin pentasaccharide in a human serum induced stasis thrombosis model. *Thromb. Res.* **43(2),** 243–248.

9. Peyrou, V., Lormeau, J. C., Caranobe, C., Gabaig, A. M., Crepon, B., Saivin, S., et al. (1994) Pharmacologic properties of CY 216 and of its ACLM and BCLM components in the rabbit. *Thromb. Haemostasis* **72(2),** 268–274.

10. Saivin, S., Caranobe, C., Petitou, M., Lormeau, J. C., Level, M., Crepon, B., et al. (1992) Antithrombotic activity, bleeding effect and pharmacodynamics of a succinyl derivative of dermatan sulfate in rabbits. *Br. J. Haematol.* **80(4),** 509–513.

11. Walenga, J. M., Petitou, M., Lormeau, J. C., Samama, M., Fareed, J., and Choay, J. (1987) Antithrombotic activity of a synthetic heparin pentasaccharide in a rabbit stasis thrombosis model using different thrombogenic challenges. *Thromb. Res.* **46(2),** 187–198.

12. Vlasuk, G. P., Ramjit, D., Fujita, T., Dunwiddie, C. T., Nutt, E. M., Smith, D. E., et al. (1991) Comparison of the in vivo anticoagulant properties of standard heparin and the highly selective factor Xa inhibitors antistasin and tick anticoagulant peptide (TAP) in a rabbit model of venous thrombosis. *Thromb. Haemostasis* **65(3),** 257–262.

13. Bacher, P., Walenga, J. M., Iqbal, O., Bajusz, S., Breddin, K., and Fareed, J. (1993) The antithrombotic and anticoagulant effects of a synthetic tripeptide and recombinant hirudin in various animal models. *Thromb. Res.* **71(4),** 251–263.

14. Millet, J., Theveniaux, J., and Brown, N. L. (1994) The venous antithrombotic profile of naroparcil in the rabbit. *Thromb. Haemostasis* **72(6),** 874–879.

15. Callas, D. D., Bacher, P., and Fareed, J. (1995) Studies on the thrombogenic effects of recombinant tissue factor. In vivo versus ex vivo findings. *Semin. Thromb. Hemost.* **21(2),** 166–176.

16. Fareed, J., Walenga, J. M., Kumar, A., and Rock, A. (1985) A modified stasis thrombosis model to study the antithrombotic actions of heparin and its fractions. *Semin. Thromb. Hemost.* **11(2),** 155–175.

17. Bacher, P., Welzel, D., Iqbal, O., Hoppensteadt, D., Callas, D., Walenga, J. M., et al. (1992) The thrombolytic potency of LMW-heparin compared to urokinase in a rabbit jugular vein clot lysis model. *Thromb. Res.* **66,** 151–158.

18. Raake, W. and Elling, H. (1989) Rat jugular vein hemostasis—a new model for testing antithrombotic agents. *Thromb. Res.* **53,** 73–77.

19. Raake, W., Klauser, R. J., Meinetsberger, E., Zeiller, P., and Elling, H. (1991) Pharmacologic profile of the antithrombotic and bleeding actions of sulfated lactobionic acid amides. *Semin. Thromb. Hemost.* **17 (Suppl. 1),** 129–135.

20. Hayes, J. M., Jeske, W., Callas, D., Iqbal, O., and Fareed, J. (1996) Comparative intravenous antithrombotic actions of heparin and site directed thrombin inhibitors in a jugular vein clamping model. *Thromb. Res.* **82(2),** 187–191.

21. Kaiser, B. (1995) Effect of tissue factor pathway inhibitor (TFPI) on venous thrombus formation and rethrombosis after lysis in the jugular veins of rabbits. *Thromb. Haemostasis* **73(6),** 944.

22. Kaiser, B., Simon, A., and Markwardt, F. (1990) Antithrombotic effects of recombinant hirudin in experimental angioplasty and intravascular thrombolysis. *Thromb. Haemostasis* **63(1),** 44–47.

23. Lyle, E. M., Fujita, T., Conner, M. W., Connolly, T. M., Vlasuk, G. P., and Lynch, J. L. (1995) Effect of inhibitors of factor Xa or platelet adhesion, heparin, and aspirin on platelet deposition in an atherosclerotic rabbit model of angioplasty injury. *J. Pharmacol. Toxicol. Methods* **33(1),** 53–61.

24. Katsuragawa, M., Fujiwara, H., Kawamura, A., Htay, T., Yoshikuni, Y., Mori, K., et al. (1993) An animal model of coronary thrombosis and thrombolysis—comparisons of vascular damage and thrombus formation in the coronary and femoral arteries after balloon angioplasty. *Jpn. Circ. J.* **57(10),** 1000–1006.

25. Kaiser, B. and Markwardt, F. (1986) Experimental studies on the antithrombotic action of a highly effective synthetic thrombin inhibitor. *Thromb. Haemostasis* **55(2),** 194–196.

26. Heras, M., Chesebro, J. H., Penny, W. J., Bailey, K. R., Lam, J. Y. T., Holmes, D. R., et al. (1988) Importance of adequate heparin dosage in arterial angioplasty in a porcine model. *Circulation* **78,** 654–660.

27. Harker, L. A. (1987) Role of platelets and thrombosis in mechanisms of acute occlusion and restenosis after angioplasty. *Am. J. Cardiol.* **60,** 20B–28B.

28. Kurz, K. D., Main, B. W., and Sandusky, G. I. (1990) Rat model of arterial thrombosis induced by ferric chloride. *Thromb. Res.* **60,** 269–280.

29. Schumacher, W. A., Heran, C. L., Steinbacher, T. E., Youssef, S., and Ogletree, M. L. (1993) Superior activity of a thromboxane receptor antagonist as compared with aspirin in rat models of arterial and venous thrombosis. *J. Cardiovasc. Pharmacol.* **22,** 526–533.

30. Elg, M., Gustafsson, D., and Carlsson, S. (1999) Antithrombotic effects and bleeding time of thrombin inhibitors and warfarin in the rat. *Thromb. Res.* **94(3),** 187–197.

31. Deschenes, I., Finkle, C. D., and Winocour, P. D. (1998) Effective use of BCH-2763, a new potent injectable direct thrombin inhibitor, in combination with tissue plasminogen activator (tPA) in a rat arterial thrombolysis model. *Thromb. Haemostasis* **80(1),** 186–191.

32. Roesken, F., Ruecker, M., Vollmar, B., Boeckel, N., Morgenstern, E., and Menger, M. D. (1997) A new model for quantitative in vivo microscopic analysis of thrombus formation and vascular recanalisation: the ear of the hairless (hr/hr) mouse. *Thromb. Haemostasis* **78(5),** 1408–1414.

33. Sanaibadi, A. R., Umemura, K., Matsimoto, N., Sakuma, S., and Nakashima, M. (1995) Vessel wall injury and arterial thrombosis induced by a photochemical reaction. *Thromb. Haemostasis* **73,** 868–872.

34. Hokamura, K., Umemura, K., Makamura, N., Watanabe, M., Takashima, T., and Nakashima, M. (1998) Effect of lipo-pro-prostaglandin EI, AS-013, on rat inner ear microcirculatory thrombosis. *Prostaglandins Leukot. Essen. Fatty Acids* **59(3),** 203–207.

35. Weichert, W. and Breddin, H. K. (1988) Effect of low-molecular-weight heparin on laser-induced thrombus formation in rat mesenteric vessels. *Haemostasis* **18S3,** 55–63.

36. Yamashita, T., Tsuda, Y., Konishi, Y., Okada, Y., Matsuoka, A., Giddings, J. C., et al. (1998) The antithrombotic effect of potent bifunctional thrombin inhibitors based on hirudin sequence, P551 and P532, on He-Ne laser-induced thrombosis in rat mesenteric microvessels. *Thromb. Res.* **90(5),** 199–206.

37. Yamamoto, J., Ishii, I., Okita, N., Sasaki, Y., Yamashita, T., Matsuoka, A., et al. (1997) The differential involvement of von Willebrand factor, fibrinogen and fibronectin in acute experimental thrombosis in rat cerebral and mesenteric microvessels. *Jpn. J. Phys.* **47(5),** 431–441.

38. Yamashita, T., Tsuji, T., Matsuoka, A., Giddings, J. C., and Yamamoto, J. (1997) The antithrombotic effect of synthetic low molecular weight human factor Xa inhibitor, DX-9065a, on He-Ne laser-induced thrombosis in rat mesenteric microvessels. *Thromb. Res.* **85(1),** 45–51.

39. Herbert, J. M., Bernat, A., and Maffrand, J. P. (1992) Importance of platelets in experimental venous thrombosis in rats. *Blood* **80,** 2281–2286.

40. Berry, C. N., Girard, D., Lochot, S., and Lecoffre, C. (1994) Antithrombotic actions of argatroban in rat models of venous, "mixed" and arterial thrombosis, and its effects on the tail transection bleeding time. *Br. J. Pharmacol.* **113,** 1209–1214.

41. Seth, P., Kumari, R., Dikshit, M., and Srimal, R. C. (1994) Effect of platelet activating factor antagonists in different models of thrombosis. *Thromb. Res.* **76,** 503–512.
42. Fu, K., Izquierdo, R., Vandevender, D., Warpeha, R. L., Wolf, H., and Fareed, J. (1997) Topical application of low molecular weight heparin in a rabbit traumatic anastomosis model. *Thromb. Res.* **86(5),** 355–361.
43. Korompilias, A. V., Chen, L. E., Seaber, A. V., and Urbaniak, J. R. (1997) Antithrombotic potencies of enoxaparin in microvascular surgery: influence of dose and administration methods on patency rate or crushed arterial anastomoses. *J. Hand Surg.* **22(3),** 540–546.
44. Stockmans, F., Stassen, J. M., Vermylen, J., Hoylaerts, M. F., and Nystrom, A. (1997) A technique to investigate mural thrombus formation in arteries and veins: II. Effects of aspirin, heparin, r-hirudin and G-4120. *Ann. Plastic Surg.* **38(1),** 63–68.
45. Van Wyk, V., Neethling, W. M. L., Badenhorst, P. N., and Kotze, H. F. (1998) r-Hirudin inhibits platelet-dependent thrombosis during cardiopulmonary bypass in baboons. *J. Cardiovasc. Surg. 39,* 633–639.
46. Dewanjee, M. K., Wu, S. M., and Hsu, L. C. (2000) Effect of heparin reversal and fresh platelet transfusion on platelet emboli post-cardiopulmonary bypass surgery in a pig model. *ASAIO J.* **46,** 313–318.
47. Dewanjee, M. K., Wu, S., Kapadvanjwala, M., et al. (1996) Reduction of platelet thrombi and emboli by L-arginine infusion during cardiopulmonary bypass in a pig model. *J. Thromb. Thrombolysis* **3,** 339–356.
48. Walenga, J. M., Bakhos, M., Messmore, H. L., Fareed, J., and Pifarre, R. (1991) Potential use of recombinant hirudin as an anticoagulant in a cardiopulmonary bypass model. *Ann. Thorac. Surg.* **51,** 271–277.
49. Henny, Ch. P., TenCate, H., TenCate, J. W., Moulijn, A. C., Sie, T. H., Warren, P., et al. (1985) A randomized blind study comparing standard heparin and a new low molecular weight heparinoid in cardiopulmonary bypass surgery in dogs. *J. Clin. Lab. Med.* **106,** 187–196.
50. Murray, W. G. (1985) A preliminary study of low molecular weight heparin in aortocoronay bypass surgery, in Low molecular weight heparin in surgical practice (Master of surgery thesis) (Murray, W. G.), University of London, London, UK, 266.

14

Arixtra® (Fondaparinux Sodium)

Shaker A. Mousa

1. Introduction

The synthetic pentasaccharide Arixtra or Fondaparinux is an indirect anti-Xa that effectively inhibits thrombin generation via its binding to anti-thrombin, the co-factor for Xa. A well-executed and designed clinical development of Fondaparinux in venous thrombosis prophylaxis demonstrated success of this agent and thus its FDA approval. Further studies are in progress in order to expand the use of this anticoagulant in various thromboembolic disorders. This represents a new challenges for the marketing of this agent vs low molecular weight heparin (LMWH) or yet to come oral direct anti-Xa or direct anti-IIa with regard to pharmacoeconomics.

Arixtra® (fondaparinux sodium) injection is a sterile solution containing fondaparinux sodium. It is a synthetic and specific inhibitor of activated Factor X (Xa). Fondaparinux sodium is methyl 0-2 deoxy-6-0-sulfo-2-(sulfoamino)-α-D-glucopyranosyl-(1-4)-0-β-D-glucopyranuronosyl-(1→4)-0-2-deoxy-3,6-di-0 sulfo-2-(sulfoamino)-α-D-glucopyranosyl-(1-4)-0-2-0-sulfo-α-L-idoPYranuronosyl-(1-~4)-2-deoxy-6-0-sulfo-2-(sulfoamino)-α-D-glucopyranoside, decasodium salt.

The molecular formula of fondaparinux sodium is $C_{31}H_{43}N_3Na_{10}O_{49}S_8$ and its molecular weight is 1728.

Arixtra® is supplied as a sterile, preservative-free injectable solution for subcutaneous (sc) use. Each single-dose, prefilled syringe of Arixtra, affixed with an automatic needle protection system, contains 2.5 mg of fondaparinux sodium in 0.5 mL of an isotonic solution of sodium chloride and water for injection. The final drug product is a clear and colorless liquid with a pH between 5.0 and 8.0 (1).

From: *Methods in Molecular Medicine, vol. 93: Anticoagulants, Antiplatelets, and Thrombolytics*
Edited by: S. A. Mousa © Humana Press Inc., Totowa, NJ

2. Clinical Pharmacology *(1)*

2.1. Mechanism of Action

The antithrombotic activity of fondaparinux sodium is the result of antithrombin III (ATIII)-mediated selective inhibition of Factor Xa. By selectively binding to ATIII, fondaparinux sodium potentiates (about 300×) the innate neutralization of Factor Xa by ATIII. Neutralization of Factor Xa interrupts the blood coagulation cascade and thus inhibits thrombin formation and thrombus development. Fondaparinux sodium does not inactivate thrombin (activated Factor II), and has no known effect on platelet function. At recommended doses, fondaparinux sodium does not affect fibrinolytic activity or bleeding time.

2.2. Anti-Xa Activity

The pharmacodynamics and pharmacokinetics of fondaparinux sodium are derived from fondaparinux plasma concentrations quantified via anti-Factor Xa activity. Only fondaparinux can be used to calibrate the anti-Xa assay. (The international standards of heparin or LMWH are not appropriate for this use.) As a result, the activity of fondaparinux sodium is expressed as milligrams (mg) of the fondaparinux calibrator. The anti-Xa activity of the drug increases with increasing drug concentration, reaching maximum values in approx 3 h.

2.3. Pharmacokinetics

Absorption: Fondaparinux sodium administered by sc injection is rapidly and completely absorbed (absolute bioavailability is 100%). Following a single sc dose of fondaparinux sodium 2.5 mg in young male subjects, Cma. of 0.34 mg/L is reached in approx 2 h. In patients undergoing treatment with fondaparinux sodium injection 2.5 mg, once daily, the peak steady-state plasma concentration is, on average, 0.39–0.50 mg/L and is reached approx 3 h post-dose. In these patients, the minimum steady-state plasma concentration is 0.14–0.19 mg/L.

2.4. Distribution

In healthy adults, intravenously or subcutaneously administered fondaparinux sodium distributes mainly in blood and only to a minor extent in extravascular fluid, as evidenced by steady state and non-steady-state apparent volume of distribution of 7–11 L. Similar fondaparinux distribution occurs in patients undergoing elective hip surgery or hip fracture surgery. In vitro, fondaparinux sodium is highly (at least 94%) and specifically bound to antithrombin III (ATIII), and does not bind significantly to other plasma proteins (including platelet Factor 4 [PF4]) or red blood cells.

2.5. Metabolism

In vivo metabolism of fondaparinux has not been investigated since the majority of the administered dose is eliminated unchanged in urine in individuals with normal kidney function.

2.6. Elimination

In individuals with normal kidney function fondaparinux is eliminated in urine mainly as unchanged drug. In healthy individuals up to 75 yr of age, up to 77% of a single sc or intravenous (iv) fondaparinux dose is eliminated in urine as unchanged drug in 72 h. The elimination half-life is 17–21 h.

3. Special Populations *(1)*

3.1. Renal Impairment

Fondaparinux elimination is prolonged in patients with renal impairment, since the major route of elimination is urinary excretion of unchanged drug. In patients undergoing elective hip surgery or hip fracture surgery, the total clearance of fondaparinux is approx 25% lower in patients with mild renal impairment (cretonne clearance 50–80 mL/min), approx 40% lower inpatients with moderate renal impairment (creatinine clearance 30–50 mL/min) and approx 55% lower in patients with severe renal impairment (<30 mL/min) compared to patients with normal renal function.

3.2. Hepatic Impairment

The pharmacokinetic properties of fondaparinux have not been studied in patients with hepatic impairment.

3.3. Elderly Patients

Fondaparinux elimination is prolonged in patients over 75 yr of age. In studies that evaluate fondaparinux sodium 2.5 mg in hip fracture surgery or elective hip surgery, the total clearance of fondaparinux was approx 25% lower in patients over 75 yr of age as compared to patients less than 65 yr of age.

3.4. Patients Weighing Less Than 50 kg

Total clearance of fondaparinux sodium is decreased by approx 30% in patients weighing less than 50 kg.

3.5. Gender

The pharmacokinetic properties of fondaparinux sodium are not significantly affected by gender.

3.6. Race

Pharmacokinetic differences resulting from race have not been studied prospectively. However, studies performed in Asian healthy subjects did not reveal a different pharmacokinetic profile compared to Caucasian healthy subjects. Similarly, no plasma clearance differences were observed between Black and Caucasian patients undergoing orthopedic surgery.

4. Clinical Studies

4.1. Prophylaxis of Thromboembolic Events Following Hip-Fracture Surgery

In a randomized, double-blind, clinical trial in patients undergoing hip fracture surgery, Arixtra (fondaparinux sodium) Injection 2.5 mg sc once daily was compared to a LMWH unapproved for use in the United States for this patient population. A total of 1711 patients were randomized and 1673 were treated. Patients ranged in age from 17–101 yr (mean age 77 yr) with 25% men and 75% women. Patients were 99% Caucasian, 1% other races. Patients with multiple trauma affecting more than one organ system, serum creatinine level more than 2 mg/dL (180 pmol/L), or platelet count less than 100,000/mm^3 were excluded from the trial. Arixtra was initiated 6 h after surgery in 88% of patients, and the comparator was initiated an average of 18 h after surgery in 74% of patients. For both drugs, treatment was continued for 7 ± 2 d. Differences in efficacy and safety between Arixtra and the comparator may have been influenced by factors such as the timing of the first dose of drug after surgery.

4.2. Prophylaxis of Thromboembolic Events Following Hip-Replacement Surgery

In two randomized, double-blind, clinical trials in patients undergoing hip replacement surgery, Arixtra 2.5 mg sc once daily was compared to either enoxaparin sodium 30 mg sc every 12 h (Study 1) or to enoxaparin sodium 40 mg sc once a day (Study 2). In Study 1, a total of 2275 patients were randomized and 2257 were treated. Patients ranged in age from 18 to 92 yr (mean age 65 yr) with 48% men and 52% women. Patients were 94% Caucasian, 4% Black, <1% Asian, and 2% other. In Study 2, a total of 2309 patients were randomized and 2273 were treated. Patients ranged in age from 24 to 97 yr (mean age 65 yr) with 42% men and 58% women. Patients were 99% Caucasian, and 1% other races. Patients with serum creatinine level more than 2 mg/dL (180 pmol/L), or platelet count less than 100,000/mm^3 were excluded from both trials. In Study 1, Arixtra was initiated 6 ± 2 h (mean 6.5 h) after surgery in 92% of patients and enoxaparin sodium was initiated 12 to 24 h (mean

20.25 h) after surgery in 97% of patients. In Study 2, Arixtra was initiated 6 ± 2 h (mean 6.25 hrs) after surgery in 86% of patients and enoxaparin sodium was initiated 12 h before surgery in 78% of patients. The first postoperative enoxaparin sodium dose was given before 12 h after surgery in 60% of patients and 12 to 24 h after surgery in 35% of patients with a mean of 13 h. For both studies, both study treatments were continued for 7 ± 2 days. Differences in efficacy and safety between Arixtra and enoxaparin may have been influenced by factors such as the timing of the first dose of the drug after surgery.

4.3. Prophylaxis of Thromboembolic Events Following Knee-Replacement Surgery

In a randomized, double-blind, clinical trial in patients undergoing knee-replacement surgery (e.g., surgery requiring resection of the distal end of the femur or proximal end of the tibia), Arixtra 2.5 mg sc once daily was compared to enoxaparin sodium 30 mg sc every 12 h. A total of 1049 patients were randomized and 1034 were treated. Patients ranged in age from 19 to 94 yr (mean age 68 yr) with 41% men and 59% women. Patients were 88% Caucasian, 8% Black, <1% Asian, and 3% other. Patients with serum creatinine level more than 2 mg/dL (180 pmol/L), or platelet count less than 100,000/mm^3 were excluded from the trial. Arixtra was initiated 6 ± 2 h (mean 6.25 h) after surgery in 94% of patients and enoxaparin sodium was initiated 12–24 h (mean 21 h) after surgery in 96% of patients. For both drugs, treatment was continued for 7 ± 2 d. Major bleeding was significantly greater in Arixtra-treated patients as compared to active enoxaparin sodium-treated patients.

5. Indications and Usage

Arixtra (fondaparinux sodium) Injection is indicated for the prophylaxis of deep venous thrombosis (DVT), which may lead to pulmonary embolism: in patients undergoing hip fracture surgery; in patients undergoing hip replacement surgery; in patients undergoing knee replacement surgery.

5.1. Contraindications

Arixtra (fondaparinux sodium) Injection is contraindicated in patients with severe renal impairment (creatinine clearance <30 mL/min). Arixtra is eliminated primarily by the kidneys, and such patients are at increased risk for major bleeding episodes. Arixtra is contraindicated in patients with body wt <50 kg. The use of Arixtra is contraindicated in patients with active major bleeding, bacterial endocarditis, patients with thrombocytopenia associated with a positive in vitro test for anti-platelet antibody in the presence of fondaparinux sodium, or in patients with known hypersensitivity to fondaparinux sodium.

5.2. Renal Impairment

The risk of hemorrhage increases with increasing renal impairment. Occurrences of major bleeding patients with normal renal function, mild renal impairment, moderate renal impairment, and severe renal impairment have been found to be 1.6% (25/1565), 2.4% (31/1288), 3.8% (19/504), and 4.8% (4/83). Therefore, Arixtra is contraindicated in patients with severe renal impairment and should be used with caution in patients with moderate renal impairment. Renal function should be assessed periodically in patients who receive the drug. Arixtra should be discontinued immediately in patients who develop severe renal impairment or labile renal function while on therapy. After discontinuation of Arixtra, its anticoagulant effects may persist for 2–4 d in patients with normal renal function (e.g., at least 3–5 half-lives). The anticoagulant effects of Arixtf may persist even longer in patients with renal impairment.

5.3. Hemorrhage

Arixtra Injection, like other anticoagulants, should be used with extreme caution in conditions with increased risk of hemorrhage, such as congenital or acquired bleeding disorders, active ulcerative gastrointestinal disease, hemorrhagic stroke, or shortly after brain, spinal surgery, or in patients who are treated concomitantly with platelet inhibitors.

5.4. Neuraxial Anesthesia and Postoperative Indwelling Epidural Catheter Use

Spinal or epidural hematomas, that may result in long-term or permanent paralysis can occur with the use of anticoagulants and neuraxial (spinal/epidural) anesthesia or spinal puncture. The risk of these events may be higher with postoperative use of indwelling epidural catheters or concomitant use of other drugs affecting haemostasis such as Naiads.

5.5. Thrombocytopenia

Thrombocytopenia can occur with the administration of Arixtra. Moderate thrombocytopenia (platelet counts between 100,000/mm^3 and 50,000/mm^3) occurred at a rate of 2.9 in patients given Arixtra 2.5 mg in clinical trials. Severe thrombocytopenia (platelet counts less than 50,000/mm^3) occurred at a rate of 0.2% in patients given Arixtra 2.5 mg in clinical trials. Thrombocytopenia of any degree should be monitored closely. If the platelet count falls below 100,000/mm^3, Arixtra should be discontinued.

5.6. Drug Interactions

In clinical studies performed with Arixtra, the concomitant use of oral anticoagulants (warfarin), platelet inhibitors (acetylsalicylic acid), nonsteroidal antiinflammatory drugs (NSAIDs) (piroxicam) and digoxin did not significantly affect the pharmacokinetics/pharmacodynamics of fondaparinux sodium. In addition, Arixtra did not influence the pharmacodynamics of warfarin, acetylsalicylic acid, piroxicam and digoxin, or the pharmacokinetics of digoxin at steady state. Agents that may enhance the risk of hemorrhage should be discontinued prior to initiation of Arixtra therapy. If co-administration is essential, close monitoring may be appropriate.

5.7. Nursing Mothers

Fondaparinux sodium was found to be excreted in the milk of lactating rats. However, it is not known whether this drug is excreted in human milk. Because many drugs are excreted in human milk, caution should be exercised when fondaparinux sodium is administered to a nursing mother.

5.8. Pediatric Use

Safety and effectiveness of Arixtra in pediatric patients have not been established.

5.9. Geriatric Use

Arixtra should be used with caution in elderly patients. Over 2300 patients, 65 yr of age and older, have received fondaparinux sodium 2.5 mg in randomized clinical trials in the orthopedic surgery program. The efficacy of Arixtra in the elderly (equal to or older than 65 yr) was similar to that seen in younger patients (younger than 65 yr). The risk of Arixtra-associated major bleeding increased with age: 1.8% (23/1253) in patients <65 yr, 2.2% (24/1111) in those? 65–74 yr of age, and 2.7% (33/1227) in those 75 yr of age. Serious adverse events increased with age for patients receiving Arixtra. Careful attention to dosing directions and concomitant medications.

Fondaparinux sodium is substantially excreted by the kidney, and the risk of toxic reactions to Arixtra may be greater in patients with impaired renal function. Because elderly patients are more likely to have decreased renal function, it may be useful to monitor renal function.

5.10. Elevations of Serum Aminotransferases

Asymptomatic increases in aspartate (AST [SGOT]) and alanine (ALT [SGPT]) aminotransferase levels greater than three times the upper limit of normal of the laboratory reference range have been reported in 1.7% and 2.6% of patients, respectively, during treatment with Arixtra 2.5-mg injection vs 3.2% and 3.9%, of patients, respectively, during treatment with enoxaparin sodium 30 mg every 12 h or 40 mg once daily or a LMWH comparator. Such elevations are fully reversible, and are rarely associated with increases in bilirubin. Since aminotransferase determinations are important in the differential diagnosis of myocardial infarction (MI), liver disease, and pulmonary emboli, elevations that might be caused by drugs such as Arixtra should be interpreted with caution.

6. Conclusions

The pentasaccharide Arixtra (fondaparinux sodium) Injection is administered by sc injection at 2.5 mg once a day to patients undergoing hip fracture, hip replacement, or knee replacement surgery. After haemostasis has been established, the initial dose should be given 6–8 h after surgery. Administration before 6 h after surgery has been associated with an increased risk of major bleeding. The usual duration of administration is 5–9 d, and up to 11 d administration has been tolerated. The role of this agent in other thromboembolic disorders is under clinical investigation.

Reference

*1. Arixtra: Prescribing information. Organon, Sanofi-Synthelabo, 2002, pp. 1–4.

---

*This report summarizes all available information on Arixtra.

15

Oral Thrombin Inhibitor Ximelagatran

Shaker A. Mousa

1. Introduction

Preclinical and initial clinical experiences with the direct oral thrombin inhibitor ximelagatran demonstrated both a short and long-term potential utility for this agent in the prevention and treatment of various thromboembolic disorders associated with both arterial and venous thrombosis. Oral administration of ximelagatran after surgery and continued for at least 6–12 d appears to be safe and effective as prophylaxis against venous thromboembolism after total knee replacement surgery. This was accomplished without laboratory monitoring of the intensity of ximelagatran anticoagulation or adjustment of the ximelagatran dose. Of the four postoperative oral ximelagatran dose regimens tested, the most effective is the 24 mg twice-daily; this regimen appears to provide at least comparable efficacy and safety as compared to postoperative low molecular weight heparin (LMWH) prophylaxis. Further testing of ximelagatran in phase III clinical trials in patients with various thromboembolic disorders is in progress.

Thrombin plays a major role in thrombus formation through its ability to rapidly activate platelets and catalyze fibrin formation *(1,2)*. The goal of anticoagulant therapy is therefore to reduce the presence and/or action of thrombin. The primary action of direct thrombin inhibitors is to directly inhibit thrombin activity without the requirement of co-factors such as antithrombin *(3)*. In addition to inhibiting thrombin activity, potent direct thrombin inhibitors have been shown to inhibit thrombin generation *(4,5)*.

A shed blood model involving incision of the skin with standardized bleeding time devices has been used to study thrombin generation in humans *(5,6)*. This model involves exposure of shed blood to subendothelial tissues, which

From: *Methods in Molecular Medicine, vol. 93: Anticoagulants, Antiplatelets, and Thrombolytics*
Edited by: S. A. Mousa © Humana Press Inc., Totowa, NJ

Table 1
Procoagulant and Inhibition of Fibrinolytic Activities of Fibrin-Bound Thrombin

Procoagulant Activity	Anti-fibrinolysis activity
Generation of fibrin from fibrinogen	Activate factor XIII (crosslinks fibrin, crosslinks $\alpha2$-antiplasmin with fibrin)
Activate platelets	Activate pro-carboxypeptidase B

are rich in tissue factor (TF) (7). TF is an important element in the activation of the coagulation cascade, and in platelet activation at sites of coronary-artery atherosclerotic plaque rupture (8–11). Thus, exposure of shed blood to TF results in immediate activation of the coagulation cascade and thrombin generation. The extent of thrombin generation can be evaluated by measuring the levels of certain markers of thrombin generation in the shed blood that is collected (5).

The mechanism by which direct thrombin inhibitors have been proposed to inhibit thrombin generation is via inhibition of thrombin's feedback activation of factors V, VIII, and XI (4,12), as well as cellular mechanisms. There is considerable variability in the degree of inhibition of thrombin generation by different thrombin inhibitors. A high affinity for thrombin (e.g., Ki <10 nm) has been suggested to be required for strong inhibition of thrombin generation (4). Additionally, a small-molecule direct thrombin inhibitor should be able to inhibit fibrin-bound thrombin that is associated with other matrices or various tumor types. See **Table 1** for the effect of fibrin-bound thrombin on coagulation and fibrinolysis.

Melagatran, the active form of the oral, direct thrombin inhibitor ximelagatran (formerly H 376/95), has a Ki of 2 nm for thrombin (13). Oral administration of ximelagatran results in rapid conversion to melagatran with low inter-individual variability in melagatran plasma levels (14–16).

A long-term follow-up of Ximelagatran as an oral anticoagulant for the prevention of stroke and systemic embolism in patients with atrial fibrillation data suggested that fixed-dose ximelagatran (36 mg bid) showed promise as an effective and well-tolerated agent for the prevention of stroke and systemic embolism, with no need for routine coagulation monitoring. Larger clinical studies to evaluate the effects of ximelagatran on the prevention of stroke in patients with NVAF are ongoing (17).

Another clinical study with a fixed-dose oral direct thrombin inhibitor ximelagatran as an alternative for dose-adjusted warfarin in patients with non-valvular atrial fibrillation (AF) concluded that fixed doses of ximelagatran of up to 60 mg bid were well-tolerated during a 3-mo treatment period in NVAF patients with a medium-to-high risk for stroke and systemic embolism *(18)*. The possible long-term beneficial effect of ximelagatran treatment justifies further exploration in large-scale clinical studies.

A randomized, double-blind, comparative study Ximelagatran (formerly H 376/95), an oral direct thrombin inhibitor, and warfarin to prevent venous thromboembolism (VTE) after total knee arthroplasty (TKA) concluded that Ximelagatran 24 mg bid starting the morning after TKA is safe, at least as effective as warfarin as prophylaxis against VTE, and does not require routine coagulation monitoring or dose adjustment *(19)*. Another randomized, double-blind comparison of Ximelagatran, an oral direct thrombin inhibitor, and enoxaparin to prevent venous thromboembolism (VTE) after total hip arthroplasty (THA) concluded that enoxaparin-treated patients had significantly fewer VTE than ximelagatran-treated patients. Bleeding rates were low and comparable between groups. Fixed-dose oral ximelagatran was well-tolerated without excess bleeding. The oral drug showed excellent efficacy compared to published literature and was used without routine coagulation monitoring or dose adjustment *(20)*.

Methro II: Dose-Response Study of the novel oral, direct thrombin inhibitor, H 376/95 and its subcutaneous (sc) formulation melagatran, compared with dalteparin as thromboembolic prophylaxis after total hip or total knee replacement demonstrated a statistically significant dose-dependent increase in efficacy was seen with melagatran/H 376/95, and the highest dose of melagatran/H 376/95 was superior to dalteparin, suggesting that the new treatment is effective and safe in the prevention of VTE *(21)*.

Results from the enhancement of fibrinolysis by melagatran via inhibition of thrombin-induced activation of PRO-CUP (TAFI) study suggested that melagatran enhances fibrinolysis by inactivating clot-bound thrombin, thus inhibiting the activation of proCPU *(22)*.

Additionally, melagatran as a safe alternative to hirudin in prevention of arterial thrombosis was demonstrated *(23)*. In this study of melagatran at equally effective antithrombotic doses, melagatran causes less bleeding than hirudin suggests that direct reversible thrombin inhibitors may be safer than irreversible thrombin inhibitors *(23)*.

2. Conclusions

Ximelagatran is the first from the class of oral direct thrombin inhibitor to continue in advanced clinical development. Further work is needed in large phase III trials to demonstrate the balance between the efficacy and safety of Ximelagatarn after long-term administration in various patient populations with thromboemobolic disorders.

References

*1. Weitz, J. I. (1997) Low-molecular-weight heparin. *N. Engl. J. Med.* **337.** 688–698.

2. Mousa, S. A. and Fareed, J. W. (2001) Advances in anticoagulant, antithrombotic, and thrombolytic drugs. *Exp. Opin. Invest. Drugs* **10(1),** 157–162.

3. Hauptmann, J. and Sturzebecher, J. (1999) Synthetic inhibitors of thrombin and factor Xa: from the bench to the bedside. *Thromb. Res.* **93,** 203–241.

4. Prasa, D., Svendsen, L., and Sturzebecher, J. (1997) The ability of thrombin inhibitors to reduce the thrombin activity generated in plasma on extrinsic and intrinsic activation. *Thromb. Haemostasis* **77,** 498–503.

5. Eichinger, S., Wolzt, M., Schneider, B., et al. (1995) Effects of recombinant hirudin on coagulation and platelet activation in vivo: comparison with unfractionated heparin and a LMWH preparation (Fragmin). *Arterioscler. Thromb. Vasc. Biol.* **15,** 886–892.

6. Kyrle, P. A., Westwick, J., Scully, M. F., et al. (1987) Investigation of the interaction of blood platelets with the coagulation system at the site of plug formation in vivo in man—Effect of low dose aspirin. *Thromb. Haemostasis* **57,** 62–66.

7. Weiss, H. J. and Lages, B. (1988) Evidence for tissue factor-dependent activation of the classic extrinsic coagulation mechanism in blood obtained from bleeding time wounds. *Blood* **71, 629–635.

8. Wilcox, J. N., Smith, K. M., Schwartz, S. M., et al. (1989) Localization of tissue factor in normal vessel wall and in the atherosclerotic plaque. *Proc. Natl. Acad. Sci. USA* **86,** 2839–2843.

9. Toschi, V., Gallo, R., Lettino, M., et al. (1997) Tissue factor modulates thrombogenicity of human atherosclerotic plaques. *Circulation* **95,** 594–599.

10. Badimon, J. J., Lettino, M., Toschi, V., et al. (1999) Local inhibition of tissue factor reduces the thrombogenicity of disrupted human atherosclerotic plaques. Effects of tissue factor pathway inhibitor on plaque thrombogenicity under flow. *Circulation* **99,** 1780–1787.

11. Tremoli, E., Camera, M., Tosch, V., et al. (1999) Tissue factor in atherosclerosis. *Atherosclerosis* **144,** 273–278.

12. Von dem Borne, P. A., Koppelman, S. J., Bouma, B. N., et al. (1994) Surface independent factor XI activation by thrombin in the presence of high molecular weight kininogen. *Thromb. Haemostasis* **72,** 397–402.

†13. Gustafsson, D., Antonsson, T., Bylund, R., et al. (1998) Effects of melagatran, a new low-molecular-weight thrombin inhibitor, on thrombin and fibrinolytic enzymes. *Thromb. Haemostasis* **79,** 110–118.

---

*This review highlights the different mechanisms involved in the inhibiting hypercoagulation states using either indirect or direct means.

**Another documentation for the role of tissue factor as a defensive mechanism in wounds.

†A comprehensive report on the influence of direct thrombin inhibitor on thrombin and the fibrinolytic system.

14. Eriksson, U. G., Johansson, L., Frison, L., et al. (1999) Single and repeated oral dosing of H 376/95, a prodrug to the direct thrombin inhibitor melagatran, to young healthy male subjects. *Blood* **94 (10 Suppl.)**, 26a.

15. Gustafsson, D., Nystrom, J.-E., Calsson, S., et al. (2001) The direct thrombin inhibitor melagatran and its oral prodrug H 376/95: Intestinal absorption properties, biochemical and pharmacodynamic effects. *Thromb. Res.* **101**, 171–181.

*16. Sarich, T. C., Eriksson, U. G., Mattsson, C., et al. (2002) Inhibition of thrombin generation by the oral direct thrombin inhibitor Ximelagatran in shed blood from healthy male subjects. *Thromb. Haemostasis* **87**, 300–305.

17. Petersen, P., on behalf of the SPORTIF II investigators. (2001) A long-term follow-up of Ximelagatran as an oral anticoagulant for the prevention of stroke and systemic embolism in patients with atrial fibrillation. *Blood* **98(11)**, 706a, 2953.

18. Olsson, B. B. and Petersen, P. (2001) Fixed-dose oral direct thrombin inhibitor ximelagatran as an alternative for dose-adjusted warfarin in patients with non-valvular atrial fibrillation. *Eur. Heart J.* **22**, 330, P1761.

19. Francis, C. W., Davidson, B. L., Berkowitz, S. D., et al. (2001) A randomized, double-blind, comparative study Ximelagatran (formerly H 376/95), an oral direct thrombin inhibitor, and warfarin to prevent venous thromboembolism (VTE) after total knee arthroplasty (TKA). *Thromb. Haemostasis* **(Suppl)**, July, OC44.

20. Colwell, W., Berkowitz, S. D., Davidson, B. L., et al. (2001) Randomized, double-blind, comparison of Ximelagatran, an oral direct thrombin inhibitor, and enoxaparin to prevent venous thromboembolism (VTE) after total hip arthroplasty (THA). *Blood* **98(11)**, 706a, 2952.

21. Eriksson, B. I., Lindbratt, I. S., Kaleboi, P., et al. (2000) Methro II: Dose-Response Study of the novel oral, direct thrombin inhibitor, H 376/95 and its subcutaneous formulation melagatran, compared with dalteparin as thromboembolic prophylaxis after total hip or total knee replacement. *Haemostasis* **30 (Suppl. 1)**, 20–21, 38.

22. Berntsson, P., Mattsson, C., Johansson, T., et al. (2001) Enhancement of fibrinolysis by melagatran via inhibition of thrombin-induced activation of PRO-CUP (TAFI). *Thromb. Haemostasis* **(Suppl.)**, July, P2014.

23. Klement, P., Carlsson, S., Liao, P., et al. (2001) Melagatran, a safe alternative to hirudin in prevention of arterial thrombosis. *Thromb. Haemostasis* **(Suppl.)**, July, P3078.

---

*This pharmacodynamic study demonstrated the effects of oral Ximelagatran on various markers of thrombin generation.

16

Pharmacogenomics and Coagulation Disorders

Omer Iqbal

1. Introduction

The term pharmacogenetics, first introduced by Vogel in 1959 (*1*) is defined as the analysis of inherited factors that define an individual's response to a drug, and generally refers to monogenetic variants that affect drug response. Pharmacogenetics refers to the monogenetic variants that affect drug response, and aims to deliver the right drug to the correct patient at the correct dosage by using DNA information. Pharmacogenomics refers to the entire library of genes that determine drug efficacy and safety. There are approx 3 billion basepairs in the human genome, which code for at least 30,000 genes. Although the majority of basepairs are identical from individual to individual, only 0.1% of the basepairs contribute to individual differences. Three consecutive basepairs form a codon that specifies the amino acids that constitute the protein, because of substantial redundancy, and two or more codons code for the same amino acid. Genes represent a series of codons that specifies a particular protein. At each gene locus, an individual carries two alleles—one from each parent. If there are two identical alleles, it is referred to as a homozygous genotype; if the alleles are different, it is heterozygous. Genetic variations usually occur as single-nucleotide polymorphisms (SNP) on average at least once every 1000 basepairs, accounting for approx 3 million basepairs distributed throughout the entire genome. Genetic variations that occur at a frequency of at least 1% in the human population are referred to as polymorphisms. Genetic polymorphisms are inherited and monogenic; they involve one locus and have interethnic differences in frequency. Rare mutations occur at a frequency of less than 1% in the human population. Other examples of genetic variations include insertion-deletion polymorphisms, tandem repeats, defective splicing, aberrant splice site, and premature stop codon polymorphisms.

From: *Methods in Molecular Medicine, vol. 93: Anticoagulants, Antiplatelets, and Thrombolytics*
Edited by: S. A. Mousa © Humana Press Inc., Totowa, NJ

The variable drug response in different patients may be the result of genetic differences in drug metabolism, drug distribution, and drug target proteins *(2)*. Pharmacogenomics may revolutionize the future practice of medicine. Through the use of a SNP test, a clinician may predict whether or not an individual will respond to a particular medication. Thus, medications can be selected or avoided based on the genetic makeup of the patient, causing a beneficial or adverse effect. Variations in a drug-metabolizing enzyme cytochrome P450 (CYP) cause interindividual differences in the plasma concentrations of narrow therapeutic drugs such as warfarin *(3)*. As patients show adverse effects, the medications may be either avoided or administered at a reduced dosage with careful monitoring. Based on the genetic control of the cellular function, new drugs may be developed to match the correct drug to the correct patient at the right dosage. Through the discovery of new genetic targets, pharmacogenomics may improve the quality of life, reduce the costs of health of care by treating specific genetic subgroups, and decrease the treatment failures and the adverse drug reactions (ADRs).

2. SNPs Mapping in Pharmacogenomics

Pharmaceutical companies are greatly interested in pharmacogenomics as a means to reduce the costs and the time involved with clinical trials, and to improve the efficacy of therapeutic compounds tailored to treat each patient at the correct dosage. Although genetic association studies are used to establish links between polymorphic variation in the coagulation Factor V gene and deep venous thrombosis (DVT), this approach of "susceptibility genes" that directly influence an individual's likelihood of developing the disease *(4)* has been extended in the identification of other gene variants. Variations in a drug-metabolizing enzyme gene, thiopurine methyltransferase (TPMT), have been linked to adverse drug reactions *(5)*; variants in a drug-target (5-lipoxygenase, ALOX5) have been linked to variations in drug response *(6)*. Through linkage disequilibrium (LD) or nonrandom association between SNPs in proximity to each other, tens of thousands of anonymous SNPs are identified and mapped. These anonymous genes may fall either within genes, susceptibility genes, or in noncoding DNA between genes. Through LD, the associations found with these anonymous SNP markers can identify a region of the genome that may harbor a particular susceptibility gene. Through positional cloning, the gene and the SNP can be revealed within, conferring the underlying associated condition or disease *(7)*. As the human genome is now completely mapped, gene-based SNP approaches will be valuable in the diagnosis of diseases. Numerous companies have now developed DNA microarrays (biochips) of different genes of interest that could be used in high-throughput sequencing in a population to detect common or uncommon genetic variants. These DNA-based diagnostic microarrays, which are targeted for patient care, must be accurate, high-throughput, reproducible, flexible, and low-cost. Thus far, there are no FDA-approved DNA microarrays on the market. Efforts should be made to improve the sensitivity as well as reduce the costs of identifying polymorphisms by direct sequencing.

It is important to understand the genetic variability in genes in relation to the safety and efficacy of an anticoagulant drug. The functional consequences of non-synonymous SNPs can be predicted by a structure-based assessment of amino acid variation *(8)*.

According to the SNP Map Working Group (Nature 2001), there are 1.42 million SNPs; one SNP per 1900 bases; 60,000 SNPs within exons; two exonic SNPs per gene (1/1080 bases); 93% of genetic loci contain two SNPs. Because each person is different at 1 in 1000–2000 bases, SNPs are responsible for human individuality. A list of genes involved in hematologic, hemostatic, and thrombotic disorders is given in **Table 1**.

3. Pharmacogenomics in Hematology

1. Coagulation Factor II (Prothrombin) G20210A: This mutation, which occurs in 2% of the population, is located in the 3′ untranslated region (UTR) of the coagulation Factor II propeptide near a putative polyadenylation site. It is associated with increased levels of prothrombin, resulting in DVT, recurrent miscarriages, and portal-vein thrombosis in cirrhotic patients *(9–12)*.
2. Coagulation factor V Leiden R506Q: This mutation (G1691A), which occurs in 8% of the population, refers to specific G to A substitution at nucleotide 1691 in the gene for factor V. It is cleaved less efficiently (10%) by activated protein C (APC), and results in DVT, recurrent miscarriages, portal-vein thrombosis in cirrhotic patients, early kidney transplant loss, and other forms of venous thromboembolism *(9,11–13)*. There is a dramatic increase in the incidence of thrombosis in women who are taking oral contraceptives.
3. Coagulation Factor IX propeptide mutations at ALA-10 (coumarin hypersensitivity): The Alanine-10> threonine and alanine-10>Valine missense mutation of factor IX propeptide is known to cause abnormal sensitivity to oral anticoagulation by reducing the affinity of the carboxylase for the vitamin K-dependent coagulation factor IX precursor, resulting in severe bleeding complications. These patients with "Coumarin hypersensitivity" bleed severely, despite the therapeutic International Normalized Ratio (INR). The increased APTT is a result of reduced factor IX. In the absence of coumarins the activated partial thromboplastin time (APTT) and factor IX levels are normal. Thus, it is important to detect the substitution G > A at position 9311 (threonine variant) or C > T at position 9312 (Valine variant) to identify the hypersensitivity before starting the patient on coumarin anticoagulation to avoid excessive bleeding complications *(14–17)*.

(text continued on page 259)

Table 1
**List of Genes Involved in Hematologic, Hemostatic,
and Thrombotic Disorders**

Clone ID	Name	Gene title
71626	ZNF268	zinc-finger protein 268
753430	ATRX	Alpha thalassemia/mental retardation syndrome X-linked RAD54 *(S. cerevisiae)* homolog
753418	VASP	Vasodilator-stimulated phosphoprotein
34778	VEGF	Vascular endothelial growth factor (VEGF)
44477	VCAM1	Vascular cell adhesion molecule 1
782789	AVPR1A	Arginine vasopressin receptor 1A
666218	TGFB2	Transforming growth factor, beta 2
212429	TF	Transferrin
810512	THBS1	Thrombospondin 1
205185	THBD	Thrombomodulin
210687	AGTR1	Angiotensin receptor 1
136821	TGFB1	Transforming growth factor, beta 1
143443	TBXAS1	Thromboxane A synthase 1
812276	SNCA	Synuclein, alpha (non A4 component of amyloid precursor)
149910	SELL	Selectin E (endothelial adhesion molecule 1)
135221	S100P	S100 calcium-binding protein P
753211	PTGER3	Prostaglandin E receptor 3 (subtype EP3)
245242	CPB2	Carboxypeptidase B2 (Plasma, carboxypeptidase U)
143287	PSG11	Pregnancy-specific beta-1 glycoprotein 11
130541	PECAM1	Platelet/endothelial-cell adhesion molecule (CD31 antigen)
40643	PDGFRB	Platelet-derived growth factor (PDGF) receptor, beta polypeptide
121218	PF4	Platelet Factor 4
66982	PLGL	Plasminogen-like
810017	PLAUR	Plasminogen activator, urokinase receptor
813841	PLAT	Plasminogen activator, tissue serine (or cysteine) proteinase inhibitor, Clade E (nexin, plasminogen activator inhibitor type 1), member 1
770670	TNFAIP3	Tumor necrosis factor (TNF), alpha-induced protein 3
142556	PSG2	Pregnancy-specific beta 1 glycoprotein 2
120189	PSG4	Pregnancy-specific beta-1-glycoprotein 4
151662	P11	Protease, serine, 22
49920	PTDSS1	Phosphatidylserine synthase 1
345430	PIK3CA	Phosphoinositide 3 kinase, catalytic, alpha polypeptide

Table 1 *(continued)*

Clone ID	Name	Gene title
194804	PITPN	Phosphotidylinositol transfer protein
809938	TACSTD2	Matrix metalloproteinase 7 (matrilysin, uterine)
22040	MMP9	Matrix metalloproteinase 9 (gelatinase B, 92-*Kd* gelatinase, 92-*Kd* type IV collagenase)
196612	MMP12	Matrix metalloproteinase 12 (macrophage elastase)
589115	MMP1	Matrix metalloproteinase 1 (interstitial collagenase)
292306	LIPC	Lipase, hepatic
160723	LAMC1	Laminin, gamma 1 (formerly LAMB2)
32609	LAMA4	Laminin, alpha 4
51447	FCGR3B	Fc fragment of IgG, low-affinity IIIb, receptor for Z(CD16)
727551	IRF2	Interferon regulatory factor 2
754080	ICAM3	Intercellular adhesion molecule 3
340644	ITGB8	Integrin, beta 8
343072	ITGB1	Integrin, beta 1 (fibronectin receptor, beta polypeptide, antigen CD29 includes MDF2, MSK12)
770859	ITGB5	Integrin, beta 5
811096	ITGB4	Integrin, beta 4
45138	VEGFC	VEGF factor C
199945	TGM2	Transglutaminase 2 (C polypeptide, protein-glutamine-gamma-glutamyltransferase)
234736	GATA6	GATA-binding protein 6
180864	ICAM5	Intercellular adhesion molecule 5, telencephalin
755054	IL18R1	Interleukin 18 receptor 1
810242	C3AR1	Complement component 3a receptor 1
41898	PTGDS	Prostaglandin D2 synthase (21 *Kd*, brain)
810124	PAFAH1B3	Platelet-activating factor acetylhydrolase, isoform 1b, gamma subunit (29 *Kd*)
810010	PDGFRL	PDGF-receptor-like
184038	SPTBN2	Spectrin, beta, non-erythrocytic 2
179276	FASN	Fatty acid synthase
776636	BHMT	Betaine-homocysteine methyltransferase
770462	CPZ	Carboxypeptidase Z
137836	PDCD10	Programmed cell death 10
127928	HBP1	HMG-box containing protein 1
138991	COL6A3	Collagen, type VI, alpha 3
212649	HRG	Histidine-rich glycoprotein
155287	HSPA1A	heatshock 70 *Kd* protein 1A
810891	LAMA5	Laminin, alpha 5

(continued)

Table 1 *(continued)*

Clone ID	Name	Gene title
811792	GSS	Glutathione synthetase
768246	G6PD	Glucose-6-phosphate dehydrogenase
260325	ALB	Albumin
131839	FOLR1	Folate receptor 1 (adult)
139009	FN1	Fibronectin 1
813757	FOLR2	Folate receptor 2 (fetal)
241788	FGB	Fibrinogen, B beta polypeptide
49509	EPOR	Erythropoietin receptor
49665	EDNRB	Endothelin receptor type B
26418	EDG1	Endothelial differentiation, sphingolipid G-protein-coupled receptor.
1813254	F2R	Coagulation factor II (thrombin) receptor
296198	CHS1	Chediak-Higashi syndrome 1
261519	TNFRSF5	TNF-receptor superfamily, member 5
243816	CD36	CD36 antigen (collagen type 1 receptor, thrombospondin receptor)
810117	ANXA11	Annexin A11
240249	APLP2	Amyloid beta (A4) precursor-like protein 2
49164	VCAM1	Vascular-cell adhesion molecule 1
714106	PLAU	Plasminogen activator, urokinase
842846	TIMP2	Tissue inhibitor of metalloproteinase 2
758266	THBS4	Thrombospondin 4
712641	PRG4	Proteoglycan 4, (megakaryocyte-stimulating factor, articular superficial-zone protein)
726086	TFPI2	Tissue-factor pathway inhibitor (TFPT) 2
67654	PDGFB	PDGF-beta polypeptide (simian sarcoma viral (v-sis) oncogene homolog
85979	PLG	Plasminogen
85678	F2	Coagulation factor II
814615	MTHFD@	Methylene tetrahydrofolate dehydrogenase (NAD-dependent), methlenetetrahydrofolate cyclohydrolase
825295	LDLR	Low-density lipoprotein-receptor (familial hypercholesterolemia)
814378	SPINT2	Serine protease inhibitor, kunitz type 2
71101	PROCR	Protein C receptor, endothelial (EPCR)
785975	F13A1	Coagulation factor XIII, A1 polypeptide
310519	F10	Coagulation factor X
840486	VWF	Von Willebrand's factor
191664	THBS2	Thrombospondin 2
788285	EDNRA	Endothelin-receptor type A

4. Platelet glycoprotein Ia C807T: Platelet glycoprotein Ia C807T gene polymorphisms is associated with nonfatal myocardial infarction (MI) in younger patients. Other platelet polymorphisms such as P-selectin, alpha 2 adrenergic receptor, and transforming growth factor beta are associated with a risk for arterial disease, or may produce a prothrombotic state *(18–21)*.
5. Platelet glycoprotein Ia G1648A (HPA-5):
6. Platelet glycoprotein IIIa T393C (HPA-1 a/b = P1A1/P1A2): HPA-1a, found on glycoprotein IIIa, has been recently found to be an inherent risk factor for coronary thrombosis, premature MI and coronary stent thrombosis. Human platelet antigen-1a (HPA-1a) is the determinant in the pathogenesis of post-transfusion purpura (PTP) and neonatal alloimmune thrombocytopenic purpura (NATP). The human platelet alloantibody P1A1 and plA2 are associated with a leucine 33/proline 33 amino acid polymorphism in membrane glycoprotein IIIa, and are distinguishable by DNA typing *(22–24)*.

4. Pharmacogenomics in Cardiovascular Disease

1. Endothelial nitric oxide synthase eNOS (E298D) (G894T). Causes increased risk for acute myocardial infarction (AMI), coronary atherosclerosis, and essential hypertension.
2. Coagulation factor II (prothrombin) (G20210A). Causes elevated prothrombin levels with increased risk of DVT.
3. Factor V Leiden (G1691A). Causes increased risk of venous thrombosis.
4. Factor XIII (V34L) (G103T) Reduced lower incidence of cardiovascular disease (CVD).
5. Methylenetetrahydrofolate reductase gene MTHFR (C677T). A major risk factor for vascular disease.

5. Pharmacogenomics in General Metabolism

1. Apolipoprotein E E2-E3-E4.
2. Butyrylcholinesterase atypic and K-variants.
3. MTHFR C677T.
4. Leukotriene C4 synthase A-444c.

6. Pharmacogenomics in Immune System and Host Response

1. Interleukin 1 beta C4336T = TaqI RFLP.
2. IL4-receptor a Q576R.
3. Interleukin 6 G-174C.
4. TNFa G-238A, G-308A.
5. TNFb A329G.
6. CD14C-260T.
7. Toll-like receptor 4 (TLR4).
8. CCR2 V641 (G190A).
9. SDF-1 3′ G810A.

7. Proposed Uses of Pharmacogenomics

7.1. Selection of Individualized and Tailored Therapy

In the future, a physician may request a genotyping test instead of a complete blood count (CBC) to come to a diagnosis and prescribe an individualized treatment because of the wide inter-patient variability in drug efficacy or response. Recent advances in molecular biological techniques will help pinpoint these mutations.

7.2. Prevention of Adverse Drug Reactions

Adverse Drug Reactions (ADRs) are the sixth leading cause of death in the United States, with an annual expenditure of $75 billion. Aside from age, sex, and nutritional status, genetic factors play a significant role in an individual's response to a drug. There are a number of inherited sequence variants (alleles) of genes that code for drug metabolizing enzymes and drug receptors that manifest as discrete drug-metabolism phenotypes. A physician would like to have a pretreatment screening for these alleles, thereby predicting a patient's response to a medication eventually helping in the selection of a drug, which is safe and efficacious. Most of the SNPs identified are present in the drug-metabolizing enzymes, receptors, and transport proteins.

1. To prevent toxicity of the drugs or adverse side effects.
2. Help pharmacists in selecting drugs with least SNPs in pathway.
3. In drug development.

7.3. SNPs in Drug-Metabolizing Enzymes

Polymorphisms in drug-metabolizing enzymes are the first-recognized and most-documented examples of genetic variations that have consequences not only in drug response, but also in drug toxicity. The drug metabolizing enzymes are divided into two phases.

7.3.1. PHASE 1: Metabolizing Enzymes

Most of these enzymes are members of the Cytochrome P450 (CYP) superfamily, and are located in the cells of the liver and gastrointestinal (GI) system. About 40 different CYP enzymes are present in humans, and they are classified by the name of the enzyme CYP, followed by the family (e.g., 2) and subfamily (e.g., D) and gene (e.g., 6) associated with the biotransformation (e.g., CYP2D6). Functional genetic polymorphisms have been discovered for CYP2A6, CYP2C9, CYP2C19, and CYP2D6 *(25)*, and more recently for CYP3A4 *(26)*. Although a polymorphism in the regulatory region of the gene that encodes for CYP1A2 has been recognized, its functional importance is unknown *(27)*. Warfarin, a narrow-therapeutic-index agent, is metabolized by CYP2C9. Because warfarin is a racemic mixture, its S-isomer (3× more potent than the r-isomer), is metabolized by CYP2C9. CYP2C9*2 and CYP2C9*3 are the most common CYP2C9 variants to exhibit single amino acid substitutions at critical positions of enzyme action *(28)*. The consequence of CYP2C9*3 homozygotes was a 90% reduction in S-warfarin clearance compared to the wild-type variant *(29)*. CYP2C9 mutant alleles were found to be overrepresented in 81% of patients who required low-dose warfarin therapy (<1.5 mg/d) *(30)*. These patients had difficulty in induction, required longer hospitalization for stabilization of the warfarin regimen, and experienced greater bleeding complications. Patients who were homozygous with CYP2C9*3 allele had a profound response to warfarin and necessitated dose reduction to 0.5 mg/d.

Polymorphisms in these genes can result in three possible phenotypes: poor, normal, and ultrafast metabolizers. Poor metabolizers lack an active form of the expressed enzyme, normals have one copy of the active gene, and the ultrafast metabolizers have duplicated copies of the active gene. Poor metabolism would lead to toxicity, and ultrafast metabolism would lead to reduced drug efficacy. More than half of the prescribed drugs are metabolized by the cytochrome P450 system; CYP3A4 account for 50% of these, CYP2D6 (20%), and CYP2D9 and CYP2D19 (15%). CYP2D6 exhibited significantly decreased or absent activity. Drug developers avoid drugs whose metabolic pathways are significantly influenced by genetic polymorphisms in the cytochrome P450 enzyme system.

7.3.2. PHASE II Metabolizing Enzymes

Examples of phase II metabolizing enzymes that exhibit genetic polymorphisms are: N-acetyltransferase, thiopurine S-methyltransferase (TPMT), and glutathione S-transferase. The relevance of genetic polymorphisms of TPMT, dihydropyrimidine dehydrogenase (DPD) and UDP-glucuronosyl transferase (UGT) have been demonstrated in cancer *(31–33)*. The TPMT gene has three mutant alleles: TPMT*3A, TPMT*2, and TPMT*3C. The most common one is TPMT*3A.

8. Drug Transporter Gene Polymorphisms

Drug transport across the GI tract, drug excretions into the bile and urine, and drug distribution across the blood–brain barrier are carried out by certain membrane proteins. Genetic variations in these proteins may result in disturbances in the distribution of drugs and alter drug concentrations affecting adequate therapeutic action and efficacy of the drug. P-glycoprotein comprises of the energy-dependent transmembrane efflux pump that is encoded by the multidrug-resistant (MDR-1) genes. It transports toxic substances out of the cells. This protein also affects the distribution of digoxin, cyclosporine, HIV protease inhibitors, dexamethasone, vinca alkaloids, and anthracyclines. The expression of this protein in cancer cells results in active cellular export of antineoplastic drugs, resulting in multidrug resistance to antineoplastic agents. Increased P-glycoprotein expression in the GI tract limits the absorption of drugs that are P-glycoprotein substrates, resulting in lower concentration of the drugs at the therapeutic sites of action. In contrast, lower p-glycoprotein expression results in supratherapeutic concentrations of the drug at sites of action. P-glycoprotein is also expressed in hepatocytes as well as renal proximal tubular cells and capillary endothelial cells (BBB).

Of the 15 MDR-1 gene polymorphisms, the most common is exon 26 of the MDR-1 (34), which influences P-glycoprotein expression in vitro (34). The homozygous form of this polymorphism in healthy volunteers resulted in significantly lower P-glycoprotein expression and in increased plasma digoxin concentrations (34). Thus, the plasma concentrations of the P-glycoprotein substrates can be predicted by the exon 26 polymorphism of the MDR-1 gene. This would also contribute to the ethnic and racial differences in the bioavailability of P-glycoprotein substrates. Identification of Exon 26 polymorphisms of the MDR-1 gene in screening tests could help in the dosing of cyclosporine, since subtherapeutic concentrations of this agent may result in organ rejection and supratherapeutic concentrations result in drug-induced nephro- and neurotoxicity.

9. Drug Target Gene Polymorphisms

Genetic polymorphisms in receptors, enzymes, and other protein genes may alter receptor function, and sensitivity and drug response to pharmacologic competitive and noncompetitive agonizes and antagonists. The apolipoprotein gene, which affects the cholinergic function of the brain, is linked to familial late-onset Alzheimer's disease. The link between the SNPs in the β-adrenergic-receptor gene and hypertension has been established (35).

10. Genetic Polymorphisms and Adverse Effects of the Drugs

Genetic polymorphisms have been linked to adverse effects of the drugs. For example, a patient with Parkinson's disease, when administered levodopa, was protected against levodopa-induced dyskinesia, because of short tandem-repeat polymorphisms in the dopamine-D2-receptor gene (36).

11. Conclusions

Pharmacogenomics-based personalized practice of medicine will reduce the number of adverse drug effects and drug failures, thereby improving the quality of medical practice and reducing the total healthcare costs. It will provide a better insight in the understanding and diagnosis of patients with drug resistance. This will ensure the administration of the correct drug to the correct patient at the right dosage. Gene therapy will be able to treat patients with the disease by altering gene expression. By correcting the genetic defects, there is a permanent restoration of normal cellular function, thereby eliminating recurrence or relapse of the disease and controlling healthcare expenditure. Although inefficient gene delivery to target cells, inadequate gene expression, and unacceptable adverse effects are major limitations of gene therapy, alternate means of a gene delivery system will offer a new approach to treatment. The use of adeno-associated viruses—human DNA-containing viruses that do not cause disease in humans or trigger immune responses upon injection—have been found to be beneficial in treating hemophilia B. Intramuscular injections of an adeno-associated virus vector that expresses the human coagulation factor IX gene were used *(37)*. In the near future, clinicians will routinely order genetic testing for identification of SNPs for finding a permanent therapeutic option. To allay public confusion, terms such as "gene mapping" instead of "genetic testing" may be used to differentiate genotyping for polymorphisms associated with drug response from genotyping for mutations linked to increased susceptibility to inherited disorders. Focusing on somatic gene transfer instead of the germline may allay the ethical concerns with gene therapy that requires transgenic manipulation of germline cells. Recently, the –33T→C polymorphism in intron 7 of the tissue-factor pathway inhibitor (TFPI) gene was reported to influence the risk of venous thromboembolism, independently of the factor V Leiden and prothrombin gene mutations *(38)*. The SNPs could be used for drug selection, dose selection, identification of disease risk, and prevention of drug toxicity, and in medical decision-making *(39)*. The effect of factor XIII VAL34LEU polymorphism on thrombolytic therapy in premature MI has been recently reported *(40)*. The pharmacogenomic basis of drug development involves target identification, target characterization and target validation to ensure the right drug for the right patient at the right time *(41)*. It is now possible to develop a fully automated method that combines bioinformatics and chemoinformatics data, for the analysis of protein-binding sites across gene families to offer a chemogenomic approach to design multiple drugs to target multi-gene families, thereby speeding up the drug discovery research and development process *(42)*. The genes encoding for Types I, II, and III nitric oxide synthase (NOS) have now been identified and localized in the human genome. Studies of knockout mice with disruption of the genes for type I, type II, and type III NOS would shed light on the functions of NO in vivo. In order to better understand the functions of NO in the body, biochemical studies of NOS inhibitors are warranted.

These studies will reveal the mechanism of synthesis of NO and the manipulation of NO in vivo as well as in vitro, and provide pharmacological tools that may be useful in studies of the function of NO.

References

1. Vogel, F. (1959) Moderne Probleme der Humangenetick. *Ergebn. Inn. Med. Klinderheilk* **12,** 52–125.
2. Evans, W. E. and Relling, M. V. (1999) Pharmacogenomics: translating functional genomics into rational therapeutics. *Science* **286,** 481–491.
3. Mamiya, K., Ieiri, I., Shimamoto, J., et al. (1999) The effects of genetic polymorphisms in the cytochrome P450 CYP2C9 with warfarin dose requirement and risk of bleeding complications. *Lancet* **353,** 717–719.
4. McCarthy, J. J. and Hilfiker, R. (2000) The use of single-nucleotide polymorphisms maps in pharmacogenomics. *Nat. Biotechnol.* **18,** 505–508.
5. Krynetski, E. Y. and Evans, W. E. (1999) Pharmacogenetics as a molecular basis of individualized drug therapy: the thiopurine S-methyltransferase paradigm. *Pharm. Res.* **16,** 342–349.
6. Drazen, J. M., et al. (1999) Pharmacogenetic association between ALOX5 promoter genotype and the response to asthma treatment. *Nat. Genet.* **22,** 168–170.
7. Collins, F. S. (1992) Positional cloning: let's not call it reverse anymore. *Nat. Genet.* **1,** 3–6.
8. Daniel Chasman, R. and Adams, M. (2001) Predicting the functional consequences of non-synonymous single nucleotide polymorphisms: structure-based assessment of amino acid variation. *J. Mol. Biol.* **307,** 683–706.
9. Manucci, P. M. (2000) The molecular basis of inherited thrombophilia. *Vox Sang.* **83 (Suppl. 2),** 39–45.
10. Soria, J. M., et al. (2000) Linkage analysis demonstrates that the prothrombin G20210A mutation jointly influences plasma prothrombin levels and risk of thrombosis. *Blood* **95(9),** 2780–2785.
11. Foka, Z. J., et al. (2000) Factor V Leiden and prothrombin G20210A mutations, but no methylenetetrahydrofolate reductase C677T, are associated with recurrent miscarriages. *Hum. Reprod.* **15(2),** 458–462.
12. Amitrano, L., et al. (2000) Inherited coagulation disorders in cirrhotic patients with portal vein thrombosis. *Hepatology* **31(2),** 345–348.
13. Ekberg, H., et al. (2000) Factor V R506Q mutation (activated protein C resistance) is additional risk factor for early renal graft loss associated with acute vascular rejection. *Transplantation* **69(8),** 1577–1581.
14. Chu, K., et al. (1996) A mutation in the propeptide of factor IX leads to warfarin sensitivity by a novel mechanism. *J. Clin. Invest.* **98(7),** 1619–1625.
15. Oldenburg, J., et al. (1997) Missense mutation at ALA-10 in the factor IX propeptide insignificant variant in normal life but a decisive cause of bleeding during oral anticoagulant therapy. *Br. J. Haematol.* **98,** 240–244.

16. Harbrecht, U., et al. (1997) Increased sensitivity of factor IX to phenprocoumon therapy a cause of severe bleeding. *Ann. Hematol.* **74 (Suppl. 2),** A106.

17. Stanley, T. B., et al. (1999) Amino acids responsible for reduced affinities of vitamin K dependent propeptides for the carboxylase. *Biochemistry* **38(47),** 15,681–15,687.

18. Santoso, S., et al. (1999) Association of the platelet glycoprotein Ia C807T gene polymorphism with nonfatal myocardial infarction in younger patients. *Blood* **93(8),** 2449–2453.

19. Bray, P. F. (2000) Platelet glycoprotein polymorphisms as risk factors for thrombosis. *Opin. Hematol.* **7(5),** 284–289.

20. Reiner, A. P., et al. (2000) Genetic variants of platelet glycoprotein receptors and risk of stroke in younger women. *Stroke* **31(7),** 1628–1633.

21. Kunicki, T. J., et al. (1997) Hereditary variation in platelet integrin a2b1 density is associated with two silent polymorphisms in the a2 gene coding sequence. *Blood* **89,** 1939.

22. Zotz, R. B., Winkelmann, B. R., Nauck, M., Giers, G., et al. (1998) Polymorphism of platelet membrane glycoprotein IIIa: human platelet antigen 1b (HPA-1b/PlA2) is an inherited risk factor for premature myocardial infarction in coronary artery disease. *Thromb. Haemostasis* **79,** 731–735.

23. Williamson, L. M., Hacket, G., Rennie, J., et al. (1998) The natural history of fetomaternal alloimmunization to the platelet-specific antigen HPA-1a (PlA1,Z) as determined by antenatal screening. *Blood* **92,** 2280–2287.

24. Newman, P. J., Derbes, R. S., and Aster, R. H. (1989) The human platelet alloantibody PlA1 and PlA2, are associated with a leucine 33/proline 33 amino acid polymorphism in membrane glycoprotein IIIa, and are distinguishable by DNA typing. *J. Clin. Investig.* **83,** 1778–1781.

25. Evans, W. E. and Relling, M. V. (1999) Pharmacogenomics: translating functional genomics into rational therapeutics. *Science* **286,** 487–491.

26. Sata, F., Sapone, A., Elizondo, G., et al. (2000) CYP3A4 allelic variants with amino acid substitution in exons 7 and 12:Evidence for an allelic variant with altered catalytic activity. *Clin. Pharmacol. Ther.* **67,** 48–56.

27. Sachse, C., Brockmoller, J., Bauer, S., et al. (1999) Functional significans of a C→A polymorphism in intron 1 of the cytochrome P450 CYP1A2 gene tested with caffeine. *Br. J. Clin. Pharmacol.* **47,** 445–449.

28. Stubbins, M. J., Harries, L. W., Smith, G., et al. (1996) Genetic analysis of the human cytochrome P450 CYP2C9 locus. *Pharmacogenetics* **6,** 429–439.

29. Takahashi, H., Kashima, T., Nomoto, S., et al. (1998) Comparisons between in vitro and in vivo metabolism of (S)-warfarin: catalytic activities of cDNA-expressed CYP2C9, its Leu359 variant and their mixture versus unbound clearance in patients with the corresponding CYP2C9 genotypes. *Pharmacogenetics* **8,** 365–373.

30. Aithal, G. P., Day, C. P., Kesteven, P. J., et al. (1999) Association of polymorphisms in the cytochrome 450 CYP2C9 with warfarin dose requirement and risk of bleeding complications. *Lancet* **353,** 717–719.

31. Relling, M. V., Hancock, M. L., Rivera, G. K., et al. (1999) Mercaptopurine therapy intolerance and heterozygosity at the thiopurine S-methyltranferase gene locus. *J. Natl. Cancer Inst.* **91**, 2001–2008.

32. Lu, Z., Zhang, R., Carpenter, J. T., et al. (1998) Decreased dihydropyrimidine dehydrogenase activity in a population of patients with breast cancer: implications for 5-flourouracil-based chemotherapy. *Clin. Cancer Res.* **4**, 325–329.

33. Ando, Y., Saka, H., Asai, G., et al. (1998) UGT1A1 genotypes and glucuronidation of SN-38, the active metabolite of irinonectan. *Ann. Oncol.* **9**, 845–847.

34. Hoffmeyer, S., Burk, O., von Richter, O., et al. (2000) Functional polymorphisms of the human multidrug-resistance gene: multiple sequence variations and correlation of one allele with P-glycoprotein expression and activity in vivo. *Proc. Natl. Acad. Sci. USA* **97**, 3473–3478.

35. Nakagawa, K. and Ishizaki, T. (2000) Therapeutic relevance of pharmacogenetic factors in cardiovascular medicine. *Pharmacol. Ther.* **86**, 1–28.

36. Oliveri, R. L., Amnesi, G., Zappia, M., et al. (1999) Dopamine-D2-receptor gene polymorphism and the risk of levodopa-induced dyskinesia in PD. *Neurology* **53**, 1425–1430.

37. Kay, M. A., Manno, C. S., Ragni, M. V., et al. (2000) Evidence for gene transfer and expression of factor IX in hemophilia B patients treated with an AAV vector. *Nat. Genet.* **24**, 257–261.

38. Amezianne, N., Seguin, C., Borgel, D., et al. (2002) The $-33T{\rightarrow}C$ polymorphism in intron 7 of the TFPI gene influences the risk of venous thromboembolism, independently of the factor V Leiden and prothrombin mutations. *Thromb. Haemostasis* **88**, 195–199.

39. Dirckx, C., Donati, M. B., and Iacovello, L. (2000) Pharmacogenetics: a molecular sophistication or a new clinical tool for cardiologist? *Ital. Heart J.* **1**, 662–666.

40. Roldan, V., Corrlal, J., Marin, F., et al. (2002) Effect of Factor XIII VAL34LEU polymorphism on thrombolytic therapy in premature Myocardial Infarction. (Letter to the Editor) *Thromb. Haemostasis* **88**, 354–355.

41. Jazwinska, E. C. (2001) Exploiting human genetic variation in drug discovery and development. *Drug Discovery Today* **6**, 198–205.

42. Edith Chan, A. W., Zuccotto, F., Dann, S. A., et al. (2002) Protein binding pocket chemogenomics. How bioinformatics tools can help. *PharmGenomics* July/August, 32–40.

17

Guidelines for Diagnosis and Treatment of Deep Venous Thrombosis and Pulmonary Embolism

Hikmat Abdel-Razeq, Mohamad Qari, Jorgen Kristensen, Hussein Alizeidah, Faisal Al-Sayegh, Mahmoud Marashi, Abdulaziz Alzeer, Omar Al-Amoudi, Hatem Qutub, Abdel-Aziz Al-Humiadi, Steen Husted, and Shaker A. Mousa, on behalf of the GCC Thrombosis Study Group

1. Introduction

Venous thromboembolism (VTE) is a term that includes both deep venous thrombosis (DVT) and pulmonary embolism (PE). Considerable progress has been made in the understanding of the risk factors for VTE. The clinical applications of molecular techniques have facilitated identification of important inherited, yet not uncommon risk factors for VTE. Factor V Leiden (*1–5*) and prothrombin G20210A mutation (*6–10*) are among the most common. Such progress raised many questions regarding the need for and duration of anticoagulation.

At the end of treatment, low molecular weight heparin (LMWH) has become the first choice and the standard of care in many instances of VTE (*11,12*).

This chapter outlines a cost-effective diagnostic approach for both suspected DVT and PE, followed by our consensus opinion on the best treatment options, using an evidence-based approach.

2. Deep Venous Thrombosis

2.1. Risk Factors for VTE

2.2.1. Inherited

2.1.1.1. COMMON

1. **Factor V Leiden (*1–5*):**
   Described in 1993 this is the most common cause of inherited thrombophilia, accounting for 20–50% of all cases. It results from a point mutation in Factor V

From: *Methods in Molecular Medicine, vol. 93: Anticoagulants, Antiplatelets, and Thrombolytics*
Edited by: S. A. Mousa © Humana Press Inc., Totowa, NJ

gene that causes a hypercoagulable state by slowing the inactivation of Factor Va by activated protein C (APC).

2. **Prothrombin G20210A mutation** *(6–10)*:
   Such point mutation results in higher level of plasma prothrombin level (Factor II activity is usually >130%), present in 2–5% of healthy individuals.

3. **Antithrombin III deficiency** *(13–15)*:
   It is the most thrombogenic of all hereditary thrombophilias with a 50% life chance of thrombosis. Luckily, the frequency of antithrombin III deficiency in the general population is low (0.02–0.17%), but is higher in patients with VTE.

4. **Protein C deficiency** *(16–18)*:
   Protein C is a vitamin K-dependent glycoprotein, synthesized in the liver and activated slowly by thrombin to APC. APC inactivates membrane-bound Factor V.

5. **Protein S deficiency** *(19,20)*:
   This is another vitamin K-dependent glycoprotein, synthesized in the liver, which acts as a cofactor for protein C. It circulates in the plasma as a free form, or is complexed with C4b-binding protein. Only the free form is the active one.

2.1.1.2. LESS COMMON

1. Congenital dysfibrinogenemia *(21)*.
2. Hyperhomocysteinemia *(22–24)*.
3. Excessive plasminogen activator inhibitor.
4. Plasminogen deficiency.
5. Dysplasminogenemia.
6. High Factor VIII *(25–29)*.
7. High Factor IX *(30)*.
8. High Factor XI *(31)*.
9. APC resistance (without factor V Leiden) *(32–34)*.

2.1.2. Acquired

1. Age *(35–37)*.
2. Antiphospholipid syndrome *(38,39)*.
3. Postphlebitic syndrome.
4. Trauma/fractures *(40,41)*.
5. Malignancy *(42–48)*.
6. Surgery *(49,50)*.
7. Prolonged immobilization (Plaster casts, bed rest, paralysis of the limbs, prolonged travel) *(51)*.
8. History of VTE *(52,53)*.
9. Central venous catheters.
10. Chronic venous insufficiency.
11. Pregnancy/puerperium *(54–57)*.
12. Nephrotic syndrome.
13. Hyperviscosity.
14. Obesity.

Table 1
Risk Factors for VTE

Persistent		Transient	
Inherited	Acquired	Mixed	
Factor V Leiden	Age	Hyperhomocysteinemia	Surgery
Prothrombin G20210A	Malignancy	High Factor VIII	Major trauma
Protein C deficiency	Antiphospholipid antibodies	High Factor IX	Pregnancy/puerperium
Protein S deficiency	History of VTE	High Factor XI	Oral contraceptives
Antithrombin deficiency		APC resistance (Without factor V Leiden)	Hormonal replacement therapy
		Dysfibrinogenemia	Prolonged immobilization

*Modified from: Martinelli (2001) Risk factors in venous thromboembolism. *Thromb. Haemostasis* **86,** 395–403.

15. Oral contraceptives and hormonal replacement therapy (HRT) *(58–63)*.
16. Heart failure.
17. Heparin-induced thrombocytopenia (HITT).
18. Myeloproliferative diseases.
19. Paroxysmal nocturnal hemoglobinurea (PNH).
20. Microangiopathic hemolytic anemia (MAHA): TTP, HUS, DIC.
21. Inflammatory bowel disease (IBD).

A simplified classification of these risk factors is shown in **Table 1**.

2.2. Signs and Symptoms

1. Asymptomatic.
2. Swelling.
3. Redness.
4. Pain and tenderness.
5. Hotness.

2.3. Differential Diagnosis

1. Ruptured Baker's cyst.
2. Cellulitis.
3. Venous insufficiency.
4. Thrombophlebitis.
5. Hematoma.
6. Postphlebitic syndrome.

2.4. Investigations

2.4.1. D-Dimer Enzyme-Linked Immunosorbent Assay (ELISA)

Has a high sensitivity, but low specificity in DVT and PE *(64–68)*.

2.4.2. Ultrasound/Doppler

Lower limb compression venous ultrasonography, an entirely noninvasive test, has a sensitivity of 97% and specificity of 98% for symptomatic proximal DVT *(69,70)*. However, it has a low sensitivity for DVT below the knee and above the groin *(71,72)*. This drawback has been overcome by serial testing *(73)*.

2.4.3. Venography

Remains the "gold standard" for diagnosing DVT. However, it is costly and invasive, and has significant interobserver variability *(74)*.

Caution: if the patient has renal impairment with creatinine >150 µmol/L.

2.4.4. Impedance Plythesmography

Less sensitive than ultrasonography, and decreasing in use *(75–77)*.

2.4.5. Laboratory Examinations

Complete blood count (CBC) diff., ESR, prothrombin time (PT), international normalized ratio (INR), aPTT and chemistry profile.

2.4.6. Hypercoagulable Assays

Examination should be done when there is a suspicion of hereditary thrombophilia (young age, positive family history), recurrent thromboembolic events, unusual localization, or extensive thrombosis. Controversies exist about the timing of the work up. Some of the functionally based assays may be low during the acute phase of the disease. If so, a repeat after 6 mo of therapy while the patient is off anticoagulants is advocated.

Note: If warfarin cannot be stopped, switch patients to LMWH for 2 wk prior to protein C or S testing. AT testing can be done while the patient is on warfarin, but not on heparin.

2.4.7. The Initial Thrombophilia Workup Should Include

1. Protein S (total and free).
2. Protein C.
3. Antithrombin.
4. APC-resistance.
5. Prothrombin mutation.
6. Lupus anticoagulant, anti-cardiolipin, and ANA.
7. Homocysteine levels.

Table 2
Clinical Model for Predicting Pretest Probability for DVT*

Clinical feature	Score
Active cancer (treatment ongoing or within previous 6 mo or palliative)	1
Paralysis, paresis, or recent plaster immobilisation of the lower extremities	1
Recently bedridden for more than 3 d or major surgery, within 4 wk	1
Localized tenderness along the distribution of the deep venous system	1
Entire leg swollen	1
Calf swelling by more than 3 cm when compared with the asymptomatic leg (measured 10 cm below tibial tuberosity)	1
Pitting edema (greater in the symptomatic leg)	1
Collateral superficial veins (non-varicose)	1
Alternative diagnosis as likely or greater than that of (DVT)	–2

*From Wells, P. S., et al. (1997) Value of assessment of pretest probability of deep-vein thrombosis in clinical management, *Lancet* **350**, 1795–1798.

2.5. Malignancy and Thrombosis

The association between cancer and thromboembolism is well-established. Patients with a first episode of unprovoked VTE have a higher chance of developing cancer during follow-up *(43–47)*. Certain types of cancer are more often associated with thromboembolism, mostly adenocarcinoma of the gastrointestinal (GI) tract, pancreatic, prostate, ovarian, and lung cancer. Examination should be done in connection with symptoms and/or findings that indicate malignancy. The examinations should include a thorough breast, rectal, and pelvic examinations and routine labs with CXR and abdominal ultrasound, prostate-specific antigen (PSA), and stool sample for occult blood. Whether or not these individuals should undergo more aggressive investigations is controversial *(42,48)*.

2.6. Cost-Effective Diagnostic Strategies for Suspected DVT

Considering the relatively high incidence of DVT and the cost implication associated with this diagnosis, several efforts have been made to establish a diagnostic strategy that is cost-effective and accurate.

1. Clinical models: Several models have been developed to help establish the clinical probability of having DVT. *Wells's model (64,79,80)* combines risk factors for DVT and clinical examination. Each element of the score is assigned one or more positive or negative points. Patients with a total score of 3 or more have a high clinical probability, and those with a total score of 0 or less have a low clinical probability. Wells's score is detailed in **Table 2**.

2. The cornerstone in diagnostic strategies of DVT is venous compression ultra-sonography, a test with limited sensitivity for distal clots that represent 15% of patients suspected of having DVTs.

   Most recent strategies rely on serial ultrasonography to rule out proximal exten-sion of the thrombus, a strategy resulted in too many repetitions of the procedure (1302 procedures in 1702 patients with low yield; only 12 DVTs in 1302 proce-dures—e.g., <1.0%) *(73)*.

3. The use of D-Dimer in addition to ultrasonography reduces the requirement for repeated ultrasounds to 9% *(81)*. The 3-mo thromboembolic risk was less than 1% in most of the studies *(79,81)*.

4. With the increasing use of D-Dimer in the initial investigation of VTE, there is little evidence to suggest that D-Dimer in its own could safely be used to rule out DVT.

5. One group from the Geneva University Hospital has recently validated an inte-grative algorithm that includes clinical evaluation, ELISA D-Dimer, and a single ultrasound in a study that included 474 patients with clinically suspected DVT *(64)*. The 3-mo thromboembolic risk in patients without DVT in that series was 2.6%.

6. Based on the published data, we propose the following algorithm: (*see* p. 273).

2.7. Treatment

2.7.1. Inpatient or Outpatient Treatment?

Most of the patients with DVT can be treated as outpatients with LMWH if the hospital has buildup routines for follow-up.

Consider hospitalization if the patient has:

1. Bleeding or risk of bleeding complication.
2. Thrombocytopenia (<100 × 10^9/L) or known heparin-induced thrombocytopenia (HIT).
3. Signs and symptoms of PE.
4. Other diseases that requires further investigations and in hospital treatment.
5. Uncontrolled hypertension (>200/110).
6. Acute ulcer (treatment initiated during the last 4 wk).
7. Impending venous gangrene.
8. Renal insufficiency requiring dialysis.
9. Serious liver disease.
10. Pregnancy.
11. Intracranial bleeding <2 mo or damage/surgery of central nervous system (CNS), eyes or ears <14 d.
12. Lack of compliance when appropriate care not available.
13. Extensive DVT.

2.7.2. Low Molecular Weight Heparin

LMWH present a number of potential advantages over unfractionated heparin (UFH): a longer half-life, improved subcutaneous (sc) bioavailability, and less variability in response to fixed doses adjusted to body wt *(82)*.

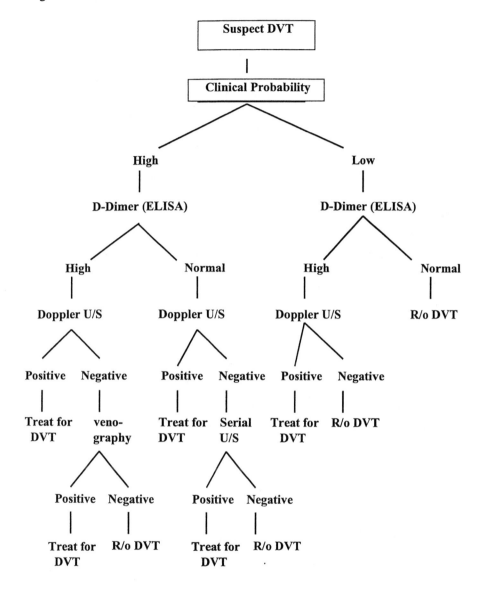

Multiple large randomized, controlled studies had suggested superiority of LMWH in terms of safety and efficacy over UFH *(83–85)*. It is to be noted that a statistically significant reduction of major bleeding was observed only with tinzaparin *(78)*.

1. Start with LMWH treatment if there is no contraindication or concerns for outpatient therapy.
2. **Table 3** shows the approved agents, doses and frequency of administration.

Table 3
LMWH Doses in VTE

LMWH	Dose
Tinzaparin	175 iu/kg sc od
Dalteparin	200 iu/kg sc daily (Max dose: 18,000 iu)
Enoxaparin	1mg/kg q 12h sc or 1.5 mg/kg/ sc od
Nadroparin	86 iu/kg sc bid or 170 iu/kg sc od
Reviparin	

Table 4
Nomogram for the Administration of iv Heparin*

APTT	Bolus U/kg	Hold (Min)	Rate Change U/kg/h	Next APTT (h)
<35	80	0	+4	6
35–45	40	0	+2	6
46–70	0	0	0	Next AM
71–90	0	0	–2	6
>90	0	60	–3	6

*To be followed 6 h after the start of the infusion.

3. Start warfarin therapy on d 1 at 5 mg and adjust the subsequent doses according to INR.
4. Check platelet count between d 3 and 5.
5. Stop LMWH after at least 4–5 d of combined therapy when INR >2.0 in two consecutive days.
6. Continue anticoagulation with warfarin for at least 3 mo. (*See* **Table 5** for duration of anticoagulation.)
7. Anti-Xa level and APTT should be checked only if the patient is bleeding.

2.7.3. UF Heparin Infusion

Heparin infusion should be given if the patient has a bleeding tendency or is a candidate for invasive procedure so as the reversal of coagulation can be easy to achieve.

1. Obtain a baseline aPTT, PT, and CBC count.
2. Check for contraindication to heparin therapy.
3. Give a bolus injection of 80 U/Kg followed by 18 U/kg/h continuous iv infusion.
4. Check the APTT 6 h after start of infusion and adjust the infusion accordingly (*see* **Table 4**).

Table 5
Duration of Anticoagulation*

3–6 mo	First event with reversible or time-limited risk factor**
>6 mo	Idiopathic VTE, first event
Lifetime	First event# with:
	1. Cancer, until resolved
	2. Anticardiolipin antibody
	3. Antithrombin deficiency
	Recurrent event, idiopathic or with any thrombophilia

*Adopted from Hyers et al. (2001) Antithrombotic Therapy for Venous Thromboembolic Disease. *Chest* **119,** 176s–193s.

**Reversible or time-limited risk factors: Surgery, trauma, immobilization, estrogen use.

#Proper duration of therapy is unclear in first event with homozygous factor V leiden, homocysetinemia, deficiency of protein C or S.

5. The APTT should be prolonged 1.5–2.0× the upper limit of the reference range.
6. Check platelet count between d 3 and 5.
7. Start warfarin therapy on d 1 at 5 mg and adjust the subsequent doses according to INR.
8. Stop UFH after at least 4–5 d of combined therapy when INR >2.0 in 2 consecutive d.
9. Continue anticoagulation with warfarin for at least 3 mo (*see* **Table 5** for duration of anticoagulation).

2.7.4. Nomograms for the Use of UFH

Heparin has a short half-life (<60 min). The current clinical practice of heparin therapy often resulted in subtherapeutic levels and inadequate anticoagulation, which may result in a higher recurrence rate of VTE. Several nomograms had been proposed *(86–88)*. Raschke et al. *(86)* and de Groot et al. *(87)* proposed and validated a weight-adjusted program for heparin infusion. The proportion of patients who achieved the therapeutic range within 24 h was >95% using this program. This Nomogram is shown in **Table 4**.

1. **Note:** Sample taken for APTT must be analyzed within 1 h; for this reason, the time of sampling must be recorded on the tube.
2. Range of APTT is variable.

2.7.5. Limitations of Unfractionated Heparin

The use of UFH requires considerable expertise, and can cause inconvenience and has limitations. Hospitalization is also required to ensure adequate heparinization. It is also associated with a higher risk of bleeding *(89,90)* and thrombocytopenia *(91)* as compared to LMWH.

2.7.6. Duration of Anticoagualtion

The duration of anticoagulation should be tailored to the individual patient according to patient age, comorbidity, and the likelihood of recurrence. In the absence of controlled studies addressing the duration of anticoagulation in special high-risk groups, we recommend following the sixth ACCP Consensus Conference on Antithrombotic Therapy *(92)* illustrated on **Table 5**.

2.7.7. VTE in Pregnancy

Two Choices:

1. Fixed dose or adjusted-dose LMWH throughout pregnancy is preferred by most clinicians *(93)*.
2. Bolus with iv UFH followed by a continuous infusion in order to maintain aPTT in the therapeutic range for 5 d followed by adjusted-dose sc UFH for the remainder of pregnancy.

Note: Adjusted-dose heparin: Give sc heparin q12 h in a dose sufficient to prolong the mid-interval APTT to 1.5–2.0× the baseline.

1. Discontinue LMWH or UFH therapy 24 h prior to elective induction of labor.
2. Postpartum anticoagulation therapy should be administered for at least 6 wk.
3. UFH, LMWH, and warfarin should be considered safe for lactating mothers *(94,95)*.
4. Long-term heparin therapy has been reported to cause osteoporosis. Most studies had reported >2% *(96)* incidence of vertebral fractures and a 30% reduction in bone density in patients receiving long-term UFH *(97)*.
5. Several studies suggest that LMWH is associated with less osteoporosis and vertebral fractures as compared to UFH *(98,99)*.

2.7.8. Thrombolytic Therapy

1. Thrombolytic agents dissolve thrombi by activating plasminogen to its active form, plasmin, which then degrades the fibrin to soluble peptides. Streptokinase, urokinase, and tissue plasminogen activator (t-PA) are the thrombolytic agents currently approved for clinical use in VTE.
2. Although the standard of care for DVT is systemic anticoagulation, thrombolytic therapy may add some benefits in special cases of DVT.
3. Thrombolytic therapy can be administered locally *(100)*—e.g., through a pedal vein for lower-extremity DVT or through systemic infusion. It can also be given via a catheter directed to the clot site (catheter-directed) *(101–106)*.
4. Reviewing the literature, we can come up with the following conclusions:
5. Thrombolytic therapy is more hazardous than standard anticoagulation because of an increased risk of major bleeding *(107–111)*.

6. Although early vein patency is an advantageous feature of thrombolytic therapy, such advantage proved to be helpful in situations such as Phlegmasia Cerulea Dolens *(105,106)*, but not in reducing the incidence of Postphlebitic Syndrome (PTS) were the available data are conflicting *(112–116)*.
7. The potential role for catheter-directed thrombolytic therapy is unknown because there are no appropriate trials.
8. Other possible indications for thrombolytic therapy include massive iliofemoral thrombosis, vena cava thrombosis, and subclavian thrombosis.

2.7.9. Venous Filters

Inferior vena cava (IVC) filters are indicated so as to prevent PE in patients with absolute contraindication to anticoagulants with recurrent VTE episode plus pulmonary hypertension, or in patients who suffer from recurrent VTE despite adequate anticoagulation *(117–122)*. Another indication is concurrent performance of surgical pulmonary embolectomy or pulmonary endarterectomy *(123–125)*. There are no long-term survival benefits because the advantage gained by less PE is offset by an increasing incidence of DVTs *(126)*. The most popular filters are Greenfield and Rutherford *(127)*.

3. Pulmonary Embolism
3.1. Clinical Findings

PE has a wide range of clinical presentations. Some PE are clinically silent and the most common signs and symptoms at presentation are:

1. Dyspnea is the most frequently reported symptom in almost 80% of the patients.
2. Tachypnoea (≥20/min) in 70% of the patients.
3. Tachycardia.
4. Pleuritic chest pain in approx 50% of the patients.
5. Syncope or shock are associated with massive PE, and is caused by a reduction in cardiac output.
6. Hemoptysis is the less frequent feature of PE.

3.2. Investigations
3.2.1. Chest X-Ray

Abnormal chest X-ray in approx 45% of the cases with plate-like atelectasis, pleural effusion, or elevation of diaphragm. However, chest X-ray is mainly useful to exclude other causes of dyspnea and chest pain, and is essential for interpreting the lung-scan findings.

3.2.2. Arterial Blood Gases (ABG)

Hypoxemia and hypo, but up to 20% of patients with PE have a normal arterial oxygen pressure.

Table 6
Findings in Lung Scan

Finding	Action
Normal LS	PE excluded
Matching changes	Probably not PE. Further work-up is needed, with clinical correlation
Mismatch	Probably PE

Caution: Arterial puncture should be avoided if massive PE is suspected and thrombolytic treatment could be indicated. If arterial puncture must be done, use the radial artery.

3.2.3. D-Dimer

A high sensitivity but non-specific test (*see* DVT). The test has a high negative predictive value for PE if the pretest probability is low, but this is not the case if the pretest probability is high *(127a)*.

3.2.4. Lung Scintigraphy

The lung scan consists of a perfusion and a ventilation component. A normal perfusion scan excludes PE, while an abnormal perfusion scan may be non-specific *(128–130)*.

3.2.5. Spiral Computed Tomography (sCT)

Spiral CT is more accurate in the demonstration of central, lobar, and segmental PE than sub-segmental PE. A negative sCT rules out clinically significant pulmonary embolism with similar accuracy as normal lung scanning or a negative pulmonary angiogram *(130a)*. The accuracy of sCT in detecting sub-segmental PE is still under debate, at the clinical relevance of such emboli is unclear, but the low rate of recurrence supports the accuracy of a negative result from sCT *(130b)*.

3.2.6. Pulmonary Angiography

Pulmonary angiography is the reference method but should be reserved for patients in whom noninvasive diagnostic tests remain indeterminate.

3.2.7. Echocardiography

Echocardiography is useful in patients with suspected massive PE. It helps both in diagnosis and determining the associated prognosis and treatment.

Dilatation of the right chamber and increased pressure is not diagnostic but can be used to make a decision of whether thrombolytic treatment is indicated or not.

3.2.8. Electrocardiogram (ECG)

ECG is frequently normal, or shows non-specific abnormalities such as T-wave abnormalities, tachycardia (exatrial fibrillation), right bundle-branch block, or right ventricular strain.

3.2.9. Venous Ultrasonography

Venous ultrasonography (VU) investigation for DVT is useful because 70% of pulmonary emboli are associated with DVT of the lower extremities and about half of the PE patients will have a DVT, which can be demonstrated by VU.

3.3. Treatment

3.3.1. Anticoagulant Therapy

In general the anticoagulant treatment strategy in the acute phase (days) of PE is similar to DVT. In most patients LMWH is preferred *(130c)*. LMWH sc once-daily *(130d)* or twice daily *(130e)* is continued for at least 5 days and until INR (2,0–3,0) has been in the therapeutic range for two days. The once daily administration of tinzaparin sc was used in a fixed weight-based dosage without the need of laboratory monitoring of the anticoagulant effect.

Also the duration of VKA follows the same rules as in DVT with calculation of recurrence risk based on clinical presentation, the presence of permanent risk factors including thrombophilia and cancer, previous VTE and the quality of the anticoagulant therapy.

Treatment in pregnancy is also identical to the treatment of DVT *(130f)* and outpatient treatment is possible in low-risk patients with a normal echocardiography. LMWH therapy can start until the diagnostic workup has confirmed the diagnosis. Thrombophilia screening is similar for PE and DVT.

UFH with intravenous infusion and APTT monitoring is used in patients receiving thrombolytic therapy.

3.3.2. Thrombolytic Therapy

Thrombolytic therapy may lower mortality from pulmonary embolism and reduce morbidity from chronic pulmonary hypertension that might complicate PE. In the absence of clinical trials demonstrating survival advantage, this therapeutic approach remains debatable *(131)*.

A recent relatively big trial showed alteplase in combination with UFH as compared to UFH alone to improve the clinical course of stable patients, who had an acute submassive PE preventing clinical deterioration requiring the escalation of therapy during the hospital stay *(131a)*. The use of thromblysis

Table 7
FDA-Approved Thrombolytic Agents*

Agent	Dose and schedule
Streptokinase	250,000 IU loading dose over 30 min, followed by 10,000 IU/h for 24 h
Urokinase	4400 IU/kg loading dose over 10 min, followed by 4400 IU/kg/h for 12–24 h
rt-PA (Alteplase)	100 mg as a continuous peripheral iv infusion over 2 h

*Modified from: Goldhaber, S. Z. (2001) Thrombolysis in pulmonary embolism: a debatable indication. *Thromb. Haemostasis* **86,** 444–451.

in submassive PE was recently debated in the Journal of Thrombosis and Haemostasis *(131b,c)*.

Risk stratification is important before deciding on thrombolytic therapy. This stratification can be based on clinical features only when PE is complicated by cardiogenic shock, systemic arterial hypotension, or respiratory failure.

Echocardiography may provide prognostic features. The presense of right ventricular dysfunction was associated with PE-related shock in 10% *(132)*. Other predictors of poor outcome in echocardiography includes patent Foramen Ovale *(133)* and free-floating thrombi in the right heart *(134)*.

More recently, troponin-I level was used to determine prognoses in PE. High levels were associated with a high frequency of right ventricular dysfunction and a high mortality. Mortality rate was 44% in a group of 56 patients with high troponin level, as compared to 3% in troponin-negative patients *(135)*.

Three agents had been approved for thrombolytic therapy in VTE (**Table 7**), while other agents, such as Reteplase and Tenecteplase, are not currently approved worldwide but have shown promise for rapid thrombolysis *(136)*. The drugs are given as IV bolus injection(s).

The following points should be considered when giving thrombolytic therapy:

1. Streptokinase and urokinase regimens are used less often. rt-PA should be your first choice.
2. No need for laboratory tests during thrombolytic infusion.
3. Concomitant heparin is not given during rt-PA infusion.
4. Obtain APTT at the conclusion of thrombolytic therapy.
5. Resume heparin infusion with no bolus once APTT is <80 s.
6. If the APTT is >80 s, repeat the test every 4 h until the results are <80.
7. The following are some of the contraindications for thrombolytic therapy:
   a. Active internal bleeding.
   b. Bleeding tendency.

Table 8
GCC—Hemostasis Study Group Members

Name	Institution	Country
Dr. Shaker A Mousa	Albany College of Pharmacy, Albany, NY	USA
Dr. Hikmat Abdel-Razeq	KFAFH-Jeddah	Saudi Arabia
Dr. Mahmoud Marashi	Rashid Hospital-Dubai	UAE
Dr. Faisal Al Sayegh	Kuwait University Hospital	Kuwait
Dr. Nabil Moshin	Royal Hospital	Oman
Dr. Samir Al Azzawi	Royal Hospital	Oman
Dr. Rajan	Royal Hospital	Oman
Dr. Mousa Othman	RKH-Riyadh	Saudi Arabia
Dr. Abdul Aziz Al Abdulaaly	RKH-Riyadh	Saudi Arabia
Dr. Saud Abu Harbesh	Security Forces Hospital-Riyadh	Saudi Arabia
Dr. Abdul Aziz Al Saif	RKH- Riyadh	Saudi Arabia
Dr. Battal Al Dosary	RKH- Riyadh	Saudi Arabia
Dr. Ali Al Shangiti	RMC-Riyadh	Saudi Arabia
Dr. AbdulAziz Al Zeer	King Khalid University Hospital-Riyadh	Saudi Arabia
Dr. Hazaa Al Zahrani	KFSH- Riyadh	Saudi Arabia
Dr. Hatem Qutub	KFTH-Dammam	Saudi Arabia
Dr. Abdulaziz Al Nwasser	KFMMC Dammam	Saudi Arabia
Dr. Wahid Al Fare	KKMCH- Dammam	Saudi Arabia
Dr. Ali M. Al-Amri	KFTH-Dammam	Saudi Arabia
Dr. Mohamed Qari	KAUH-Jeddah	Saudi Arabia
Dr. Mohamed Abdelaal	KKNGH-Jeddah	Saudi Arabia
Dr. Abdulaziz Al Homaidhi	KFSH-Jeddah	Saudi Arabia
Dr. Mubarak H. Zafer	ASSER Hospital	Saudi Arabia
Dr. Omar Al Amoudi	KAUH-Jeddah	Saudi Arabia
Dr. Jamal Al Hashemy	KAUH-Jeddah	Saudi Arabia
Dr. Usama Al Homsi	Hamad Medical Center	Qatar
Dr. Abdulla Al Ajmi		Bahrain
Dr. Jorgen Kristensen	Tawam Hospital-Al Ain	UAE
Dr. Hussein Alizadeh	Tawam Hospital-Al Ain	UAE
Dr. Steen Husted	Aarhus University Hospital	Denmark

    c. Operation and trauma within the last 10 d.
    d. Stroke within 6 mo and CNS trauma/surgery within 2 mo.
    e. Other major bleeding within the last 2 mo.
    f. Uncontrolled hypertension >180/110.
    g. Endocarditis and pericarditis.
    h. Acute pancreatitis.
    i. Previous treatment with streptokinase.

3.3.3. Surgical Embolectomy

A high-risk procedure has operative mortality rates that range between 10 and 75%, and with reported postoperative complications that include ARDS, mediastitis, acute renal failure, and severe neurological sequelae.

Before attempting embolectomy, the following criteria must be met *(92)*:

1. Massive PE.
2. Hemodynamic instability despite heparin and resuscitative efforts.
3. Failure of thrombolytic therapy or a contraindication to its use.
4. An experienced cardiac surgical team must be immediately available.

Acknowledgment

Our appreciation and thanks for the secretarial support of Ms. Esper Anonuevo, Ms. Gigi Palado, and Ms. Lamya Hibshi, and for Leo Pharmaceutical for the sponsoring all the meeting to come up with these guidelines.

References

1. Bertina, R. M., Koeleman, R. P. C., Koster, T., Rosendaal, F. R., Dirven, R. J., De Ronde, H., et al. (1994) Mutation in blood coagulation factor V associated with resistance to activated protein C. *Nature* **369,** 64–67.
2. Rees, D. C., Cox, M., and Clegg, J. B. (1995) World distribution of factor V Leiden. *Lancet* **346,** 1133–1134.
3. Svensson, P. J. and Dahlback, B. (1994) Resistance to activated protein C as a basis for venous thrombosis. *N. Engl. J. Med.* **330,** 517–522.
4. Koster, T., Rosendaal, F. R., de Ronde, H., Briet, E., Vandenbroucke, J. P., and Bertina, R. M. (1993) Venous thrombosis due to a poor anticoagulant response to activated protein C: leiden thrombophilia study. *Lancet* **342,** 1503–1506.
5. Rosendaal, F. R., Koster, T., Vandenbroucke, J. P., and Reitsma, P. H. (1995) High risk of thrombosis in patients homozygous for factor V Leiden (activated protein C resistance). *Blood* **85,** 1504–1508.
6. Kyrle, P. A., Mannhalter, C., Beguin, S., Stumpflen, A., Hirschl, M., Weltermann, A., et al. (1998) Clinical studies and thrombin generation in patients homozygous or heterozygous for the G20210A mutation in the prothrombin gene. *Arterioscler. Thromb. Vasc. Biol.* **18,** 1287–1291.
7. Rosendaal, F. R., Doggen, C. J. M., Zivelin, A., Arruda, V. R., Aiach, M., Siscovick, D. S., et al. (1998) Geographic distribution of the 20210G to A prothrombin variant. *Thromb. Haemostasis* **79,** 706–708.
8. Hillarp, A., Zoller, B., Svensson, P. J., and Dahlback, B. (1997) The 20210A allele of the prothrombin gene is a common risk factor among Swedish outpatients with verified deep venous thrombosis. *Thromb. Haemostasis* **78,** 990–992.
9. Leroyer, C., Mercier, B., Oger, E., Chenu, E., Abgrall, J. F., Ferec, C., et al. (1998) Prevalence of the 202a0A allele of the prothrombin gene in venous thromboembolism patients. *Thromb. Haemostasis* **80,** 49–51.

10. Margaglione, M., Brancaccio, V., Guiliani, N., D'Andrea, G., Cappucci, G., Iannaccone, L., et al. (1998) Increased risk for venous thrombosis in carriers of the prothrombin G20210A gene variant. *Ann. Intern. Med.* **129,** 89–93.

11. Merli, G., Spiro, T. E., Olsson, G. C., et al. (2001) Subcutaneous Enoxaparin once or twice daily compared with intravenous unfractionated heparin for treatment of venous thromboembolitic disease. *Ann. Intern. Med.* **134,** 191–202.

12. The Columbus Investigators (1997) Low-molecular-weight heparin in the treatment of patient with venous thromboembolism. *N. Engl. J. Med.* **337,** 657–662.

13. Finazzi, G. and Barbui, T. (1994) Different incidence of venous thrombosis in patients with inherited deficiencies of antithrombin III, protein C and protein S. *Thromb. Haemostasis* **71,** 15–18.

14. Demers, C., Ginsberg, J. S., Hirsh, J., Henderson, P., and Blajchman, M. A. (1992) Thrombosis in antithrombin III-deficient persons: report of a large kindred and literature review. *Ann. Intern. Med.* **116,** 754–761.

15. Tait, R. C., Walker, I. D., Perry, D. J., Islam, S. I., Daly, M. E., McCall, F., et al. (1994) Prevalence of antithrombin deficiency in the healthy population. *Br. J. Haematol.* **87,** 106–112.

16. Tait, R. C., Walker, I. D., Reitsma, P. H., Islam, S. I., McCall, F., Poor, S. R., et al. (1995) Prevalence of protein C deficiency in the healthy population. *Thromb. Haemostasis* **73,** 87–93.

17. Griffin, J. H., Evatt, B., Zimmerman, T. S., Kleiss, A. J., and Wideman, C. (1981) Deficiency of protein C in congenital thrombotic disease. *J. Clin. Invest.* **68,** 1370–1373.

18. Broekmans, A. W., Veltkamp, J. J., and Bertina, R. M. (1983) Congenital protein C deficiency and venous thromboembolism: a study of three Dutch families. *N. Engl. J. Med.* **309,** 340–344.

19. Schwarz, H. P., Fischer, M., Hopmeier, P., Batard, M. A., and Griffin, J. H. (1984) Plasma protein S deficiency in familial thrombotic disease. *Blood* **64,** 1297–1300.

20. Sanson, B. J., Simioni, P., Tormene, D., Moia, M., Friederick, P. W., Huisman, M. V., et al. (1999) The incidence of venous thromboembolism in asymptomatic carriers of deficiency of antithrombin, protein C, or protein S: a prospective cohort study. *Blood* **94,** 3702–3706.

21. Haverkate, F. and Samama, M. (1995) Familial dysfibrinogenemia and thrombophilia. Report on a study of the SSC Subcommittee on fibrinogen. *Thromb. Haemostasis* **73,** 151–161.

22. Cattaneo, M. (1999) Hyperhomocysteinemia, atherosclerosis and thrombosis. *Thromb. Haemostasis* **81,** 165–176.

23. Falcon, C. R., Cattaneo, M., Panzeri, D., Martinelli, I., and Mannucci, P. M. (1994) High prevalence of hyperhomocyst(e)inemia in patients with juvenile venous thrombosis. *Arterioscler. Thromb.* **14,** 1080–1083.

24. Ridker, P. M., Hennekens, C. H., Selhub, J., Miletich, J. P., Malinow, M. R., and Stampfer, M. J. (1997) Interrelation of hyperhomocyt(e)inemia, factor V Leiden, and the risk of future venous thromboembolism. *Circulation* **95,** 1777–1782.

25. Koster, T., Blann, A. D., Briet, E., Vandenbroucke, J. P., and Rosendaal, F. R. (1995) Role of clotting factor VIII in effect of von Willebrand factor an occurrence of deep-vein thrombosis. *Lancet* **345,** 152–155.

26. O'Donnell, J., Tuddenham, E. G., Manning, R., Kemball-Cook, G., Johnson, D., and Laffan, M. (1997) High prevalence of elevated factor VIII levels in patients referred for thrombophilia screening: role of increased synthesis and relationship to acute phase reaction. *Thromb. Haemostasis* **77,** 825–828.

27. Kraaijenhagen, R. A., in't Anker, P. S., Koopman, M. M., Reitsma, P. H., Prins, M. H., van den Ende, A., et al. (2000) High plasma concentration of factor VIIIc is a major risk factor for venous thromboembolism. *Thromb. Haemostasis* **83,** 5–9.

28. O'Donnell, J., Mumford, A. D., Manning, R. A., and Laffan, M. (2000) Elevation of FVIII:C in venous thromboembolism is persistent and independent of the acute phase response. *Thromb. Haemostasis* **83,** 10–13.

29. Kyrle, P. A., Minar, E., Hirschl, M., Bialonczyk, C., Stain, M., Schneider, B., et al. (2000) High plasma levels of factor VIII and the risk of recurrent venous thromboembolism. *N. Engl. J. Med.* **343,** 457–462.

30. van Hylckama, V. A., van der Linden, I. K., Bertina, R. M., and Ronsendaal, F. R. (2000) High levels of factor IX increase the risk of venous thrombosis. *Blood* **95,** 3678–3682.

31. Meijers, C. M. J., Tekelenburg, L. H. W., Bouma, N. B., Bertina, R. M., and Rosendaal, F. R. (2000) High levels of coagulation factor XI as a risk factor for venous thrombosis. *N. Engl. J. Med.* **343,** 696–701.

32. Zoller, Svensson, P. J., He, X., and Dahlback, B. (1994) Identification of the same factor V gene mutation in 47 out of 50 thrombosis-prone families with inherited resistance to activated protein C. *J. Clin. Invest.* **94,** 2521–2524.

33. Bernardi, F., Faioni, E. M., Castoldi, E., Lunghi, B., Castaman, G., Sacchi, E., et al. (1997) A factor V genetic component differing from factor V R506Q contributed to the activated protein C resistance phenotype. *Blood* **90,** 1552–1557.

34. Williamson, D., Brown, K., Luddington, R., Baglin, C., and Baglin, T. (1998) Factor V Cambridge: a new mutation (Arg306®Thr) associated with resistance to activated protein C. *Blood* **91,** 1140.4.

35. Nordstrom, M., Lindblad, B., Bergqvist, D., and Kjellstrom, T. (1992) A prospective study of the incidence of deep-vein thrombosis within a defined urban population. *J. Intern. Med.* **232,** 155–160.

36. Anderson, F. A., Wheeler, H. G., Goldberg, R. J., Hosmer, D. W., Patwardhan, N. A., Jovanovic, B., et al. (1991) A population based perspective of the hospital incidence and case-fatality rates deep vein thrombosis and pulmonary embolism. The Worcester DVT study. *Arch. Intern. Med.* **151,** 933–938.

37. Ridker, P. M., Glynn, R. J., Miletich, J. P., Goldhaber, S. Z., Stampfer, M. J., and Hennekens, C. H. (1997) Age-specific incidence rates of venous thromboembolism among heterozygous carriers of factor V Leiden mutation. *Ann. Intern. Med.* **126,** 528–531.

38. Ginsberg, J. S., Wells, P. S., Brill-Edwards, P., Donovan, D., Moffatt, K., Johnston, M., et al. (1995) Antiphospholipid antibodies and venous thromboembolism. *Blood* **86,** 3685–3691.
39. Simioni, P., Prandoni, P., Zanan, E., Saracino, M. A., Scudeller, A., Villalta, S., et al. (1986) Deep venous thrombosis and lupus anticoagulant. *Thromb. Haemostasis* **76,** 187–189.
40. Geerts, W. H., Code, K. I., Jay, R. M., Chen, E., and Szalai, J. P. (1994) A prospective study of venous thromboembolism after major trauma. *N. Engl. J. Med.* **331,** 1601–1606.
41. Geerts, W. H., Jay, R. M., Code, K. I., Chen, E., Szalai, J. P., Saibil, E. A., et al. (1996) A comparison of low-dose heparin with low molecular weight heparin as prophylaxis against venous thromboembolism after major trauma. *N. Engl. J. Med.* **335,** 701–707.
42. Prandoni, P., Lensing, A. W. A., Buller, H. R., Cogo, A., Prins, M. H., Cattelan, A. M., et al. (1992) Deep-vein thrombosis and the incidence of subsequent symptomatic cancer. *N. Engl. J. Med.* **327,** 1128–1133.
43. Monreal, M., Lafoz, E., Casals, A., Inaraja, L., Montserrat, E., Callejas, J. M., et al. (1991) Occult cancer in patients with deep venous thrombosis. *Cancer* **67,** 541–545.
44. Cornuz, J., Pearson, S. D., Creager, M. A., Cook, E. F., and Goldman, L. (1996) Importance of findings on the initial evaluation for cancer in patients with symptomatic idiopathic deep venous thrombosis. *Ann. Intern. Med.* **125,** 785–793.
45. Piccioli, A., Prandoni, P., Ewenstein, B. M., and Goldhaber, S. Z. (1996) Cancer and venous thromboembolism. *Am. Heart J.* **132,** 850–855.
46. Goldberg, R. J., Seneff, M., Gore, J. M., Anderson, F. A., Jr., Greene, H. L., Wheeler, H. B., et al. (1987) Occult malignant neoplasm in patients with deep venous thrombosis. *Arch. Intern. Med.* **147,** 251–253.
47. Hettiarachchi, R. J., Lok, J., Prins, M. H., Buller, H. R., and Prandoni, P. (1998) Undiagnosed malignancy in patients with deep vein thrombosis: incidence, risk indicators, and diagnosis. *Cancer* **83,** 180–185.
48. Sorensen, H. T., Mellemkjaer, L., Steffenssen, F. H., Olsen, J. H., and Nielsen, G. L. (1998) The risk of diagnosis of cancer after primary deep venous thrombosis or pulmonary embolism. *N. Engl. J. Med.* **338,** 1169–1173.
49. Clagett, G. P. (1994) Prevention of postoperative venous thromboembolism: an update. *Am. J. Surg.* **168,** 515–522.
50. Hull, R. D. and Raskob, G. E. (1986) Prophylaxis of venous thromboembolic disease following hip and knee surgery. *J. Bone Jt. Surg.* **68,** 146–150.
51. Gibbs, N. M. (1957) Venous thrombosis of the lower limbs with particular reference to bed rest. *Br. J. Surg.* **54,** 209.
52. Sigel, B., Ipse, J., and Felix, W. R. (1974) The epidemiology of lower extremity deep venous thrombosis in surgical patient. *Ann. Surg.* 179–278.
53. Hull, R., Delmore, T., Carter, C., Hirsh, J., Genton, E., Gen, M.. et al. (1982) Adjusted subcutaneous heparin versus Warfarin sodium in the long-term treatment of venous thrombosis. *N. Engl. J. Med.* **306,** 189–194.

54. Andersen, B. S., Steffensen, F. H., Sorensen, H. T., Nielsen, G. L., and Olsen, J. (1998) The cumulative incidence of venous thromboembolism during pregnancy and puerperium. *Acta Obstet. Gynecol. Scand.* **77,** 170–173.

55. Lindqvist, P., Dahlback, B., and Marsal, K. (1999) Thrombotic risk during pregnancy: a population study. *Obstet. Gynecol.* **94,** 595–59.

56. Treffers, P. E., Huidekoper, B. L., Weenink, G. H., and Kloosterman, G. J. (1983) Epidemiological observations of thromboembolic disease during pregnancy and in the puerperium, in 56,022 women. *Int. J. Gynaecol. Obstet.* **21,** 327–331.

57. Ray, J. G. and Chan, W. S. (1999) Deep vein thrombosis during pregnancy and the puerperium. *Obstet. Gynecol. Surv.* **54,** 265–271.

58. Gerstmann, B. B., Piper, J. M. Tomita, D. K., Ferguson, W. J., Stadel, B. V., and Lundin, F. E. (1991) Oral contraceptive estrogen dose and the risk for deep venous thromboembolic disease. *Am. J. Epidemiol.* **133,** 32–37.

59. Helmerhorst, F. M., Bloemenkamp, K. W., Rosendaal, F. R., and Vandenroucke, J. P. (1997) Oral contraceptives and thrombotic disease: risk of venous thromboembolism. *Thromb. Haemostasis* **78,** 327–333.

60. WHO Study Group (1995) Effect of different progestagens in low estrogen oral Contraceptives on venous thromboembolic disease. World Health Organization Collaborative Study of Cardiovascular Disease and Steroid Hormone Contraception. *Lancet* **346,** 1582–1588.

61. Spitzer, W. O., Lewis, M. A., Heinemann, L. A., Thorogood, M., and Mac Rae, K. D. (1996) Third generation oral contraceptives and risk of venous thromboembolic disorders: an international case-control study. Transnational Research Group on Oral Contraceptives and the Health of Young Women. *Br. Med. J.* **312,** 83–88.

62. Farmer, R. D., Lawrenson, R. A., Thompson, C. R., Kennedy, J. G., and Hambleton, I. R. (1997) Population-based study of risk of venous thromboembolism associated with various oral contraceptives. *Lancet* **349,** 83–88.

63. Bloemenkamp, K. W., Rosendaal, F. R., Helmerhorst, F. M., Buller, H. R., Colly, L. P., and Vandenbroucke, J. P. (1999) The association between oral contraceptives and venous thrombosis: the myth of the diagnostic suspicion and referral bias. *Arch. Intern. Med.* **159,** 65–70.

64. Perrier, A., Desmarais, S., Miron, M. J., de Moerloose, P., Lepage, R., Slosman, D., et al. (1999) Non-invasive diagnosis of venous thromboembolism in outpatients. *Lancet* **353,** 190–195.

65. Bounameaux, H., de Moerloose, P., Perrier, A., and Miron, M. J. (1997) D-dimer testing in suspected venous thromboembolism: an update. *QJM* **90,** 437–442.

66. Becker, D. M., Philbrick, J. T., Bachhuber, T. L., and Humphries, J. E. (1996) D-dimer testing and acute venous thromboembolism. A shortcut to accurate diagnosis? *Arch. Intern. Med.* **156,** 939–946.

67. Janssen, M. C., Wollersheim, H., Verbruggen, B., and Novakova, I. R. (1998) Rapid D-dimer assays to exclude deep venous thrombosis and pulmonary embolism: current status and new developments. *Semin. Thromb. Hemost.* **24,** 393–400.

68. Borg, J. Y., Levesque, H., Cailleux, N., Franc, C., Hellot, M. F., and Courtois, H. (1997) Rapid quantitative D-dimer assay and clinical evaluation for the diagnosis of clinical suspected deep vein thrombosis. *Thromb. Haemostasis* **77,** 602–603.

69. Becker, D. M., Philbrick, J. T., and Abbitt, P. L. (1989) Real-time ultrasonography for the diagnosis of lower extremity deep venous thrombosis. The wave of the future? *Arch. Intern. Med.* **149,** 173–174.

70. Lensing, A. W. A., Pandoni, P., Brandjes, D., Huisman, P. M., Vigo, M., Tomasella, G., et al. (1989) Detection of deep-vein thrombosis by real-time B-mode ultrasonography. *N. Engl. J. Med.* **320,** 342–345.

71. Cogo, A., Lensing, A. W. A., Koopman, M. M. W., Piovella, F., Siragusa, S., Wells, P. S., et al. (1998) Compression ultrasonography for diagnostic management of patients with clinically suspected deep vein thrombosis: prospective cohort study. The Multicenter Italian D-dimer Ultrasound Study Investigators Group. *BMJ* **317,** 1037–1040.

72. Kearon, C., Ginsberg, J. S., and Hish, J. (1998) The role of venous ultrasonography in the diagnosis of suspected deep venous thrombosis and pulmonary embolism. *Ann. Intern. Med.* **129,** 1044–1049.

73. Cogo, A., Lensing, A. W. A., Koopman, M. M. W., Piovella, F., Siragusa, S., Wells, P. S., et al. (1998) Compression ultrasonography for diagnostic management of patients with clinically suspected deep vein thrombosis: prospective cohort study. The Multicentre Italian D-dimer Ultrasound Study Investigators Group. *BMJ* **317,** 1037–1040.

74. Wells, P. S., Hirsh, J., Andreson, D. R., Lensing, A. W., Foster, G., Kearon, C., et al. (1995) Accuracy of clinical assessment of deep vein thrombosis. *Lancet* **345,** 1326–1330.

75. Wells, P. S., Hirsch, J., Anderson, D. R., Lensing, A. W., Foster, G., Kearon, C., et al. (1995) Accuracy of clinical assessment of deep-vein thrombosis. *Lancet* **345,** 1326–1330.

76. Anderson, D. R., Lensing, A. W. A., Wells, P. S., Levine, M. N., Weitz, J. R., and Hirsh, J. (1993) Limitations of impedance plethysmography in the diagnosis of clinical suspected deep-vein thrombosis. *Ann. Intern. Med.* **118,** 25–30.

77. Ginserg, J. S., Wells, P. S., Hirsh, J., Panju, A. A., Patel, M. A., Malone, D. E., et al. (1994) Reevaluation of the sensitivity of impedance plethysmography for the detection of proximal deep vein thrombosis. *Arch. Intern. Med.* **154,** 1930–1933.

78. Hull, R. D., Raskob, G. E., Pinco, G. F., et al. (1992) Subcutaneous low molecular weight heparin compared with continuous intravenous heparin in the treatment of proximal vein thrombosis. *N. Engl. J. Med.* **326,** 975–982.

79. Wells, P. S., Anderson, D. R., Bormani, J., Guy, F., Mitchell, M., Gray, L., et al. (1997) Value of assessment of pretest probability of deep-vein thrombosis in clinical management. *Lancet* **350,** 1795–1798.

80. Bigaroni, A., Perrier, A., and Bounameaux, H. (2000) Is clinical probability assessment of deep vein thrombosis by a score really standardized? *Thromb. Haemostasis* **83,** 788–789.

81. Heijboer, H., Buller, H. R., Lensing, A. W. A., Turpie, A. G. G., Colly, L. P., and ten Cate, J. W. (1993) A comparison of real-time compression ultrasonography with impedance plethysmography for the diagnosis of deep-vein thrombosis in symptomatic outpatients. *N. Engl. J. Med.* **329,** 1365–1369.

82. Weitz, J. I. (1997) Low-molecular-weight heparins. *N. Engl. J. Med.* **337,** 688–698.

83. Lensing, A. W. A., Orins, M. H., Davidson, B. L., et al. (1995) Treatment of deep venous thrombosis with low-molecular-weight heparin: a meta-analysis. *Arch. Intern. Med.* **155,** 601–607.

84. Siragusa, S., Cosmi, B., Piovella, F., et al. (1996) Low-molecular-weight heparins and unfractionated heparin in the treatment of patients with acute venous thromboembolism: results of a meta-analysis. *Am. J. Med.* **100,** 269–277.

85. Leizorovicz, A., Simonneau, G., Decousus, H., et al. (1994) Comparison of efficacy and safety of low-molecular-weight heparins and unfractionated heparin in the initial treatment of deep venous thrombosis: a meta-analysis. *Br. Med. J.* **309,** 299–304.

86. Raschke, R. A., Reilly, B. M., Guidry, J. R., et al. (1993) The weight-based heparin dosing normogram compared with a "standard care" normogram. A randomized controlled trial. *Ann. Intern. Med.* **119,** 874–881.

87. de Groot, M. R., Büller, H. R., ten Cate, J. W., et al. (1998) Use of a heparin nomogram for treatment of patients with venous thromboembolism in a community hospital. *Thromb. Haemostasis* **80,** 70–73.

88. Cruickshank, M. K., Lering, M. N., Hirsh, J., et al. (1991) A standard heparin normogram for the management of Heparin therapy. *Arch. Intern. Med.* **151,** 333–337.

89. Campbell, N. R. C., Hull, R. D., Brant, R., et al. (1996) Aging and heparin-related bleeding. *Arch. Intern. Med.* **156,** 857–860.

90. Zidane, M., Schram, M. T., Planken, E. W., et al. (2000) Frequency of major hemorrhage in patients treated with unfractionated intravenous heparin for deep venous thrombosis or pulmonary embolism. *Arch. Intern. Med.* **160,** 2369–2373.

91. Nand, S., Wong, W., Yuen, B., et al. (1997) Heparin-induced thrombocytopenia with thrombosis: incidence analysis of risk factors and clinical outcomes in 108 consecutive patients treated at a single institution. *Am. J. Hematol.* **56,** 12–16.

92. Hyers, et al. (2001) Antithrombotic therapy for venous thromboembolic disease. *Chest* **119,** 176s–193s.

93. Dulitzki, M., Pauzner, R., Langevitz, P., et al. (1996) Low molecular weight heparin during pregnancy and delivery: preliminary experience with 41 pregnancies. *Obstet. Gynecol.* **87,** 380–383.

94. Orme, L'E., Lewis, M., de Swiet, M., et al. (1977) May mothers given warfarin breast-feed their infants? *BMJ* **1,** 1564–1565.

95. McKenna, R., Cole, E. R., and Vasan, V. (1983) Is warfarin sodium contraindicated in the lactating mother? *J. Pediatr.* **103,** 325–327.

96. Dahlman, T. C. (1993) Osteoporotic fractures and the recurrence of thromboembolism during pregnancy and the puerperium in 184 women undergoing thromboprophylaxis with heparin. *Am. J. Obstet. Gynecol.* **168,** 1265–1270.

97. Douketies, J. D., Ginsberg, J. S., Burrows, R. F., et al. (1996) The effects of long-term heparin therapy during pregnancy on bone density. *Thromb. Haemostasis* **75,** 254–257.

98. Monreal, M., Iafoz, E., Olive, A., et al. (1994) Comparison of subcutaneous unfractionated heparin with a low molecular weight heparin (Fragmin) in patients with venous thromboembolism and contraindications to coumarin. *Thromb. Haemostasis* **71,** 7–11.

99. Muir, J. M., Hirsh, J., Weitz, J. I., et al. (1997) A histomorphometric comparison of the effects of heparin and low-molecular-weight heparin on cancellous bone in rats. *Blood* **89,** 3236–3242.

100. Schwieder, G., Grimm, W., Siemens, H., Flor, B., Hilden, A., and Gmelin, E. (1995) Intermittent regional therapy with rt-PA is not superior to systemic thrombolysis in deep vein thrombosis (DVT): a German multi-center trial. *Thromb. Haemostasis* **74,** 1240–1243.

101. Grossman, C. and McPherson, S. (1999) Safety and efficacy of catheter-directed thrombolysis for iliofemoral venous thrombosis. *Am. J. Roentgenol.* **172,** 667–672.

102. Mewissen, M. W., Seabrook, G. R., Meissner, M. H., Cynamon, J., Labropoulos, N., and Haughton, S. H. (1999) Catheter-directed thrombolysis for lower extremity deep venous thrombosis: report of a national multi-center registry. *Radiology* **211,** 39–49.

103. Comerota, A. J., Throm, R. C., Matias, S. D., Haughton, S., and Mewisson, M. W. (2000) Catheter-directed thrombolysis for iliofemoral deep venous thrombosis improves health-related quality of life. *J. Vasc. Surg.* **32,** 130–137.

104. Tarry, W. C., Makhoul, R. G., Tisnado, J., Posner, M. P., Sober, M., and Lee, H. M. (1994) Catheter-directed thrombolysis following vena cava filtration for severe deep venous thrombosis. *Ann. Vasc. Surg.* **8,** 583–590.

105. Patel, N. H., Plorde, J. J., and Meisner, M. (1998) Catheter directed thrombolysis in the treatment of phlegmasia cerulea dolens. *Ann. Vasc. Surg.* **12,** 471–475.

106. Centeno, R. F., Nguyen, A. H., Ketterer, C., Stiller, G., Chait, A., and Fallahnejad, M. (1999) An alternative approach: antegrade catheter-directed thrombolysis in a case of phlegmasia cerulea dolens. *Am. Surg.* **65,** 229–231.

107. Arnesen, H., Hoiseth, A., and Ly, B. (1982) Streptokinase or heparin in the treatment of deep vein thrombosis. Follow-up results of a prospective study. *Acta Med. Scand.* **211,** 65–68.

108. Ng, C. M. and Rivera, J. O. (1998) Meta-analysis of streptokinase and heparin in deep vein thrombosis. *Am. J. Health Syst. Pharm.* **55,** 1995–2001.

109. Goldhaber, S. Z., Hirsch, D. R., MacDougall, R. C., Polak, J. F., and Creager, M. A. (1996) Bolus recombinant urokinase versus heparin in deep vein thrombosis: a randomized controlled trial. *Am. Heart J.* **132,** 314–318.

110. Goldhaber, S. Z., Meyerovits, M. F., Green, D., Vogelzang, R. L., Citrin, P., and Heit, J. (1990) Randomized controlled trial of tissue plasminogen activator in proximal deep venous thrombosis. *Am. J. Med.* **88,** 235–240.

111. Turpie, A. G. G., Levine, M., Hirsh, J., Ginsberg, J. S., Cruikshank, M., and Jay, R. (1990) Tissue plasminogen activator (rt-PA) vs heparin in deep vein thrombosis: results of a randomized trial. *Chest* **97,** 1728–1758.

112. Arnesen, H., Hoiseth, A., and Ly, B. (1982) Streptokinase or heparin in the treatment of deep vein thrombosis: follow-up results of a prospective trial. *Acta Med. Scand.* **211,** 65.

113. Johanson, L., Nylander, G., Hedner, U., et al. (1979) Comparison of streptokinase with heparin: late results in the treatment of deep vein thrombosis. *Acta Med. Scand.* **206,** 93–98.

114. Watz, R. and Savidge, G. F. (1979) Rapid thrombolysis and preservation of valvular venous function in high deep vein thrombosis. *Acta Med. Scand.* **205,** 293–298.

115. Kakkar, V. V. and Lawrence, D. (1985) Hemodynamic and clinical assessment after therapy of acute deep vein thrombosis. *Am. J. Surg.* **10,** 54–63.

116. Prandoni, P., Lensing, A. W. A., Cogo, A., et al. (1996) The long-term clinical course of acute deep venous thrombosis. *Ann. Intern. Med.* **125,** 1–7.

117. Stewart, J. R. and Greenfield, L. J. (1982) Transvenous vena caval filtration and pulmonary embolectomy. *Surg. Clin. North Am.* **62,** 411–430.

118. Greenfield, L. J. and Langham, M. R. (1984) Surgical approaches to thromboembolism. *Br. J. Surg.* **71,** 968–970.

119. Dorfman, G. S. (1990) Percutaneous inferior vena caval filters. *Radiology* **174,** 987–992.

120. Leach, T. A., Pastena, J. A., Swan, K. G., et al. (1994) Surgical prophylaxis for pulmonary embolism. *Am. Surg.* **60,** 292–295.

121. Linsenmaier, U., Rieger, J., Schenk, F., et al. (1998) Indications, management, and complications of temporary inferior vena cave filters. *Cardiovasc. Interv. Radiol.* **21,** 464–469.

122. Spence, L. K., Gironta, M. G., Malde, H. M., et al. (1999) Acute upper extremity deep venous thrombosis: safety and effectiveness of superior vena caval filters. *Radiology* **210,** 53–58.

123. Meyer, G., Tamisier, D., Sors, H., et al. (1991) Pulmonary embolectomy a 20-year experience at one center. *Ann. Thorac. Surg.* **51,** 232–236.

124. Gray, H. H., Morgan, J. M., Paneth, M., et al. (1988) Pulmonary embolectomy for acte massive pulmonary embolism: an analysis of 71 cases. *Br. Heart J.* **60,** 196–200.

125. Clarke, D. B. and Abrams, L. D. (1986) Pulmonary embolectomy: a 25-year experience. *J. Thorac. Cardiovasc. Surg.* **92,** 442–445.

126. Decousus, H., Leizorovicz, A., Parent, F., et al. (1998) A clinical trial of vena caval filters in the prevention of pulmonary embolism in patients with prevention of pulmonary embolism in patients with proximal deep-vein thrombosis. *N. Engl. J. Med.* **338,** 409–415.

127. Greenfield, L. J. and Rutherford, R. B. (1999) Recommended reporting standards for vena caval filter placement and patient follow-up: Vena Caval Filter Consensus Conference. *J. Vasc. Interv. Radiol.* **10,** 1013–1019.

127a. Kruip, M. J. H., Slob, M. J., Schijen, J. H., van der Heul, C., Böller, H. (2002) Use of a clinical decision rule in combination with D-dimer concentration in diagnostic workup of patients with suspected pulmonary embolism. *Arch. Intern. Med.* **162**, 1631–1635.

128. Hull, R. D., Hirsh, J., Carter, C., et al. (1983) Pulmonary angiography, ventilation, lung scanning and venography for clinically suspected pulmonary embolism with abnormal perfusion lung scan. *Ann. Intern. Med.* 98–891.

129. Hull, R. D., Hirsh, J., Carter, C., et al. (1985) Diagnostic value of ventilation-perfusion in patients with suspected pulmonary embolism and abnormal perfusion lung scans. *Chest* **88**, 819.

130. PIOPED Investigatiors (1990) Value of the ventilation/perfusion scan in acute pulmonary embolism: results of the prospective investigation of pulmonary embolism diagnosis (PIOPED). *JAMA* **263**, 2753.

130a. Gottsöter, A., Berg, A., Centergard, J., Frennby, B., Nirhov, N., Nyman, U. (2001) Clinically suspected pulmonary embolism: is it safe to withhold anti-coagulation after a negative sCT? *Eur. Radiol.* **11**, 65–72.

130b. Van Beck, E. J. R., Brouwers, E. M. J., Song, B., Stein, P., Oudkerk, M. (2001) Clinical validation of a normal pulmonary angiogram in patients with suspected pulmonary embolism a critical review. *Clin. Radiol.* **56**, 838–842.

130c. Goldhaber, S. Z. LMWH in combination with a vitamin K antagonist (VKA).

130d. Simonneau, G., Sors, H., Charbonnier, B, Page Y, Laaban J-P, Azarian R, et al. for the THSE Study Group. (1997) A comparison of low-molecular weight heparin with unfractionated heparin for acute pulmonary embolism. *N. Engl. J. Med.* **337**, 663–669.

130e. The Columbus Investigators. (1997) Low-molecular weight heparin in the treatment of patients with venous thromboembolism. *N. Engl. J. Med.* **337,** 657–662.

130f. Ginsberg, J. S., Bates, S. M. (2003) Management of venous thromboembolism during pregnancy. *J. Thrombos. Haemostas.* **1**, 1435–1442.

131. Goldhaber (2001) Thrombolysis in pulmonary embolism, a debatable indication. *Thromb. Haemostasis* **86**, 444–451.

131a. Konstantinides, S., Geibel, A., Heusel, G., Heinrich, F., Kasper, W. (2002) for the Management Strategies and Prognosis of Pulmonary Embolism-3 Trial Investigators. *N. Engl. J. Med.* **347**, 1143–1150.

131b. Konstantinides, S. (2003) Thrombolysis in submassive pulmonary embolism? Yes. *J. Thromb. Haemostas.* **1**, 1127–1129.

131c. Dalen, J. E. (2003) Thrombolysis in submassive pulmonary embolism? No. *J. Thrombos. Haemostas.* **1**, 1130–1132.

132. Grifoni, S., Olivotto, I., Cecchini, P., Pieralli, F., Camaiti, A., Santoro, G., et al. (2000) Short-term clinical outcome of patients with acute pulmonary embolism, normal blood pressure, and echocardiographic right ventricular dysfunction. *Circulation* **101**, 2817–2822.

133. Konstantinides, S., Geibel, A., Kasper, W., Olschewski, M., Blumel, L., and Just, H. (1998) Patent foramen ovale is an important predictor of adverse outcome in patients with major pulmonary embolism. *Circulation* **97**, 1946–1951.

134. Chartier, L., Bera, J., Delomez, M., Asseman, P., Beregi, J. P., Bauchart, J. J., et al. (1999) Free-floating thrombi in the right heart: diagnosis, management, and prognostic indices in 38 consecutive patients. *Circulation* **99,** 2779–2783.

135. Giannitsis, E., Muller-Bardorff, M., Kurowski, V., Weidtmann, B., Wiegand, U., Kampmann, M., et al. (2000) Independent prognostic value of cardiac troponin T in patients with confirmed pulmonary embolism. *Circulation* **102,** 211–217.

136. Tebbe, U., Graf, A., Kamke, W., et al. (1999) Hemodynamic effects of double bolus reteplase versus alteplase infusion in massive pulmonary embolism. *Am. Heart J.* **138,** 39–44.

Index